Death and Dying
Dying
SOURCEBOOK

Third Edition

Health Reference Series

Third Edition

Death and Dying

SOURCEBOOK

Basic Consumer Health Information about End-of-Life Care and Related Perspectives and Ethical Issues, Including End-of-Life Symptoms and Treatments, Pain Management, Quality-of-Life Concerns, the Use of Life Support, Patients' Rights and Privacy Issues, Advance Directives, Physician-Assisted Suicide, Care Giving, Organ and Tissue Donation, Funeral Arrangements, and Grief

Along with Statistical Data, Information about the Leading Causes of Death, a Glossary, and Directories of Support Groups and Other Resources

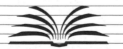

OMNIGRAPHICS

615 Griswold, Ste. 901, Detroit, MI 48226

Bibliographic Note
Because this page cannot legibly accommodate all the copyright notices, the Bibliographic Note portion of the Preface constitutes an extension of the copyright notice.

* * *

Health Reference Series
Keith Jones, *Managing Editor*
***

OMNIGRAPHICS
A PART OF RELEVANT INFORMATION
***

Library of Congress Cataloging-in-Publication Data

Names: Omnigraphics, Inc.

Title: Death and dying sourcebook: basic consumer health information about end-of-life care and related perspectives and ethical issues, including end-of-life symptoms and treatments,pain management, quality-of-life concerns, the use of life support, patients' rights and privacy issues, advance directives, physician-assisted suicide, caregiving, organ and tissue donation, autopsies, funeral arrangements, and grief along with statistical data, information about the leading causes of death, a glossary, and directories of support groups and other resources.

Description: Third edition. | Detroit, MI: Omnigraphics, [2017] | Series: Health reference series | Includes bibliographical references and index.

Identifiers: LCCN 2016044060 (print) | LCCN 2016044865 (ebook) | ISBN 9780780814967 (hardcover: alk. paper) | ISBN 9780780814974 (ebook) | ISBN 9780780814974 (eBook)

Subjects: LCSH: Death. | Terminal care.

Classification: LCC R726.8 .D3785 2017 (print) | LCC R726.8 (ebook) | DDC 362.17/5--dc23

LC record available at https://lccn.loc.gov/2016044060

Table of Contents

Part IV: End-of-Life Care Facilities

Part V: End-of-Life Caregiving

Part VIII: Final Arrangements

Part IX: Mortality Statistics

Part X: Additional Help and Information

Preface

About This Book

Although people are living healthier and longer lives, more than 2.6 million Americans die annually according to the Centers for Disease Control and Prevention (CDC). Some die suddenly; others pass away after long-term struggles with chronic disabilities or disease. Considering the dying process in advance allows people to talk about their choices concerning end-of-life medical preferences. Discussing these topics can be difficult, but appropriate planning allows people to remain in charge of their health care even after they are no longer able to make decisions. Additionally, knowledge about loved ones' wishes can help friends and families cope with the shock and grief of death.

Death and Dying Sourcebook, Third Edition, provides information about end-of-life perspectives and the medical management of symptoms that can occur as death draws near. It discusses palliative care and describes issues surrounding life support choices, the termination of life-sustaining treatment, and the donation process for organs and tissues. The book also addresses caregiver concerns and provides information about children and death. Facts about legal and economic issues at the end of life, funerals and other final arrangements, and grief are also included, along with statistical data, a glossary, and directories of support groups and other resources.

How to Use This Book

This book is divided into parts and chapters. Parts focus on broad areas of interest. Chapters are devoted to single topics within a part.

Part I: End-of-Life Perspectives begins by defining end-of-life and discusses the importance of end-of-life planning. Cultural and spiritual concerns that impact end-of-life decisions are discussed, and research findings about end-of-life care are also described.

Part II: Medical Management of End-of-Life Symptoms begins with an explanation of palliative care. Pain management and assessment is discussed in detail, and information on managing and treating fatigue is also provided. It describes wound care, and cognitive disorders common at the end of life. Specific information for cancer and dementia patients is also included.

Part III: Medical Decisions Surrounding the End of Life presents facts about life support choices, termination of treatments, organ and tissue donation, and physician-assisted suicide. It also provides specific information for commonly experienced end-of-life issues related to Alzheimer disease, advanced cancer, and HIV/AIDS.

Part IV: End-of-Life Care Facilities offers guidelines for evaluating care facilities and selecting options based on the needs of patients and caregivers. Hospice care, long-term care, home care, and other alternatives are described.

Part V: End-of-Life Caregiving has practical information for caregivers about coordinating communications among patients, families, and healthcare and support service providers. Topics include how to help at the end of life, the dying process, what to do when death occurs, and self-care tips for caregivers.

Part VI: Death and Children: Information for Parents provides advice about caring for terminally ill children and grieving the death of a child. Guidance for helping children cope with death, funerals, and grief is also presented.

Part VII: Legal and Economic Issues at End of Life presents guidelines for advance directives, powers of attorney for healthcare, financial assistance, taxes, and social security issues. It also describes patients' legal rights, the Family and Medical Leave Act (FMLA), and the duties of an executor.

Part VIII: Final Arrangements offers practical information about planning funerals or memorial services, certification of death, and how to facilitate arrangements if death occurs while traveling. Information on planning a military funeral is also provided. Chapters on grief which address bereavement, how to help grieving people, and tips for working through grief are also included.

Part IX: Mortality Statistics includes global and national mortality trends and statistics on the leading causes of death in the United States, life expectancy at birth, and common causes of fatalities. Disparities in deaths from suicide, alcohol, and stroke are also discussed.

Part X: Additional Help and Information includes a glossary of end-of-life terms, a directory of support groups for end-of-life concerns, and a directory of organizations able to provide more information about death and dying.

Bibliographic Note

This volume contains documents and excerpts from publications issued by the following U.S. government agencies:

Bureau of Land Management (BLM); Centers for Disease Control and Prevention (CDC); Centers for Medicare and Medicaid Services (CMS); *Eunice Kennedy Shriver* National Institute of Child Health and Human Development (NICHD); Federal Trade Commission (FTC); Internal Revenue Service (IRS); National Cancer Institute (NCI); National Heart, Lung, and Blood Institute (NHLBI); National Institute of Nursing Research (NINR); National Institute on Aging (NIA); National Institutes of Health (NIH); Office on Women's Health (OWH); U.S. Department of Health and Human Services (HHS); U.S. Department of Labor (DOL); U.S. Department of Veterans Affairs (VA); U.S. Environmental Protection Agency (EPA); U.S. Food and Drug Administration (FDA); U.S. Government Accountability Office (GAO); and U.S. Social Security Administration (SSA)

In addition, this volume contains copyrighted documents from the following organization: The Nemours Foundation

It may also contain original material produced by Omnigraphics and reviewed by medical consultants.

About the Health Reference Series

The *Health Reference Series* is designed to provide basic medical information for patients, families, caregivers, and the general public. Each volume takes a particular topic and provides comprehensive coverage. This is especially important for people who may be dealing with a newly diagnosed disease or a chronic disorder in themselves or in a family member. People looking for preventive guidance, information about disease warning signs, medical statistics, and risk factors for health problems will also find answers to their questions in the *Health Reference Series*. The *Series*, however, is not intended to serve as a tool for diagnosing illness, in prescribing treatments, or as a substitute for the physician/patient relationship. All people concerned about medical symptoms or the possibility of disease are encouraged to seek professional care from an appropriate health care provider.

A Note about Spelling and Style

Health Reference Series editors use *Stedman's Medical Dictionary* as an authority for questions related to the spelling of medical terms and the *Chicago Manual of Style* for questions related to grammatical structures, punctuation, and other editorial concerns. Consistent adherence is not always possible, however, because the individual volumes within the *Series* include many documents from a wide variety of different producers, and the editor's primary goal is to present material from each source as accurately as is possible. This sometimes means that information in different chapters or sections may follow other guidelines and alternate spelling authorities.

Medical Review

Omnigraphics contracts with a team of qualified, senior medical professionals who serve as medical consultants for the *Health Reference Series*. As necessary, medical consultants review reprinted and originally written material for currency and accuracy. Citations including the phrase, "Reviewed (month, year)" indicate material reviewed by this team. Medical consultation services are provided to the *Health Reference Series* editors by:

Dr. Senthil Selvan, MBBS, DCH, MD
Dr. K. Sivanandham, MBBS, DCH, MS (Research), PhD

Our Advisory Board

We would like to thank the following board members for providing initial guidance on the development of this series:

- Dr. Lynda Baker, Associate Professor of Library and Information Science, Wayne State University, Detroit, MI

- Nancy Bulgarelli, William Beaumont Hospital Library, Royal Oak, MI

- Karen Imarisio, Bloomfield Township Public Library, Bloomfield Township, MI

- Karen Morgan, Mardigian Library, University of Michigan-Dearborn, Dearborn, MI

- Rosemary Orlando, St. Clair Shores Public Library, St. Clair Shores, MI

Health Reference Series *Update Policy*

The inaugural book in the *Health Reference Series* was the first edition of *Cancer Sourcebook* published in 1989. Since then, the *Series* has been enthusiastically received by librarians and in the medical community. In order to maintain the standard of providing high-quality health information for the layperson the editorial staff at Omnigraphics felt it was necessary to implement a policy of updating volumes when warranted.

Medical researchers have been making tremendous strides, and it is the purpose of the *Health Reference Series* to stay current with the most recent advances. Each decision to update a volume is made on an individual basis. Some of the considerations include how much new information is available and the feedback we receive from people who use the books. If there is a topic you would like to see added to the update list, or an area of medical concern you feel has not been adequately addressed, please write to:

Managing Editor
Health Reference Series
Omnigraphics
615 Griswold, Ste. 901
Detroit, MI 48226

Part One

End-of-Life Perspectives

Chapter 1

Defining End of Life

Preparing for the End of Life

Few of us are comfortable talking about death, whether our own or a loved one's. It is a scary, even taboo, subject for many. The end of a life, no matter how long and well lived, can bring with it a sense of loss and sadness. It can also be a reminder of our own mortality, so we may avoid even thinking about death.

This is normal—but death is normal, too. All of us will face it at some point.

Defining the End of Life

The end of life and how people die has changed a great deal in the past century. Thanks in large part to advances in public health, medicine, and healthcare, most Americans no longer die suddenly from injury or infection. Instead, we live longer and, more often than not, die after a period of chronic illness.

As a result, it is hard to know when the dying process begins. Some people pass quickly, while others recover from severe illness several times before death. Even people who are the same age and sex, with the same disease and state of health, are unlikely to reach the end of life at the same time.

Text in this chapter is excerpted from "End of Life," NIHSeniorHealth, National Institute on Aging (NIA), March 26, 2014.

We often rely on healthcare providers to tell us when the end of life is near. But even the most experienced healthcare provider may find it hard to predict when someone will die. An expert may say the end is within weeks or months, but the dying person slips away much sooner or survives for a year or more.

Preferences for the End of Life

Because the end of life is hard to predict, it is best to plan ahead. You might want to start by asking yourself or a loved one, "What is the best way to plan for the end of life?"

The answer will differ from person to person. Some people want to spend their final days at home, surrounded by family and friends. Others may prefer to be alone, or to be in a hospital receiving treatments for an illness until the very end.

The answer may also change over time—the person who wanted everything possible done to prolong life may decide to change focus to comfort. Someone else who originally declined treatment may agree to an experimental therapy that may benefit future patients with the same condition.

No matter how a person chooses to approach the end of their life, there are some common hopes—nearly everyone says they do not want to die in pain or to lose their dignity. Planning for end-of-life care, also known as advance care planning, can help ensure such hopes are fulfilled.

Chapter 2

Cultural Response to Death

Coping with a Loss of a Loved One

People cope with the loss of a loved one in different ways. Most people who experience grief will cope well. Others will have severe grief and may need treatment. There are many things that can affect the grief process of someone who has lost a loved one to cancer. They include:

- The personality of the person who is grieving.

- The relationship with the person who died.

- The loved one's cancer experience and the way the disease progressed.

- The grieving person's coping skills and mental health history.

- The amount of support the grieving person has.

- The grieving person's cultural and religious background.

- The grieving person's social and financial position.

Bereavement and Grief

Bereavement is the period of sadness after losing a loved one through death. Grief and mourning occur during the period of bereavement.

This chapter includes text excerpted from "Grief, Bereavement, and Coping with Loss (PDQ®)—Patient Version," National Cancer Institute (NCI), March 6, 2013.

Grief and mourning are closely related. Mourning is the way we show grief in public. The way people mourn is affected by beliefs, religious practices, and cultural customs. People who are grieving are sometimes described as bereaved.

Grief is the normal process of reacting to the loss. Grief is the emotional response to the loss of a loved one. Common grief reactions include the following:

- Feeling emotionally numb.

- Feeling unable to believe the loss occurred.

- Feeling anxiety from the distress of being separated from the loved one.

- Mourning along with depression.

- A feeling of acceptance.

Cultural Responses to Grief and Loss

Cultures have different ways of coping with death. Grief felt for the loss of loved ones occurs in people of all ages and cultures. Different cultures, however, have different myths and mysteries about death that affect the attitudes, beliefs, and practices of the bereaved.

Individual, personal experiences of grief are similar in different cultures. The ways in which people of all cultures feel grief personally are similar. This has been found to be true even though different cultures have different mourning ceremonies and traditions to express grief.

Cultural issues that affect people who are dealing with the loss of a loved one include rituals, beliefs, and roles. Helping family members cope with the death of a loved one includes showing respect for the family's culture and the ways they honor the death. The following questions may help caregivers learn what is needed by the person's culture:

- What are the cultural rituals for coping with dying, the deceased person's body, and honoring the death?

- What are the family's beliefs about what happens after death?

- What does the family feel is a normal expression of grief and the acceptance of the loss?

- What does the family consider to be the roles of each family member in handling the death?

- Are certain types of death less acceptable (for example, suicide), or are certain types of death especially hard for that culture (for example, the death of a child)?

Death, grief, and mourning are normal life events. All cultures have practices that best meet their needs for dealing with death. Caregivers who understand the ways different cultures respond to death can help patients of these cultures work through their own normal grieving process.

Chapter 3

Spirituality in End-of-Life Care

General Information about Spirituality

Studies have shown that religious and spiritual values are important to Americans. Most American adults say that they believe in God and that their religious beliefs affect how they live their lives. However, people have different ideas about life after death, belief in miracles, and other religious beliefs. Such beliefs may be based on gender, education, and ethnic background.

Many patients with serious illnesses rely on spiritual or religious beliefs and practices to help them cope with their disease. This is called spiritual coping. Many caregivers also rely on spiritual coping. Each person may have different spiritual needs, depending on cultural and religious traditions. For some seriously ill patients, spiritual well-being may affect how much anxiety they feel about death. For others, it may affect what they decide about end-of-life treatments. Some patients and their family caregivers may want doctors to talk about spiritual concerns, but may feel unsure about how to bring up the subject.

Some studies show that doctors' support of spiritual well-being in very ill patients helps improve their quality of life. Healthcare providers who treat patients coping with serious illnesses are looking at new ways to help them with religious and spiritual concerns. Doctors

This chapter includes text excerpted from "Spirituality in Cancer Care (PDQ®)—Patient Version," National Cancer Institute (NCI), May 18, 2015.

may ask patients which spiritual issues are important to them during treatment as well as near the end of life. When patients with advanced cancer receive spiritual support from the medical team, they may be more likely to choose hospice care and less aggressive treatment at the end of life.

Spirituality and Religion May Have Different Meanings

The terms spirituality and religion are often used in place of each other, but for many people they have different meanings. Religion may be defined as a specific set of beliefs and practices, usually within an organized group. Spirituality may be defined as an individual's sense of peace, purpose, and connection to others, and beliefs about the meaning of life. Spirituality may be found and expressed through an organized religion or in other ways. Patients may think of themselves as spiritual or religious or both.

Serious Illness, Such as Cancer, May Cause Spiritual Distress

Serious illnesses like cancer may cause patients or family caregivers to have doubts about their beliefs or religious values and cause much spiritual distress. Some studies show that patients with cancer may feel that they are being punished by God or may have a loss of faith after being diagnosed. Other patients may have mild feelings of spiritual distress when coping with cancer.

Spirituality and Quality of Life

It is not known for sure how spirituality and religion are related to health. Some studies show that spiritual or religious beliefs and practices create a positive mental attitude that may help a patient feel better and improve the well-being of family caregivers. Spiritual and religious well-being may help improve health and quality of life in the following ways:

- Decrease anxiety, depression, anger, and discomfort.
- Decrease the sense of isolation (feeling alone) and the risk of suicide.
- Decrease alcohol and drug abuse.
- Lower blood pressure and the risk of heart disease.

- Help the patient adjust to the effects of cancer and its treatment.
- Increase the ability to enjoy life during cancer treatment.
- Give a feeling of personal growth as a result of living with cancer.
- Increase positive feelings, including:
- Hope and optimism.
- Freedom from regret.
- Satisfaction with life.
- A sense of inner peace.

Spiritual and religious well-being may also help a patient live longer.

Spiritual Distress May Also Affect Health

Healthcare providers may encourage patients to meet with experienced spiritual or religious leaders to help deal with their spiritual issues. This may improve their health, quality of life, and ability to cope.

Spiritual Assessment

A spiritual assessment is a method or tool used by doctors to understand the role that religious and spiritual beliefs have in the patient's life. This may help the doctor understand how these beliefs affect the way the patient responds to the diagnosis and decisions about cancer treatment. Some doctors or caregivers may wait for the patient to bring up spiritual concerns. Others may use an interview or a questionnaire.

A Spiritual Assessment Explores Religious Beliefs and Spiritual Practices

A spiritual assessment may include questions about the following:

- religious denomination, if any
- beliefs or philosophy of life
- important spiritual practices or rituals
- using spirituality or religion as a source of strength

11

- being part of a community of support

- using prayer or meditation

- loss of faith

- conflicts between spiritual or religious beliefs and cancer treatments

- ways that healthcare providers and caregivers may help with the patient's spiritual needs

- concerns about death and afterlife

- planning for the end of life

Meeting the Patient's Spiritual and Religious Needs

To help patients with spiritual needs, medical staff will listen to the wishes of the patient. Spirituality and religion are very personal issues. Patients should expect doctors and caregivers to respect their religious and spiritual beliefs and concerns. Patients with cancer who rely on spirituality to cope with the disease should be able to count on the healthcare team to give them support. This may include giving patients information about people or groups that can help with spiritual or religious needs. Most hospitals have chaplains, but not all outpatient settings do. Patients who do not want to discuss spirituality should also be able to count on the healthcare team to respect their wishes.

Doctors and caregivers will try to respond to their patients' concerns, but may not take part in patients' religious practices or discuss specific religious beliefs.

The Healthcare Team Will Help with a Patient's Spiritual Needs When Setting Goals and Planning Treatment

The healthcare team may help with a patient's spiritual needs in the following ways:

- Suggest goals and options for care that honor the patient's spiritual and/or religious views.

- Support the patient's use of spiritual coping during the illness.

- Encourage the patient to speak with his/her religious or spiritual leader.

- Refer the patient to a hospital chaplain or support group that can help with spiritual issues during illness.

- Refer the patient to other therapies that have been shown to increase spiritual well-being. These include mindfulness relaxation, such as yoga or meditation, or creative arts programs, such as writing, drawing, or music therapy.

Chapter 4

Chronic Illness in Old Age

Addressing Chronic Illness among Old Age People

In the United States, 45 million adults—14% of the population—are 65 or older. By 2050, that number is expected to climb to about 80 million, or 20% of the population. This growth in the number and proportion of older adults is unprecedented. Americans are living longer than ever before.

Quick Stats

- Americans are at higher risk of chronic conditions—such as heart disease, cancer, and diabetes—as they age.
- Much of the illness, disability, and premature death from these conditions is preventable.
- The prevalence of Alzheimer disease is rising with the aging of the U.S. population and is the 5th leading cause of death for people aged 65 or older.
- Less than half of adults aged 65 or older are up to date on clinical preventive services, such as cancer screenings.

Public Health Problem

Chronic diseases—such as heart disease, cancer, and diabetes—account for most deaths in the United States, and Americans are at

This chapter includes text excerpted from "Healthy Aging," Centers for Disease Control and Prevention (CDC), September 9, 2015.

higher risk of these conditions as they age. In 2012, 63% of Medicare beneficiaries aged 65 to 74, 78% of those aged 75 to 84, and 83% of those aged 85 or older had multiple chronic conditions.

Age also brings with it a higher risk of dementia and infectious diseases:

- Alzheimer disease is the 6th leading cause of death in the United States and the 5th leading cause for adults aged 65 or older.

- Infectious diseases such as flu and pneumonia affect older adults at higher rates than their younger counterparts. For example, during most flu seasons in the United States, an estimated 90% of flu-related deaths and 50% to 60% of flu-related illness occur in people aged 65 or older.

Much of the illness, disability, and premature death from these conditions can be prevented with healthier behaviors, more supportive environments, and better access to preventive health services.

Environmental and Social Supports

Centers for Disease Control and Prevention (CDC)'s Healthy Aging Research Network has defined healthy aging as "the development and maintenance of optimal physical, mental (cognitive and emotional), spiritual, and social well-being and function in older adults."

Research has shown that people can achieve healthy aging most easily when:

- Physical environments and communities are safe and support attitudes and behaviors, such as regular walking, that promote health and well-being.

- Health services and community programs are used effectively to prevent or minimize the impact of acute and chronic disease on function.

Public health efforts for older adults are beginning to address the total spectrum of health. The value of this broader perspective is that it accounts for challenges such as confusion and memory loss, difficulty performing the activities of daily living, or isolation from friends and family.

Public Health Strategies

The most effective public health strategies for improving the health and quality of life of older adults are:

- Promoting healthy environments and lifestyles.

- Closing gaps in the delivery of clinical preventive services.

- Meeting the needs of older adults with cognitive impairment and their caregivers.

Promoting Healthy Environments and Lifestyles

Despite the benefits of being physically active, one-third of older adults do not get regular physical activity. People who are physically active, eat a healthy diet, and do not use tobacco decrease their risk of developing heart disease, cancer, diabetes, and other chronic conditions.

Healthy communities are those that make it easier for people to pursue healthy behaviors. For example, in communities that provide safe walking and biking trails, residents are more likely to get out and walk or bike regularly.

Closing Gaps in the Delivery of Clinical Preventive Services

Clinical preventive services, including cancer screenings and immunizations for flu and pneumonia, can prevent disease or find disease early, when treatment is more effective. Greater use of these services could prevent thousands of deaths among older Americans each year. However, only about one-third of adults aged 50 to 64 and less than half of those aged 65 or older are up to date on a selected set of recommended screenings and immunizations.

Meeting the Needs of Older Adults with Cognitive Impairment and Their Caregivers

Cognitive impairment, defined as a decline in the ability to think, concentrate, and remember, affects the health of millions of older adults. Moderate or severe impairment can also have a substantial impact on their families. In most cases, family members care for people with Alzheimer disease or other dementias. Given longer lifespans and the growing prevalence of such conditions, the need for caregivers, both informal (e.g., family members) and formal, will likely increase significantly as the U.S. population ages.

Chapter 5

Research Findings about End-of-Life Care and Outcomes

Chapter Contents

Section 5.1

NIH Research on Palliative and End-of-Life Care

This section includes text excerpted from "End of Life:
Research Efforts," NIHSeniorHealth, National
Institute on Aging (NIA), March 2014.

Research Efforts

As the lead National Institutes of Health (NIH) Institute for end-of-life research, the National Institute of Nursing Research (NINR) supports science to assist individuals, families, and healthcare professionals in managing the symptoms of advanced illness and planning for end-of-life decisions.

Research in Palliative and End-of-Life Care

NINR also recognizes that high-quality, evidence-based palliative care is a critical component of maintaining quality of life at any stage of illness, including the end of life.

To advance palliative and end-of-life care, NINR supports research to:

- relieve symptoms and suffering

- better understand how care needs differ according to setting, culture, and location

NINR-supported research has found that end-of-life care varies largely in different settings, especially in the provision of hospice care and withdrawal of life support. End-of-life care is beginning to be provided in nursing homes, intensive care units, and in hospice settings, yet standards and quality of care vary across these settings.

Health Disparities and End-of-Life Care

NINR-supported researchers are also examining health disparities at the end of life, especially the impact of culture, ethnicity and geographic location on end-of-life care. Their studies have found that families who speak limited English receive less information and support in the intensive care unit during conferences between clinicians and family members. They have also found geographic differences in the accessibility of hospice care, with rural areas often having limited access.

Nursing Home Care at End of Life

While the number of seniors dying in nursing homes is steadily increasing, few studies have examined the quality of end-of-life care in these facilities, or determined if there are differences between rural and urban areas in terms of quality of end-of-life care. A recent research finding indicates that quality may differ, with nursing home residents more likely to have in-hospital death and less hospice use. Understanding the role of hospice-use practices in the quality-of-care problems in nursing homes is essential to overcoming geographic and quality challenges.

Depression and End of Life

In another NINR-funded study, systematic assessment for depression was added to the usual care provided in hospice; the patient's caregivers were also assessed. The researchers found that when this assessment was reported to the interdisciplinary team that cared for the patients and their caregivers, patient depression rates were lower, and quality of life improved without any additional assessment or intervention.

Decision Making at the End of Life

Decision making at the end of life, including withdrawal of life support, is a very stressful time for families and decision makers for the terminally ill. One NINR-supported project found that family satisfaction with the decision-making process was associated with how the intensive care unit (ICU) clinician recommended withdrawing life support, if he or she discussed the patient's wishes and the family's spiritual needs, and if the family felt supported during the decision-making process.

Research in end-of-life care continues to be an important part of NINR's scientific agenda. The significance of this research area is highlighted in the NINR strategic plan. As such, "The Science of Compassion: Enhancing End-of-Life and Palliative Care" is recognized as one of four key themes that will guide the future growth of NINR-supported science.

Section 5.2

Prognosis Discussions Improve Understanding of Illness for Patients with Terminal Cancer

This section includes text excerpted from "Prognosis Discussions Improve Understanding of Illness for Patients with Terminal Cancer," National Cancer Institute (NCI), June 27, 2016.

The study results show that many patients with advanced, incurable cancer have a poor understanding of their prognosis or life expectancy. Fewer than one in four patients in the study reported having a recent discussion about prognosis with their oncologist, although those who did were more likely to understand the serious nature of their illness, the study showed.

"To our knowledge, our study is the first to directly address and demonstrate these associations between the timing of patient-reported prognostic discussions and improvements in illness understanding by patients," the study authors wrote in a paper published May 23 in the Journal of Clinical Oncology.

The findings suggest that many people with terminal cancer "don't understand basic information about where they are in the illness trajectory and have unrealistic expectations of treatment outcome," said study leader Holly Prigerson, Ph.D., of Weill Cornell Medicine in New York.

"Patients have a right to know the status of their illness and the likely outcomes of treatment so that they can make informed decisions about their care," continued Dr. Prigerson, who directs the Center for Research on End-of-Life Care at Weill Cornell.

Assessing Illness Understanding

To evaluate how well patients understand their prognosis, Dr. Prigerson's team interviewed 178 adults with advanced solid cancers before and after they met with their oncologists to discuss the results of recent scans done to assess disease progression. The patients, recruited from nine U.S. cancer centers, were participants in the NCI-funded Coping with Cancer II study. Most had either lung or gastrointestinal cancer, and all had a life expectancy of 6 months or less, as estimated by their oncologists.

At both pre- and post-scan interviews, the researchers asked the patients four questions that assessed whether they understood that they had a terminal illness, that the disease was incurable, that they had advanced disease, and that their life expectancy was months, not years. During the post-scan interviews, patients also were asked whether they had discussed their prognosis or life expectancy at their recent oncology visit or during past visits.

The researchers assigned a score of 0 or 1 for inaccurate or accurate responses to each of the four questions and added the scores to give a maximum "illness understanding score" of 4. The difference in scores between pre- and post-scan visits was used to define changes in illness understanding.

Overall, the researchers found, study participants had improvements in illness understanding after the post-scan appointment. However, improvements in understanding were statistically significant only if patients reported having at least a recent discussion about prognosis or life expectancy with their oncologist.

Of the 178 participants, 24 (13%) reported both recent and past discussions about prognosis with their oncologist, 18 (10%) had only recent discussions, and 68 (38%) had only past discussions. The remaining 68 (38%) reported never having such discussions.

A follow-up analysis of the same study, presented earlier this month at the American Society of Clinical Oncology annual meeting in Chicago, showed that "the messenger matters, too," Dr. Prigerson said. Patients who reported discussing their scan results with an oncologist versus another member of their care team were approximately four times more likely to recognize that their disease was at a late or end stage.

Overcoming Communication Challenges

"Dr. Prigerson's team showed not only how important these prognosis conversations are, but also how often they don't happen," commented Wen-Ying Sylvia Chou, Ph.D., M.P.H., of NCI's Division of Cancer Control and Population Sciences.

Dr. Chou oversees NCI-funded projects on patient-provider communication and health literacy. "In research that has delved into these clinical interactions," she said, "it has become clear that the key issue is about patients' understanding of the goals of care. And you can't adequately understand the goals of care without knowing your diagnosis and your prognosis."

The delicate task of conveying a terminal cancer prognosis to patients and their loved ones is difficult, for a variety of reasons. "Palliative care, hospice, and talking about quality of life are important topics, but I think often these topics are stigmatized, and that's a more societal and cultural issue that we need to address," Dr. Chou said.

Furthermore, some oncologists worry that conveying bad news will make patients anxious or depressed. However, Dr. Prigerson said, she and others have shown that patients don't have worse depression, anxiety, or quality of life as a result of such conversations. Nor do these discussions appear to harm the doctor-patient relationship.

But not all patients are ready to have such discussions. For instance, Dr. Prigerson said, "There are cultural groups in which discussing death and cancer are taboo." In addition, many religiously devout patients believe their fate is in God's hands and are less likely to accept bad news from their doctor.

To help address ethnic and racial differences in readiness to discuss death, Dr. Prigerson's team is developing videos in which patients and their families share stories about the impact that different treatment options had on their own quality of life. The goal of the videos is to help inform the decisions of other patients who may be more likely to accept information from people like themselves.

Section 5.3

Too Few Patients with Cancer Communicate Preferences for End-of-Life Care

This section includes text excerpted from "Too Few Patients with Cancer Communicate Preferences for End-of-Life Care," National Cancer Institute (NCI), August 10, 2015.

Many patients with cancer are not communicating their preferences for end-of-life medical care either through written documents or discussions with loved ones, a study suggests. The study also found a large increase in the number of people receiving intensive treatment in the last days and weeks of their lives.

The results, published online July 9 in JAMA Oncology, underscore the need for patients to share their end-of-life care wishes before they are too sick to do so, the study authors said.

Near the end of life, many patients with advanced cancer rely on loved ones—as well as legal documents such as living wills and durable power of attorney—to ensure that their medical care reflects their values, goals, and care preferences.

The study describes trends in the use of advance care planning. Amol K. Narang, M.D., of the Johns Hopkins School of Medicine, and his colleagues analyzed survey data on the use of advance care plans and end-of-life care discussions from nearly 2,000 participants in the prospective Health and Retirement Study who died from cancer between 2000 and 2012.

The Health and Retirement Study includes biennial interviews with a representative sample of Americans who are older than 50 years of age. Within two years of a participant's death, a study investigator interviews a knowledgeable proxy (often the participant's next of kin) about the individual's end-of-life care.

Over the study period, the use of living wills and participation in discussions about end-of-life care did not change significantly among the study population, the researchers found.

By contrast, from 2000 to 2012, the percentage of patients with cancer who designated durable power of attorney privileges to a loved one increased from 52 percent to 74 percent. However, nearly 40 percent of the survey respondents said their loved ones had not discussed end-of-life care preferences with them. And the percentage of patients who received "all care possible" near the end of life rose from 7 percent to 58 percent during the study period.

Assigning durable power of attorney was associated with lower chances of patients dying in the hospital rather than in a hospice facility or their own home. And patients who had a living will and had also engaged in end-of-life discussions were far more likely to have limited treatment at the end of life than those who had neither.

The survey results underscore the need to "find ways that prompt clinicians to have discussions with patients and caregivers about their end-of-life preferences," Dr. Narang said in a news release.

If a patient's treatment preferences have not been communicated explicitly, either through writing or discussions, then surrogates "may default to providing all care possible instead of limiting potentially intensive, life-prolonging care," the researchers noted.

The study had several limitations, including the use of subjective survey questions and the potential for recall errors among respondents to the survey, the study authors noted.

Cancer care in the United States continues to be "intensive, with evidence of increasing rates of hospitalizations, intensive care unit stays, and emergency department visits in the last month of life, along with persistently high rates of terminal hospitalizations, late hospice referrals, and burdensome transitions near death," the authors wrote.

In the study population, between 20 percent and 25 percent of terminally ill patients with cancer died in the hospital, which is consistent with previous reports.

For patients and families, determining and articulating their values and preferences for end-of-life care can be "a difficult and emotional exercise, sometimes fraught with legalistic elements, and it is often avoided," noted Michael J. Fisch, M.D., of AIM Specialty Health, in an accompanying editorial. "For many, the task seems daunting and the reward nebulous."

The path to progress starts with "better communication by proactive, prepared clinician teams," wrote Dr. Fisch. "Advance directives have inherent limitations and might be regarded as sometimes necessary but rarely sufficient for achieving optimal cancer care toward the end of life for each individual patient."

The primary focus of healthcare providers, Dr. Fisch continued, should be "on fostering prognostic awareness, focusing on goals of care rather than specific treatments, and responding to emotions."

The Institute of Medicine has called for the development of evidence-based standards for clinician-patient communication and advance care planning, which should lead to progress in the field, he noted.

Part Two

Medical Management of End-of-Life Symptoms

Chapter 6

What Is Palliative Care?

Dealing with the symptoms of any painful or serious illness is difficult. However, special care is available to make you more comfortable right now. It's called palliative care. You receive palliative care at the same time that you're receiving treatments for your illness. Its primary purpose is to relieve the pain and other symptoms you are experiencing and improve your quality of life. Palliative care is a central part of treatment for serious or life-threatening illnesses. The information in this brochure will help you understand how you or someone close to you can benefit from this type of care.

Palliative care is comprehensive treatment of the discomfort, symptoms and stress of serious illness. It does not replace your primary treatment; palliative care works together with the primary treatment you're receiving. The goal is to prevent and ease suffering and improve your quality of life.

If you need palliative care, does that mean you're dying?

The purpose of palliative care is to address distressing symptoms such as pain, breathing difficulties or nausea, among others. Receiving palliative care does not necessarily mean you're dying.

Palliative Care Gives You a Chance to Live Your Life More Comfortably

Palliative care provides relief from distressing symptoms including pain, shortness of breath, fatigue, constipation, nausea, loss of

---

This chapter includes text excerpted from "Palliative Care the Relief You Need When You're Experiencing the Symptoms of Serious Illness," National Institute of Nursing Research (NINR), May 2011. Reviewed October 2016.

appetite, problems with sleep and many other symptoms. It can also help you deal with the side effects of the medical treatments you're receiving. Perhaps, most important, palliative care can help improve your quality of life. Palliative care also provides support for you and your family and can improve communication between you and your healthcare providers. Palliative care strives to provide you with:

- Expert treatment of pain and other symptoms so you can get the best relief possible.

- Open discussion about treatment choices, including treatment for your disease and management of your symptoms.

- Coordination of your care with all of your healthcare providers.

- Emotional support for you and your family.

Palliative Care Can Be Very Effective

Researchers have studied the positive effects palliative care has on patients. Recent studies show that patients who receive palliative care report improvement in:

- pain and other distressing symptoms, such as nausea or shortness of breath

- communication with their healthcare providers and family members

- emotional support

Other studies also show that palliative care:

- Ensures that care is more in line with patients' wishes.

- Meets the emotional and spiritual needs of patients.

Palliative Care Is Different from Hospice Care

Palliative care is available to you at any time during your illness. Remember that you can receive palliative care at the same time you receive treatments that are meant to cure your illness. Its availability does not depend upon whether or not your condition can be cured. The goal is to make you as comfortable as possible and improve your quality of life. You don't have to be in hospice or at the end of life to receive palliative care. People in hospice always receive palliative care, but hospice focuses on a person's final months of life. o qualify for some hospice programs, patients must no longer be receiving treatments to cure their illness.

A Palliative Care Can Improve Your Quality of Life in a Variety of Ways

Together with your primary healthcare provider, your palliative care team combines vigorous pain and symptom control into every part of your treatment. Team members spend as much time with you and your family as it takes to help you fully understand your condition, care option and other needs. They also make sure you experience a smooth transition between the hospital and other services, such as home care or nursing facilities.

This results in well-planned, complete treatment for all of your symptoms throughout your illness-treatment that takes care of you in your present condition and anticipates your future needs.

A team approach to patient-centered care.

Palliative care is provided by a team of specialists that may include:

- palliative care doctors
- palliative care nurses
- social workers
- chaplains
- pharmacists
- nutritionists
- counselors and others

Palliative care supports you and those who love you by maximizing your comfort. It also helps you set goals for the future that lead to a meaningful, enjoyable life while you get treatment for your illness.

How Do You Know If You Need Palliative Care?

Many adults and children living with illnesses such as cancer, heart disease, lung disease, kidney failure, AIDS and cystic fibrosis, among others, experience physical symptoms and emotional distress related to their diseases. Sometimes these symptoms are related to the medical treatments they are receiving.

31

You may want to consider palliative care if you or your loved one:

- suffers from pain or other symptoms due to ANY serious illness
- experiences physical or emotional pain that is NOT under control
- needs help understanding your situation and coordinating your care

Getting Palliative Care Is as Easy as Asking for It

In most cases, palliative care is provided in the hospital. The process begins when either your healthcare provider refers you to the palliative care team or you ask your healthcare provider for a referral. In the hospital, palliative care is provided by a team of professionals, including medical and nursing specialists, social workers, pharmacists, nutritionists, clergy and others.

Insurance Pays for Palliative Care

Most insurance plans cover all or part of the palliative care treatment you receive in the hospital, just as they would other services. Medicare and Medicaid also typically cover palliative care. If you have concerns about the cost of palliative care treatment, a social worker from the palliative care team can help you.

Start Palliative Care as Soon as You Need It

It's never too early to start palliative care. In fact, palliative care occurs at the same time as all other treatments for your illness and does not depend upon the course of your disease. There is no reason to wait. Serious illnesses and their treatments can cause exhaustion, anxiety and depression. Palliative care teams understand that pain and other symptoms affect your quality of life and can leave you lacking the energy or motivation to pursue the things you enjoy. They also know that the stress of what you're going through can have a big impact on your family. And they can assist you and your loved ones as you cope with the difficult experience.

Working Together as a Team

Patients who are considering palliative care often wonder how it will affect their relationships with their current healthcare providers.

Some of their questions include:

- Will I have to give up my primary healthcare provider?
- What do I say if there is resistance to referring me for palliative care services?
- Will I offend my healthcare provider if I ask questions?

Most important, you do NOT give up your own healthcare provider in order to get palliative care. The palliative care team and your healthcare provider work together.

Most clinicians appreciate the extra time and information the palliative care team provides to their patients. Occasionally a clinician may not refer a patient for palliative care services. If this happens to you, ask for an explanation. Let your healthcare provider know why you think palliative care could help you.

What Happens When You Leave the Hospital

When you leave the hospital, your palliative care team will help you make a successful move to your home, hospice or other healthcare setting.

Chapter 7

Pain Management and Assessment

Chapter Contents

Section 7.1

Pain and Pain Management

This section includes text excerpted from "Health and Aging," National Institute on Aging (NIA), National Institutes of Health (NIH), May 2015.

Acute Pain and Chronic Pain

There are two kinds of pain. Acute pain begins suddenly, lasts for a short time, and goes away as your body heals. You might feel acute pain after surgery or if you have a broken bone, infected tooth, or kidney stone.

Pain that lasts for several months or years is called chronic (or persistent) pain. This pain often affects older people. Examples include rheumatoid arthritis (RA) and sciatica. In some cases, chronic pain follows after acute pain from an injury or other health issue has gone away, like postherpetic neuralgia after shingles.

Living with any type of pain can be very hard. It can cause many other problems. For instance, pain can:

- Get in the way of your daily activities
- Disturb your sleep and eating habits
- Make it difficult to continue working
- Cause depression or anxiety

Describing Pain

Many people have a hard time describing pain. Think about these questions when you explain how the pain feels:

- Where does it hurt?
- When did it start? Does the pain come and go?
- What does it feel like? Is the pain sharp, dull, or burning? Would you use some other word to describe it?
- Do you have other symptoms?

- When do you feel the pain? In the morning? In the evening? After eating?

- Is there anything you do that makes the pain feel better or worse? For example, does using a heating pad or ice pack help? Does changing your position from lying down to sitting up make it better? Have you tried any over-the-counter medications for it?

- Your doctor or nurse may ask you to rate your pain on a scale of 0 to 10, with 0 being no pain and 10 being the worst pain you can imagine. Or, your doctor may ask if the pain is mild, moderate, or severe. Some doctors or nurses have pictures of faces that show different expressions of pain. You point to the face that shows how you feel.

Cancer Pain

Some people with cancer are more afraid of the pain than of the cancer. But, most pain from cancer or cancer treatments can be controlled. As with all pain, it's best to start managing cancer pain early. It might take a while to find the best approach. Talk with your doctor so the pain management plan can be corrected to work for you.

One special concern in managing cancer pain is "breakthrough pain." This is a pain that comes on quickly and can take you by surprise. It can be very upsetting. After one attack, many people worry it will happen again. This is another reason why it is so important to talk with your doctor about having a pain management plan in place.

Alzheimer Disease and Pain

People who have Alzheimer disease may not be able to tell you when they're in pain. When you're caring for someone with Alzheimer disease, watch for clues. A person's face may show signs of being in pain or feeling ill. You may also notice sudden changes in behavior such as increased yelling, striking out, or spending more time in bed. It's important to find out if there is something wrong. If you're not sure what to do, call the doctor for help.

Pain at the End of Life

Not everyone who is dying is in pain. But if a person has pain at the end of life, there are ways to help. Experts often believe it's best to focus on making the person comfortable, without worrying about possible addiction or drug dependence.

Speak to a palliative care or pain management specialist if you are concerned about pain for yourself or a loved one. These specialists are trained to manage pain and other symptoms for people with serious illnesses.

Treating Pain

Treating, or managing, chronic pain is important. The good news is that there are ways to care for pain. Some treatments involve medications, and some do not. Your doctor may make a treatment plan that is specific for your needs.

Most treatment plans do not just focus on reducing pain. They also include ways to support daily function while living with pain.

Pain doesn't always go away overnight. Talk with your doctor about how long it may take before you feel better. Often, you have to stick with a treatment plan before you get relief. It's important to stay on a schedule. Sometimes this is called "staying ahead" or "keeping on top" of your pain. As your pain lessens, you can likely become more active and will see your mood lift and sleep improve.

Medicines to Treat Pain

Your doctor may prescribe one or more of the following pain medications:

- Acetaminophen

- Nonsteroidal anti-inflammatory drugs (NSAIDs)

- Narcotics

- Other medications

As people age, they are at risk for developing more serious side effects from medication. It's important to take exactly the amount of pain medicine your doctor prescribes.

Mixing any pain medication with alcohol or other drugs, such as tranquilizers, can be dangerous. Make sure your doctor knows all the medicines you take, including over-the-counter drugs and herbal supplements, as well as the amount of alcohol you drink.

Pain Specialist

Some doctors receive extra training in pain management. If you find that your regular doctor can't help you, ask him or her for the name of a pain medicine specialist. You also can ask for suggestions from friends and family, a nearby hospital, or your local medical society.

What Other Treatments Help with Pain?

In addition to drugs, there are a variety of complementary and alternative approaches that may provide relief. Talk to your doctor about these treatments. It may take both medicine and other treatments to feel better.

- Acupuncture uses hair-thin needles to stimulate specific points on the body to relieve pain.

- Biofeedback helps you learn to control your heart rate, blood pressure, and muscle tension. This may help reduce your pain and stress level.

- Cognitive behavioral therapy is a form of short-term counseling that may help reduce your reaction to pain.

- Distraction can help you cope with pain by learning new skills that may take your mind off your discomfort.

- Electrical nerve stimulation uses electrical impulses in order to relieve pain.

- Guided imagery uses directed thoughts to create mental pictures that may help you relax, manage anxiety, sleep better, and have less pain.

- Hypnosis uses focused attention to help manage pain.

- Massage therapy can release tension in tight muscles.

- Physical therapy uses a variety of techniques to help manage everyday activities with less pain and teaches you ways to improve flexibility and strength.

Helping Yourself

There are things you can do yourself that might help you feel better. Try to:

- Keep a healthy weight. Putting on extra pounds can slow healing and make some pain worse. Keeping a healthy weight might help with knee pain, or pain in the back, hips, or feet.

- Be active. Try to keep moving. Pain might make you inactive, which can lead to a cycle of more pain and loss of function. Mild activity can help.

- Get enough sleep. It will improve healing and your mood.

- Avoid tobacco, caffeine, and alcohol. They can get in the way of your treatment and increase your pain.

- Join a pain support group. Sometimes, it can help to talk to other people about how they deal with pain. You can share your ideas and thoughts while learning from others.

- Participate in activities you enjoy. Taking part in activities that you find relaxing, like listening to music or doing art, might help take your mind off of some of the pain.

Section 7.2

Pain Assessment in Cancer Patients

This section includes text excerpted from "Cancer Pain (PDQ®)—Patient Version," National Cancer Institute (NCI), September 23, 2016.

General Information about Cancer Pain

Cancer, treatment for cancer, or diagnostic tests may cause you to feel pain. Pain is one of the most common symptoms in cancer patients. Pain can be caused by cancer, treatment for cancer, or a combination of factors. Tumors, surgery, intravenous chemotherapy, radiation therapy, targeted therapy, supportive care therapies such as bisphosphonates, and diagnostic procedures may cause you pain.

Younger patients are more likely to have cancer pain and pain flares than older patients. Patients with advanced cancer have more severe pain, and many cancer survivors have pain that continues after cancer treatment ends.

Pain Control Can Improve Your Quality of Life

Pain can be controlled in most patients who have cancer. Although cancer pain cannot always be relieved completely, there are ways to lessen pain in most patients. Pain control can improve your quality of life all through your cancer treatment and after it ends.

Pain Can Be Managed before, during, and after Diagnostic and Treatment Procedures

Many diagnostic and treatment procedures are painful. It helps to start pain control before the procedure begins. Some drugs may be used to help you feel calm or fall asleep. Treatments such as imagery or relaxation can also help control pain and anxiety related to treatment. Knowing what will happen during the procedure and having a relative or friend stay with you may also help lower anxiety.

Different Cancer Treatments May Cause Specific Types of Pain

Patients may have different types of pain depending on the treatments they receive, including:

- Spasms, stinging, and itching caused by intravenous chemotherapy.

- Mucositis (sores or inflammation in the mouth or other parts of the digestive system) caused by chemotherapy or targeted therapy.

- Skin pain, rash, or hand-foot syndrome (redness, tingling, or burning in the palms of the hands and/or the soles of feet) caused by chemotherapy or targeted therapy.

- Pain in joints and muscles throughout the body caused by paclitaxel or aromatase inhibitor therapy.

- Osteonecrosis of the jaw caused by bisphosphonates given for cancer that has spread to the bone.

- Pain syndromes caused by radiation, including mucositis, pain flares, and dermatitis.

Cancer Pain May Affect Quality of Life and Ability to Function Even after Treatment Ends

Pain that is severe or continues after cancer treatment ends increases the risk of anxiety and depression. Patients may be disabled

41

by their pain, unable to work, or feel that they are losing support once their care moves from their oncology team back to their primary care team. Feelings of anxiety and depression can worsen cancer pain and make it harder to control.

Each Patient Needs a Personal Plan to Control Cancer Pain

Each person's diagnosis, cancer stage, response to pain, and personal likes and dislikes are different. For this reason, each patient needs a personal plan to control cancer pain. You, your family, and your healthcare team can work together to manage your pain. As part of your pain control plan, your healthcare provider can give you and your family members written instructions to control your pain at home. Find out who you should call if you have questions.

Assessment of Cancer Pain

You and your healthcare team work together to assess cancer pain. It's important that the cause of the pain is found early and treated quickly. Your healthcare team will help you measure pain levels often, including at the following times:

- After starting cancer treatment.
- When there is new pain.
- After starting any type of pain treatment.

To learn about your pain, the healthcare team will ask you to describe the pain with the following questions:

- When did the pain start?
- How long does the pain last?
- Where is the pain? You will be asked to show exactly where the pain is on your body or on a drawing of a body.
- How strong is the pain?
- Have there been changes in where or when the pain occurs?
- What makes the pain better or worse?
- Is the pain worse during certain times of the day or night?
- Is there breakthrough pain (intense pain that flares up quickly even when pain control medicine is being used)?

- Do you have symptoms, such as trouble sleeping, fatigue, depression, or anxiety?
- Does pain get in the way of activities of daily life, such as eating, bathing, or moving around?

Your healthcare team will also take into account:

- Past and current pain treatments.
- Prognosis (chance of recovery).
- Other conditions you may have, such as kidney, liver, or heart disease.
- Past and current use of nicotine, alcohol, or sleeping pills.
- Personal or family history of substance abuse.
- Personal history of childhood sexual abuse.
- Your own choices.

A family member or caregiver may be asked to give answers for a patient who has a problem with speech, language, or understanding.

Physical and neurological exams will be done to help plan pain control.

The following exams will be done:

- **Physical exam and history:** An exam of the body to check general signs of health, including checking for signs of disease, such as lumps or anything else that seems unusual. A history of your health habits and past illnesses and treatments will also be taken.
- **Neurological exam:** A series of questions and tests to check the brain, spinal cord, and nerve function. The exam checks your mental status, coordination, and ability to walk normally, and how well the muscles, senses, and reflexes work. This may also be called a neuro exam or a neurologic exam.

Your healthcare team will also assess your psychological, social, and spiritual needs.

Using Drugs to Control Cancer Pain

The doctor will prescribe drugs based on whether the pain is mild, moderate, or severe. Your doctor will prescribe drugs to help relieve your pain. These drugs need to be taken at scheduled times to keep a constant level of the drug in the body to help keep the pain from coming back. Drugs may be taken by mouth or given in other ways, such as by infusion or injection.

Your doctor may prescribe extra doses of a drug that can be taken as needed for pain that occurs between scheduled doses of the drug. The doctor will adjust the drug dose for your needs.

A scale from 0 to 10 is used to measure how severe the pain is and decide which pain medicine to use. On this scale:

- 0 means no pain

- 1 to 3 means mild pain

- 4 to 6 means moderate pain

- 7 to 10 means severe pain

Acetaminophen and nonsteroidal anti-inflammatory drugs (NSAIDs) help relieve mild pain. They may be given with opioids for moderate to severe pain.

Pain relievers of this type include:

- Acetaminophen
- Ibuprofen
- Celecoxib
- Ketoprofen
- Diclofenac
- Ketorolac

Patients, especially older patients, who are taking acetaminophen or NSAIDs need to be closely watched for side effects.

Other Treatments for Cancer Pain

Most cancer pain can be controlled with drug treatments, but some patients have too many side effects from drugs or have pain in a certain part of the body that needs to be treated in a different way. You can talk to your doctor to help decide which methods work best to relieve your pain. These other treatments include:

Nerve Blocks

A nerve block is the injection of either a local anesthetic or a drug into or around a nerve to block pain. Nerve blocks help control pain that can't be controlled in other ways. Nerve blocks may also be used to find where the pain is coming from, to predict how the pain will respond to long-term treatments, and to prevent pain after certain procedures.

Neurological Treatments

Surgery can be done to insert a device that delivers drugs or stimulates the nerves with mild electric current. In rare cases, surgery may be done to destroy a nerve or nerves that are part of the pain pathway.

Cordotomy

Cordotomy is a less common surgical procedure that is used to relieve pain by cutting certain nerves in the spinal cord. This blocks pain and also hot/cold feelings. This procedure may be chosen for patients who are near the end of life and have severe pain that cannot be relieved in other ways.

Palliative Care

Certain patients are helped by palliative care services. Palliative care providers may also be called supportive care providers. They work in teams that include doctors, nurses, mental health specialists, social workers, chaplains, pharmacists, and dietitians. Some of the goals of palliative care are to:

- Improve quality of life for patients and their families.

- Manage pain and non-pain symptoms.

- Support patients who need higher doses of opioids, have a history of substance abuse, or are coping with emotional and social problems.

Radiation Therapy

Radiation therapy is used to relieve pain in patients with skin lesions, tumors, or cancer that has spread to the bone. This is called palliative radiation therapy. It may be given as local therapy directly to the tumor or to larger areas of the body. Radiation therapy helps drugs and other treatments work better by shrinking tumors that are causing pain. Radiation therapy may help patients with bone pain move more freely and with less pain.

Physical Medicine and Rehabilitation

Patients with cancer and pain may lose their strength, freedom of movement, and ability to manage their daily activities. Physical therapy or occupational therapy may help these patients.

Physical medicine uses physical methods, such as exercise and machines to prevent and treat disease or injury.

Physical methods to treat weakness, muscle wasting, and muscle and bone pain include the following:

- Exercise to strengthen and stretch weak muscles, loosen stiff joints, help coordination and balance, and strengthen the heart.

- Changing position (for patients who are not able to move on their own).

- Limiting the movement of painful areas or broken bones.

Some patients may be referred to a physiatrist (a doctor who specializes in physical medicine) who can develop a personal plan for them. Some physiatrists are also trained in procedures to treat and manage pain.

Complementary Therapies

Complementary and alternative therapies combined with standard treatment may be used to treat pain. They may also be called integrative therapies. Acupuncture, support groups, and hypnosis are a few integrative therapies that have been used to relieve pain.

Treating Cancer Pain in Older Patients

Certain factors affect cancer pain treatment in older adults. Some problems are more likely in patients 65 years and older. For caregivers of these patients, the following should be kept in mind:

Lower Doses

Pain medicine should be started at lower doses in older patients and adjusted slowly to allow for differences in their pain threshold and the ways they respond and function. Older patients may need lower doses of opioids since they are more sensitive to their effects. Side effects of opioids, such as drowsiness and constipation, are more likely in older patients. Opioid doses may need to be lower in older patients for either acute or chronic pain. Lower doses may give older patients better pain relief that lasts longer than in younger patients. Meperidine, and some drugs often used with opioids, are not given to certain older patients.

More than one chronic disease and source of pain.

Older patients may have more than one chronic disease and take several drugs for different conditions. This can increase the risk of drug interactions. Drugs taken together can change how they work in the body and can affect the patient's chronic diseases.

Section 7.3

Pain Assessment in Patients with Dementia

This section includes text excerpted from "Prevalence and Management of Pain, by Race and Dementia among Nursing Home Residents: United States, 2004," Centers for Disease Control and Prevention (CDC), November 6, 2015.

Pain and Dementia

Pain is common among nursing home residents, and effective pain management has an impact on improving quality of life. Previous research has shown race differences in pain reporting and management in various settings, with racial and ethnic minority groups less likely than white residents to report pain and receive adequate treatment. Other studies have documented cognitive impairment as a barrier in the detection and self-report of pain, with the underreporting likely resulting in under treatment. However, the relationships among race, dementia, and pain reporting and management remain understudied. This section explores the combined impact of race and a diagnosis of dementia on reporting or showing signs of pain and pain management among nursing home residents.

Does Pain Vary by Race? Does Pain Vary by a Diagnosis of Dementia?

Overall among nursing home residents, 23% reported or showed signs of pain in the 7 days prior to the interview.

Nonwhite residents were less likely to report or show signs of pain than white residents. Nursing home residents with dementia were also less likely to report or show signs of pain compared with residents who did not have dementia.

47

Among all residents, 17% of nonwhite residents compared with 24% of white residents reported or showed signs of pain.

Seventeen percent of those with dementia reported or showed signs of pain in the 7 days prior to the interview compared with 29% of those without dementia.

A similar association between dementia status and reporting of pain existed among both white and nonwhite residents, with a significantly greater proportion of residents without dementia reporting or showing signs of pain compared with residents with dementia. Nonwhite residents with dementia (12%) were least likely to report or show signs of pain, and white residents without dementia (31%) were most likely to report or show signs of pain.

Did Residents with Pain Receive Appropriate Pain Management?

Although the use of medications for pain management may vary by age, sex, and clinical condition, appropriate care for pain is either standing orders for pain medication or receipt of services from a special program for pain management, particularly among nursing home residents with moderate to severe pain. Among nursing home residents with pain, 44% neither had standing orders nor received special services for pain management, 46% either had standing orders or received special services, and another 10% had both standing orders and received special services for pain management.

Among Residents with Pain, Does Appropriate Pain Management Vary by Race or Diagnosis of Dementia?

There were no statistically significant differences in lack of appropriate pain management by dementia diagnosis (44% of those with dementia and 45% of those without dementia) or race (45% of white residents and 48% of nonwhite residents).

If one considers race and dementia diagnosis simultaneously, a similar percentage of white residents with or without dementia and nonwhite residents without dementia lacked appropriate pain management (43%, 46%, and 44%, respectively).However, lack of appropriate pain management differed between nonwhite residents with dementia and white residents with dementia; 56% of nonwhite residents with dementia lacked appropriate pain management compared with 43% of white residents with dementia ($p<.05$).

Summary

About one-quarter of nursing home residents reported or showed signs of pain. Prevalence of pain among residents varied by race and dementia diagnosis. Consistent with previous research, these nationally representative results suggest that non-white residents were less likely to report or show signs of pain than white residents, and residents with dementia were less likely to report or show signs of pain than residents without dementia. As a group, white residents without dementia appear at one end of the spectrum with the highest likelihood of reporting or showing signs of pain. At the other end of the spectrum are nonwhite residents with dementia, who are least likely to report or show signs of pain.

Over 40% of all nursing home residents with pain received neither standing orders for pain medication nor special services for pain management. Among residents with dementia and pain, there were differences in appropriate pain management between nonwhite and white residents, with non-white residents being more likely than white residents to lack appropriate pain management. Because questions about pain management were asked only if a resident reported or showed signs of pain, residents whose pain was controlled were not included in this analysis. Therefore, residents without reported or noted pain because it was controlled, may have received pain management, and the estimates of receipt of pain management approaches presented in this report may be underestimated.

In light of national goals to reduce racial disparities in healthcare quality, these findings contribute to the literature by exploring the complex associations among race, dementia, and pain management.

49

Chapter 8

Managing and Treating Fatigue

Chapter Contents

Section 8.1

Fatigue: More than Being Tired

This section includes text excerpted from "Fatigue: More
than Being Tired," National Institute on Aging (NIA),
National Institutes of Health (NIH), July 2016.

Some Illnesses Cause Fatigue

Feeling fatigued can be like an alarm going off in your body. It may
be the first sign that something is wrong. But, fatigue itself is not
a disease. For example, people with rheumatoid arthritis, a painful
condition that affects the joints, often complain of other symptoms,
including fatigue. People with cancer may feel fatigued from the disease, treatments, or both.

Many medical problems and treatments can add to fatigue. These
include:

- Taking certain medications, such as antidepressants, antihistamines, and medicines for nausea and pain

- Having medical treatments, like chemotherapy and radiation

- Recovery from major surgery

What Role Do Emotions Play in Feeling Fatigued?

Are you fearful about the future? Do you worry about your health
and who will take care of you? Are you afraid you are no longer needed?
Emotional worries like these can take a toll on your energy. Fatigue
can be linked to many emotions, including:

- Anxiety

- Depression

- Grief from loss of family or friends

- Stress from financial or personal problems

- Feeling that you no longer have control over your life

Regular physical activity or exercise may help reduce feelings of depression and stress while improving your mood and overall well-being.

What Else Causes Fatigue?

Some lifestyle habits can make you feel tired. Here are some things that may be draining your energy:

- **Staying up too late.** A good night's sleep is important to feeling refreshed and energetic. Try going to bed and waking up at the same time every day.

- **Having too much caffeine.** Drinking caffeinated drinks like soda, tea, or coffee late in the day can keep you from getting a good night's sleep. Limit the amount of caffeine you have during the day, and avoid it in the evening.

- **Drinking too much alcohol.** Alcohol changes the way you think and act. It may also interact with your medical treatments.

- **Eating junk food.** Say "no thanks" to food with empty calories, like fried foods and sweets, which have few nutrients and are high in fat and sugars. Nutritious foods will give you the energy you need to do the things you enjoy.

Can Boredom Cause Fatigue?

Being bored can also make you feel tired. That may sound strange, but it's true. If you were very busy during your working years, you may feel lost about how to spend your time when you retire. When you wake up in the morning, you may see long days stretching before you with nothing planned. It doesn't have to be that way.

Engaging in social and productive activities that you enjoy, like volunteering in your community, may help maintain your well-being. Think about what interests you and what skills or knowledge you have to offer, and look for places to volunteer.

How Can I Feel Less Tired?

Some changes to your lifestyle can make you feel less tired. Here are some suggestions:

- **Keep a fatigue diary** to help you find patterns throughout the day when you feel more or less tired.

53

- **Exercise regularly.** Almost anyone, at any age, can do some type of physical activity. If you have concerns about starting an exercise program, ask your doctor if there are any activities you should avoid. Moderate exercise may improve your appetite, energy, and outlook. Some people find that exercises combining balance and breathing (for example, tai chi or yoga) improve their energy.

- **Try to avoid long naps** (over 30 minutes) late in the day. Long naps can leave you feeling groggy and may make it harder to fall asleep at night.

- **Stop smoking.** Smoking is linked to many diseases and disorders, such as cancer, heart disease, and breathing problems, which can drain your energy.

- **Ask for help if you feel swamped.** Some people have so much to do that just thinking about their schedules can make them feel tired. Working with others may help a job go faster and be more fun.

When Should I See a Doctor for Fatigue?

If you've been tired for several weeks with no relief, it may be time to call your healthcare provider. He or she will ask questions about your sleep, daily activities, appetite, and exercise, and will likely give you a physical exam and order lab tests.

Your treatment will be based on your history and the results of your exam and lab tests. Your doctor may prescribe medications to target underlying health problems, such as anemia or irregular thyroid activity. He or she may suggest that you eat a well-balanced diet and begin an exercise program.

Section 8.2

Cancer and Fatigue

This section includes text excerpted from "Fatigue (PDQ®)—Patient Version," National Cancer Institute (NCI), May 7, 2015.

General Information about Fatigue

Fatigue is the most common side effect of cancer treatment. Cancer treatments such as chemotherapy, radiation therapy, and biologic therapy can cause fatigue in cancer patients. Fatigue is also a common symptom of some types of cancer. Patients describe fatigue as feeling tired, weak, worn-out, heavy, slow, or that they have no energy or get-up-and-go. Fatigue in cancer patients may be called cancer fatigue, cancer-related fatigue, and cancer treatment-related fatigue.

Fatigue related to cancer is different from fatigue that healthy people feel. When a healthy person is tired by day-to-day activities, their fatigue can be relieved by sleep and rest. Cancer-related fatigue is different. Cancer patients get tired after less activity than people who do not have cancer. Also, cancer-related fatigue is not completely relieved by sleep and rest and may last for a long time. Fatigue usually decreases after cancer treatment ends, but patients may still feel some fatigue for months or years.

Fatigue can decrease a patient's quality of life. Fatigue can affect all areas of life by making the patient too tired to take part in daily activities, relationships, social events, and community activities. Patients may miss work or school, spend less time with friends and family, or spend more time sleeping. In some cases, physical fatigue leads to mental fatigue and mood changes. This can make it hard for the patient to pay attention, remember things, and think clearly. Money may become a problem if the patient needs to take leave from a job or stop working completely. Job loss can lead to the loss of health insurance. All these things can lessen the patient's quality of life and self-esteem. Getting help with fatigue may prevent some of these problems and improve quality of life.

Causes of Fatigue in Cancer Patients

Fatigue in cancer patients may have more than one cause. Doctors do not know all the reasons cancer patients have fatigue. Many conditions may cause fatigue at the same time. Fatigue in cancer patients may be caused by the following:

- cancer treatment with chemotherapy, radiation therapy, and some biologic therapies
- anemia (a lower than normal number of red blood cells)
- hormone levels that are too low or too high
- trouble breathing or getting enough oxygen
- heart trouble
- infection
- pain
- stress
- loss of appetite or not getting enough calories and nutrients
- dehydration (loss of too much water from the body, such as from severe diarrhea or vomiting)
- changes in how well the body uses food for energy
- loss of weight, muscle, and/or strength
- medicines that cause drowsiness
- problems getting enough sleep
- being less active
- other medical conditions

Fatigue is common in people with advanced cancer who are not receiving cancer treatment.

How Cancer Treatments Cause Fatigue Is Not Known

Doctors are trying to better understand how cancer treatments such as surgery, chemotherapy, and radiation therapy cause fatigue. Some studies show that fatigue is caused by:

- The need for extra energy to repair and heal body tissue damaged by treatment.

- The build-up of toxic substances that are left in the body after cells are killed by cancer treatment.

- The effect of biologic therapy on the immune system.

- Changes in the body's sleep-wake cycle.

When they begin cancer treatment, many patients are already tired from medical tests, surgery, and the emotional stress of coping with the cancer diagnosis. After treatment begins, fatigue may get worse. Patients who are older, have advanced cancer, or receive more than one type of treatment (for example, both chemotherapy and radiation therapy) are more likely to have long-term fatigue.

Different cancer treatments have different effects on a patient's energy level. The type and schedule of treatments can affect the amount of fatigue caused by cancer therapy.

Fatigue Caused by Chemotherapy

Patients treated with chemotherapy usually feel the most fatigue in the days right after each treatment. Then the fatigue decreases until the next treatment. Fatigue usually increases with each cycle. Some studies have shown that patients have the most severe fatigue about mid-way through all the cycles of chemotherapy. Fatigue decreases after chemotherapy is finished, but patients may not feel back to normal until a month or more after the last treatment. Many patients feel fatigued for months or years after treatment ends.

Fatigue during chemotherapy may be increased by the following:

- Pain.

- Depression.

- Anxiety.

- Anemia. Some types of chemotherapy stop the bone marrow from making enough new red blood cells, causing anemia (too few red blood cells to carry oxygen to the body).

- Lack of sleep caused by some anticancer drugs.

Fatigue Caused by Radiation Therapy

Many patients receiving radiation therapy have fatigue that keeps them from being as active as they want to be. After radiation therapy begins, fatigue usually increases until mid-way through the course of treatments and then stays about the same until treatment ends. For many patients, fatigue improves after radiation therapy stops. However, in some patients, fatigue will last months or years after treatment ends. Some patients never have the same amount of energy they had before treatment.

Cancer-related fatigue has been studied in patients with breast cancer and prostate cancer. The amount of fatigue they felt and the time of day the fatigue was worst was different in different patients.

In men with prostate cancer, fatigue was increased by having the following symptoms before radiation therapy started:

- poor sleep
- depression

In women with breast cancer, fatigue was increased by the following:

- working while receiving radiation therapy
- having children at home
- depression
- anxiety
- trouble sleeping
- younger age
- being underweight
- having advanced cancer or other medical conditions

Fatigue Caused by Biologic Therapy

Biologic therapy often causes flu-like symptoms. These symptoms include being tired physically and mentally, fever, chills, muscle pain, headache, and not feeling well in general. Some patients may also have problems thinking clearly. Fatigue symptoms depend on the type of biologic therapy used.

Fatigue Caused by Surgery

Fatigue is often a side effect of surgery, but patients usually feel better with time. However, fatigue caused by surgery can be worse when the surgery is combined with other cancer treatments.

Anemia Is a Common Cause of Fatigue

Anemia affects the patient's energy level and quality of life. Anemia may be caused by the following:

- cancer

- cancer treatments

- a medical condition not related to the cancer

The effects of anemia on a patient depend on the following:

- how quickly the anemia occurs

- the patient's age

- the amount of plasma (fluid part of the blood) in the patient's blood

- other medical conditions the patient has

Side Effects Related to Nutrition May Cause or Increase Fatigue

The body's energy comes from food. Fatigue may occur if the body does not take in enough food to give the body the energy it needs. For many patients, the effects of cancer and cancer treatments make it hard to eat well. In people with cancer, three major factors may affect nutrition:

- A change in the way the body is able to use food. A patient may eat the same amount as before having cancer, but the body may not be able to absorb and use all the nutrients from the food. This is caused by the cancer or its treatment.

- A decrease in the amount of food eaten because of low appetite, nausea, vomiting, diarrhea, or a blocked bowel.

- An increase in the amount of energy needed by the body because of a growing tumor, infection, fever, or shortness of breath.

Anxiety and Depression Are the Most Common Psychological Causes of Fatigue in Cancer Patients

The emotional stress of cancer can cause physical problems, including fatigue. It's common for cancer patients to have changes in moods and attitudes. Patients may feel anxiety and fear before and after a cancer diagnosis. These feelings may cause fatigue. The effect of the disease on the patient's physical, mental, social, and financial well-being can increase emotional distress.

About 15% to 25% of patients who have cancer get depressed, which may increase fatigue caused by physical factors. The following are signs of depression:

- feeling tired mentally and physically

- loss of interest in life

- problems thinking

- loss of sleep

- feeling a loss of hope

Some patients have more fatigue after cancer treatments than others do.

Fatigue may be increased when it is hard for patients to learn and remember. During and after cancer treatment, patients may find they cannot pay attention for very long and have a hard time thinking, remembering, and understanding. This is called attention fatigue. Sleep helps to relieve attention fatigue, but sleep may not be enough when the fatigue is related to cancer. Taking part in restful activities and spending time outdoors may help relieve attention fatigue.

Not Sleeping Well May Cause Fatigue

Some people with cancer are not able to get enough sleep. The following problems related to sleep may cause fatigue:

- waking up during the night

- not going to sleep at the same time every night

- sleeping during the day and less at night

- not being active during the day

Poor sleep affects people in different ways. For example, the time of day that fatigue is worse may be different. Some patients who have trouble sleeping may feel more fatigue in the morning. Others may have severe fatigue in both the morning and the evening.

Even in patients who have poor sleep, fixing sleep problems does not always improve fatigue. A lack of sleep may not be the cause of the fatigue.

Medicines Other than Chemotherapy May Add to Fatigue

Patients may take medicines for cancer symptoms, such as pain, or conditions other than the cancer. These medicines may cause the patient to feel sleepy. Opioids, antidepressants, and antihistamines have this side effect. If many of these medicines are taken at the same time, fatigue may be worse.

Taking opioids over time may lower the amount of sex hormones made in the testicles and ovaries. This can lead to fatigue as well as sexual problems and depression.

Fatigue after Cancer Treatment Ends

Fatigue continues to be a problem for many cancer survivors long after treatment ends and the cancer is gone. Studies show that some patients continue to have moderate-to-severe fatigue years after treatment. Long-term therapies such as tamoxifen can also cause fatigue. In children who were treated for brain tumors and cured, fatigue may continue after treatment.

The causes of fatigue after treatment ends are different than the causes of fatigue during treatment. Treating fatigue after treatment ends also may be different from treating it during cancer therapy.

Since fatigue may greatly affect the quality of life for cancer survivors, long-term follow-up care is important.

Section 8.3

Assessment and Treatment of Fatigue

This section includes text excerpted from "Fatigue (PDQ®)—Patient Version," National Cancer Institute (NCI), May 7, 2015.

Assessment of Fatigue

An assessment is done to find out the level of fatigue and how it affects the patient's daily life. There is no test to diagnose fatigue, so it is important for the patient to tell family members and the healthcare team if fatigue is a problem. To assess fatigue, the patient is asked to describe how bad the fatigue is, how it affects daily activities, and what makes the fatigue better or worse. The doctor will look for causes of fatigue that can be treated. An assessment of fatigue includes a physical exam and blood tests. The assessment process may include the following:

- **Physical exam**: This is an exam of the body to check general signs of health or anything that seems unusual. The doctor will check for problems such as trouble breathing or loss of muscle strength. The patient's walking, posture, and joint movements will be checked.

- **Rating the level of fatigue**: The patient is asked to rate the level of fatigue (how bad the fatigue is). There is no standard way to rate fatigue. The doctor may ask the patient to rate the fatigue on a scale from 0 to 10. Other ways to rate fatigue check for how much the fatigue affects the patient's quality of life.

- A series of questions about the following:
  - When the fatigue started, how long it lasts, and what makes it better or worse.
  - Symptoms or side effects, such as pain, the patient is having from the cancer or the treatments.
  - Medicines being taken.
  - Sleeping and resting habits.
  - Eating habits and changes in appetite or weight.
  - How the fatigue affects daily activities and lifestyle.
  - How the fatigue affects being able to work.
  - Whether the patient has depression, anxiety, or pain.
  - Health habits and past illnesses and treatments.

- **Blood tests to check for anemia**:

  The most common blood tests to check if the number of red blood cells is normal are:

- Complete blood count (CBC) with differential: A procedure in which a sample of blood is taken and checked for the following:
  - The number of red blood cells and platelets.
  - The number and type of white blood cells.

- The amount of hemoglobin (the protein that carries oxygen) in the red blood cells.

- The portion of the blood sample made up of red blood cells.

- Peripheral blood smear: A procedure in which a sample of blood is checked for the number and kinds of white blood cells, the number of platelets, and changes in the shape of blood cells.

- Other blood tests may be done to check for other conditions that affect red blood cells. These include a bone marrow aspiration and biopsy or a Coombs' test. Blood tests to check the levels of vitamin B12, iron, and erythropoietin may also be done.

- Checking for other causes of fatigue that can be treated.

A fatigue assessment is repeated at different times to see if there are patterns of fatigue. A fatigue assessment is repeated to see if there is a pattern for when fatigue starts or becomes worse. Fatigue may be worse right after a chemotherapy treatment, for example. The same method of measuring fatigue is used at each assessment. This helps show changes in fatigue over time.

Treatments for Fatigue

Fatigue in cancer patients is often treated by relieving related conditions such as anemia and depression. Treatment of fatigue depends on the symptoms and whether the cause of fatigue is known. When the cause of fatigue is not known, treatment is usually given to relieve symptoms and teach the patient ways to cope with fatigue.

Treatment of Anemia

Treating anemia may help decrease fatigue. When known, the cause of the anemia is treated. When the cause is not known, treatment for anemia is supportive care and may include the following:

- **Change in diet.** Eating more foods rich in iron and vitamins may be combined with other treatments for anemia.

- **Transfusions of red blood cells.** Transfusions work well to treat anemia. Possible side effects of transfusions include an allergic reaction, infection, graft-versus-host disease, immune system changes, and too much iron in the blood.

- **Medicine.** Drugs that cause the bone marrow to make more
  red blood cells may be used to treat anemia-related fatigue in
  patients receiving chemotherapy. Epoetin alfa and darbepoe-
  tin alfa are two of these drugs. This type of drug may shorten
  survival time, increase the risk of serious heart problems, and
  cause some tumors to grow faster or recur. The U.S. Food and
  Drug Administration (FDA) has not approved these drugs for
  the treatment of fatigue. Discuss the risks and benefits of these
  drugs with your doctor.

Treatment of Pain

If pain is making fatigue worse, the patient's pain medicine may
be changed or the dose may be increased. If too much pain medicine
is making fatigue worse, the patient's pain medicine may be changed
or the dose may be decreased.

Treatment of Depression

Fatigue in patients who have depression may be treated with antidepressant drugs. Psychostimulant drugs may help some patients have
more energy and a better mood, and help them think and concentrate.
The use of psychostimulants for treating fatigue is still being studied.
The U.S. Food and Drug Administration (FDA) has not approved psychostimulants for the treatment of fatigue.

Psychostimulants have side effects, especially with long-term use.
Different psychostimulants have different side effects. Patients who
have heart problems or who take anticancer drugs that affect the heart
may have serious side effects from psychostimulants. These drugs have
warnings on the label about their risks. Talk to your doctor about the
effects these drugs may have and use them only under a doctor's care.
Some of the possible side effects include the following:

- trouble sleeping

- euphoria (feelings of extreme happiness)

- headache

- nausea

- anxiety

- mood changes

- loss of appetite

- nightmares

- paranoia (feelings of fear and distrust of other people)

- serious heart problems

The doctor may prescribe low doses of a psychostimulant to be used for a short time in patients with advanced cancer who have severe fatigue. Talk to your doctor about the risks and benefits of these drugs. Certain drugs are being studied for fatigue related to cancer.

The following drugs are being studied for fatigue related to cancer:

- Bupropion is an antidepressant that is being studied to treat fatigue in patients with or without depression.

- Dexamethasone is an anti-inflammatory drug being studied in patients with advanced cancer. In one clinical trial, patients who received dexamethasone reported less fatigue than the group that received a placebo. More trials are needed to study the link between inflammation and fatigue.

Certain dietary supplements are being studied for fatigue related to cancer.

The following dietary supplements are being studied for fatigue related to cancer:

- L-carnitine is a supplement that helps the body make energy and lowers inflammation that may be linked to fatigue.

- Ginseng is an herb used to treat fatigue which may be taken in capsules of ground ginseng root. In a clinical trial, cancer patients who were either in treatment or had finished treatment, received either ginseng or placebo. The group receiving ginseng had less fatigue than the placebo group.

Section 8.4

Coping with Fatigue

This section includes text excerpted from "Fatigue (PDQ®)—Patient Version," National Cancer Institute (NCI), May 7, 2015.

Exercise

Exercise (including walking) may help people with cancer feel better and have more energy. The effect of exercise on fatigue in cancer patients is being studied. One study reported that breast cancer survivors who took part in enjoyable physical activity had less fatigue and pain and were better able to take part in daily activities. In clinical trials, some patients reported the following benefits from exercise:

- More physical energy

- Better appetite

- More able to do the normal activities of daily living

- Better quality of life

- More satisfaction with life

- A greater sense of well-being

- More able to meet the demands of cancer and cancer treatment

Moderate activity for 3 to 5 hours a week may help cancer-related fatigue. You are more likely to follow an exercise plan if you choose a type of exercise that you enjoy. The healthcare team can help you plan the best time and place for exercise and how often to exercise. Patients may need to start with light activity for short periods of time and build up to more exercise little by little. Studies have shown that exercise can be safely done during and after cancer treatment.

Mind and body exercises such as qigong, tai chi, and yoga may help relieve fatigue. These exercises combine activities like movement, stretching, balance, and controlled breathing with spiritual activity such as meditation.

A Schedule of Activity and Rest

Changes in daily routine make the body use more energy. A regular routine can improve sleep and help the patient have more energy to be active during the day. A program of regular times for activity and rest help to make the most of a patient's energy. A healthcare professional can help patients plan an exercise program and decide which activities are the most important to them.

The following sleep habits may help decrease fatigue:

- Lie in bed for sleep only.

- Take naps for no longer than one hour.

- Avoid noise (like television and radio) during sleep.

Cancer patients should not try to do too much. Health professionals have information about support services to help with daily activities and responsibilities.

Talk Therapy

Therapists use talk therapy (counseling) to treat certain emotional or behavioral disorders. This kind of therapy helps patients change how they think and feel about certain things. Talk therapy may help decrease a cancer patient's fatigue by working on problems related to cancer that make fatigue worse, such as:

- Stress from coping with cancer.

- Fear that the cancer may come back.

- Feeling hopeless about fatigue.

- Not enough social support.

- A pattern of sleep and activity that changes from day to day.

Self-Care for Fatigue

Fatigue is often a short-term side effect of treatment, but in some patients it becomes chronic (continues as a long-term condition). Managing chronic fatigue includes adjusting to life with fatigue. Learning the facts about cancer-related fatigue may help you cope with it better and improve quality of life. For example, some patients in treatment worry that having fatigue means the treatment is not working. Anxiety over this can make fatigue even worse. Some patients may feel that reporting fatigue is complaining. Knowing that fatigue is a normal side effect that should be reported and treated may make it easier to manage.

Working with the healthcare team to learn about the following may help patients cope with fatigue:

- How to cope with fatigue as a normal side effect of treatment.

- The possible medical causes of fatigue such as not enough fluids, electrolyte imbalance, breathing problems, or anemia.

- How patterns of rest and activity affect fatigue.

- How to schedule important daily activities during times of less fatigue, and give up less important activities.

- The kinds of activities that may help you feel more alert (walking, gardening, bird-watching).

- The difference between fatigue and depression.

- How to avoid or change situations that cause stress.

- How to avoid or change activities that cause fatigue.

- How to change your surroundings to help decrease fatigue.

- Exercise programs that are right for you and decrease fatigue.

- The importance of eating enough food and drinking enough fluids.

- Physical therapy for patients who have nerve problems or muscle weakness.

- Respiratory therapy for patients who have trouble breathing.

- How to tell if treatments for fatigue are working.

Chapter 9

Palliative Wound Care

Whereas typical medical treatment focuses on healing, the aim of palliative care is to treat symptoms and improve the quality of life for terminally ill patients and their families. More than one-third of hospice patients and other individuals with serious illnesses suffer from such issues as pressure ulcers (bedsores), surgical wounds, and other skin problems as a result of the deterioration of the body and multi-organ systems failure. Palliative wound care is an effective method for relieving pain, treating infection, preventing new wounds from developing, and helping the patient and his or her family make the most of the remaining time they have together.

Management of Palliative Wound Care

Palliative care takes a coordinated approach to treating wounds and lessening symptoms, with the ultimate goal of ensuring patient comfort and sense of well-being. Generally, this means local wound care (treatment of the wound itself) and pain management.

Local Wound Care

Although healing is not always possible in palliative care, proper treatment of wounds can help prevent infection and improve the patient's state of mind. Wound care addresses such issues as:

- **Bleeding.** The repeated dressing and re-dressing of wounds often results in the tearing of tissue, which can lead to bleeding, increased discomfort, and infection. Topical vasoconstrictors are often used to stem blood flow, and a variety of sealants or barriers may be applied to the surface. Dressings with silicone adhesives may be used, since they are less likely to cause trauma to the wound with repeated applications.

- **Exudates.** These are clear or pus-like liquids that ooze out of cuts or areas of inflammation. Normally exudates are beneficial and central to the healing process, but in the case of chronic wounds they can cause problems such as infection of the wound or inflammation of the surrounding skin. The most common ways to manage exudates are through the use of the proper dressings and the application of topical steroids.

- **Infection.** Open wounds can easily become contaminated with bacteria, often leading to infection, which can spread and cause additional problems. And in the case of chronically ill patients, who frequently have compromised immune systems, this can be particularly dangerous. The best practice is to prevent infection in the first place. This is accomplished by using wound dressings with antimicrobial agents, applying topical antibiotics, and cleansing and debriding (removing dead tissue) the area when changing dressings.

- **Odor.** Unpleasant odor is a common problem with wounds, particularly those in which infection has set in, and in additional to being a sign of physical issues this has a tendency to negatively affect the patient's mental state. The first step in addressing or preventing odor is the proper cleansing of the wound, along with the application of topical antibiotics to treat infection and the use of specialized dressings.

Pain Management

Pressure ulcers and other skin problems can be especially painful, and unfortunately they are extremely common among terminally ill patients and others requiring palliative care. Therefore, controlling pain is one of the most important components in palliative wound care and is perhaps the one with the most impact on the patient's well-being and quality of life. Pain management may include:

- **Prevention.** The best way to manage pain is to prevent it as much as possible in the first place. This often means using special dressings that don't stick to wounds and training care-givers in the proper way to change dressings. Bedridden patients are usually turned frequently to prevent pressure ulcers, but in some cases, as when certain wounds are present, this procedure can increase pain, so less frequent turning may be called for. Debridement, although necessary, can be extremely painful, so in some cases medical professionals may need to administer a local anesthetic prior to the procedure.

- **Assessment.** Since pain is a subjective experience, assessing the degree to which it affects any given individual can be difficult. But since palliative care includes involving the patient in decision-making, his or her own description of pain must be taken into account by care-givers. In addition, a variety of tools — numerical scales, charts, and drawings — are often used, as are physiological and behavior observations by medical professionals.

- **Topical anesthetics.** The application of pain-relief medication directly to the wound has the advantage of bypassing the circulatory system, thus avoiding many side effects and often allowing for lower doses. Common topical anesthetics include lidocaine, benzydamine, sucralfate, and morphine gel, sometimes with antibiotics added to help prevent infection. Dressings that contain slow-release pain-relief pain medication, such as ibuprofen, have also proven effective.

- **Systemic analgesics.** These medications can be administered orally, by injection, or though an IV, and work by being absorbed into the bloodstream where they affect the body's pain receptors. Generally, the treatment of moderate pain will begin with such medications as acetaminophen and nonsteroidal anti-inflammatory drugs. More severe pain often requires the use of opioid (narcotic) analgesics, such as morphine, meperidine, nalbuphine, butorphanol, and fentanyl. Although these medications relieve pain, they tend to reduce the patient's mental status or, in large doses, make him or her sleep most of the time, so doctors need to balance their benefits against quality of life.

- **Alternative methods.** A number of methods for controlling pain without medication — or with lower doses of medication — have proven effective in some cases. These include gentle massage, physical therapy, acupuncture, and relaxation techniques, such as biofeedback and hypnosis. Transcutaneous electrical nerve stimulation, or TENS, which employs low-voltage electrical current for pain relief, has also been used with good results. And many patients respond well to pet therapy, as the presence of an animal and stoking its fur can have a very soothing effect.

Locations for Palliative Wound Care

Palliative wound care can take place in a hospital, an outpatient clinic (if the patient is ambulatory), at home, or in a hospice. In all cases, the palliative-care team will typically consist of doctors, nurses, and social workers, as well as the patient and family members, who are integral part of the management process. In some cases, other specialists, including massage therapists, pharmacists, and nutritionists, may be part of the team. Each location has its advantages and disadvantages, which depend on the illness, the severity of symptoms, the patient's preferences, and access to qualified care-givers.

- **Hospital care.** During the early stages of an illness, patients are generally treated in a hospital. And even when treatment is completed or discontinued, many hospitals now have specialists on staff to provide palliative-care, although unless the hospital has a hospice or other dedicated facility, this is usually only available for a limited time.

- **Outpatient palliative care.** If a patient is ambulatory, specialized wound care may be provided at a clinic that is outfitted and staffed for palliative care. The advantage of this type of care is that the patient and family are able to maintain close to their normal routines, while the illness is managed as required by a team of professionals.

- **Palliative care at home.** Most patients prefer to live at home, rather than in a care facility. And with the many types of professional support available through a variety of hospital programs, government agencies, and private sources, many individuals with serious illnesses are able to do so. Generally, this means working with a team of visiting nurses, social workers, and other professionals—as well as the cooperation of family members—to ensure that adequate care is available as needed.

- **Hospice care.** When illnesses have progressed too far for home or outpatient care, palliative care in a hospice may be recommended. In most instances, hospices are for terminally ill patients who may have only months to live. Here, although the

72

level of care is not as intense as in a hospital, the patient can be observed more closely and professional help is generally more readily available. But, as with all palliative care, the emphasis is on patient comfort and quality of life.

References

1. Graves, Marilyn L., MSN, RN, CHPN, CWOCN, and Virginia Sun, PhD, RN. "Providing Quality Wound Care at the End of Life," Medscape.com, n.d.

2. Hughes, Ronda G. PhD, MHS, RN, et al. "Palliative Wound Care at the End of Life," Home Health Care Management and Practice, April 2005.

3. "Managing Pain Beyond Drugs," Web MD, August 14, 2015.

4. Tippett, Aletha W., MD. "Palliative Wound Treatment Promotes Healing," Wounds, January 2015.

5. Woo, Kevin Y., PhD, RN, ACNP, GNC(C), FAPWCA, et al. "Palliative Wound Care Management Strategies for Palliative Patients and Their Circles of Care," Clinical Management, March 2015.

Chapter 10

Acute Respiratory Distress Syndrome (ARDS)

What Is Acute Respiratory Distress Syndrome (ARDS)?

ARDS, or acute respiratory distress syndrome, is a lung condition that leads to low oxygen levels in the blood. ARDS can be life threatening because your body's organs need oxygen-rich blood to work well. People who develop ARDS often are very ill with another disease or have major injuries. They might already be in the hospital when they develop ARDS.

To understand ARDS, it helps to understand how the lungs work. When you breathe, air passes through your nose and mouth into your windpipe. The air then travels to your lungs' air sacs. These sacs are called alveoli. Small blood vessels called capillaries run through the walls of the air sacs. Oxygen passes from the air sacs into the capillaries and then into the bloodstream. Blood carries the oxygen to all parts of the body, including the body's organs.

In ARDS, infections, injuries, or other conditions cause fluid to build up in the air sacs. This prevents the lungs from filling with air and moving enough oxygen into the bloodstream. As a result, the body's organs (such as the kidneys and brain) don't get the oxygen they need. Without oxygen, the organs may not work well or at all.

This chapter includes text excerpted from "What Is ARDS?" National Heart, Lung, and Blood Institute (NHLBI), January 12, 2012. Reviewed October 2016.

People who develop ARDS often are in the hospital for other serious health problems. Rarely, people who aren't hospitalized have health problems that lead to ARDS, such as severe pneumonia. If you have trouble breathing, call your doctor right away. If you have severe shortness of breath, call 9–1–1.

More people are surviving ARDS now than in the past. One likely reason for this is that treatment and care for the condition have improved. Survival rates for ARDS vary depending on age, the underlying cause of ARDS, associated illnesses, and other factors. Some people who survive recover completely. Others may have lasting damage to their lungs and other health problems. Researchers continue to look for new and better ways to treat ARDS.

What Causes ARDS?

Many conditions or factors can directly or indirectly injure the lungs and lead to ARDS. Some common ones are:

- Sepsis. This is a condition in which bacteria infect the bloodstream.
- Pneumonia. This is an infection in the lungs.
- Severe bleeding caused by an injury to the body.
- An injury to the chest or head, like a severe blow.
- Breathing in harmful fumes or smoke.
- Inhaling vomited stomach contents from the mouth.

It's not clear why some very sick or seriously injured people develop ARDS and others don't. Researchers are trying to find out why ARDS develops and how to prevent it.

Who Is at Risk for ARDS?

People at risk for ARDS have a condition or illness that can directly or indirectly injure their lungs.

Direct Lung Injury

Conditions that can directly injure the lungs include:

- Pneumonia. This is an infection in the lungs.
- Breathing in harmful fumes or smoke.
- Inhaling vomited stomach contents from the mouth.

- Using a ventilator. This is a machine that helps people breathe; rarely, it can injure the lungs.
- Nearly drowning.

Indirect Lung Injury

Conditions that can indirectly injure the lungs include:

- Sepsis. This is a condition in which bacteria infect the bloodstream.
- Severe bleeding caused by an injury to the body or having many blood transfusions.
- An injury to the chest or head, such as a severe blow.
- Pancreatitis. This is a condition in which the pancreas becomes irritated or infected. The pancreas is a gland that releases enzymes and hormones.
- Fat embolism. This is a condition in which fat blocks an artery. A physical injury, like a broken bone, can lead to a fat embolism.
- Drug reaction.

What Are the Signs and Symptoms of ARDS?

The first signs and symptoms of ARDS are feeling like you can't get enough air into your lungs, rapid breathing, and a low blood oxygen level. Other signs and symptoms depend on the cause of ARDS. They may occur before ARDS develops. For example, if pneumonia is causing ARDS, you may have a cough and fever before you feel short of breath.

Sometimes people who have ARDS develop signs and symptoms such as low blood pressure, confusion, and extreme tiredness. This may mean that the body's organs, such as the kidneys and heart, aren't getting enough oxygen-rich blood. People who develop ARDS often are in the hospital for other serious health problems. Rarely, people who aren't hospitalized have health problems that lead to ARDS, such as severe pneumonia.

If you have trouble breathing, call your doctor right away. If you have severe shortness of breath, call 9-1-1.

Complications from ARDS

If you have ARDS, you can develop other medical problems while in the hospital.

77

The most common problems are:

- **Infections**. Being in the hospital and lying down for a long time can put you at risk for infections, such as pneumonia. Being on a ventilator also puts you at higher risk for infections.

- **Pneumothorax** (collapsed lung). This is a condition in which air or gas collects in the space around the lungs. This can cause one or both lungs to collapse. The air pressure from a ventilator can cause this condition.

- **Lung scarring**. ARDS causes the lungs to become stiff (scarred). It also makes it hard for the lungs to expand and fill with air. Being on a ventilator also can cause lung scarring.

- **Blood clots**. Lying down for long periods can cause blood clots to form in your body. A blood clot that forms in a vein deep in your body is called a deep vein thrombosis. This type of blood clot can break off, travel through the bloodstream to the lungs, and block blood flow. This condition is called pulmonary embolism.

How Is ARDS Diagnosed?

Your doctor will diagnose ARDS based on your medical history, a physical exam, and test results.

Medical History

Your doctor will ask whether you have or have recently had conditions that could lead to ARDS. Your doctor also will ask whether you have heart problems, such as heart failure. Heart failure can cause fluid to build up in your lungs.

Physical Exam

ARDS may cause abnormal breathing sounds, such as crackling. Your doctor will listen to your lungs with a stethoscope to hear these sounds. He or she also will listen to your heart and look for signs of extra fluid in other parts of your body. Extra fluid may mean you have heart or kidney problems. Your doctor will look for a bluish color on your skin and lips. A bluish color means your blood has a low level of oxygen. This is a possible sign of ARDS.

Diagnostic Tests

You may have ARDS or another condition that causes similar symptoms. To find out, your doctor may recommend one or more of the following tests.

- An arterial blood gas test
- Chest X-ray
- Blood tests
- Sputum culture

How Is ARDS Treated?

ARDS is treated in a hospital's intensive care unit. Current treatment approaches focus on improving blood oxygen levels and providing supportive care. Doctors also will try to pinpoint and treat the underlying cause of the condition.

Oxygen Therapy

One of the main goals of treating ARDS is to provide oxygen to your lungs and other organs (such as your brain and kidneys). Your organs need oxygen to work properly. Oxygen usually is given through nasal prongs or a mask that fits over your mouth and nose. However, if your oxygen level doesn't rise or it's still hard for you to breathe, your doctor will give you oxygen through a breathing tube. He or she will insert the flexible tube through your mouth or nose and into your windpipe. Before inserting the tube, your doctor will squirt or spray a liquid medicine into your throat (and possibly your nose) to make it numb. Your doctor also will give you medicine through an intravenous (IV) line in your bloodstream to make you sleepy and relaxed. The breathing tube will be connected to a machine that supports breathing (a ventilator). The ventilator will fill your lungs with oxygen-rich air.

Your doctor will adjust the ventilator as needed to help your lungs get the right amount of oxygen. This also will help prevent injury to your lungs from the pressure of the ventilator. You'll use the breathing tube and ventilator until you can breathe on your own. If you need a ventilator for more than a few days, your doctor may do a tracheotomy.

This procedure involves making a small cut in your neck to create an opening to the windpipe. The opening is called a tracheostomy.

Your doctor will place the breathing tube directly into the windpipe. The tube is then connected to the ventilator.

Supportive Care

Supportive care refers to treatments that help relieve symptoms, prevent complications, or improve quality of life. Supportive approaches used to treat ARDS include:

- Medicines to help you relax, relieve discomfort, and treat pain.

- Ongoing monitoring of heart and lung function (including blood pressure and gas exchange).

- Nutritional support. People who have ARDS often suffer from malnutrition. Thus, extra nutrition may be given through a feeding tube.

- Treatment for infections. People who have ARDS are at higher risk for infections, such as pneumonia. Being on a ventilator also increases the risk of infections. Doctors use antibiotics to treat pneumonia and other infections.

- Prevention of blood clots. Lying down for long periods can cause blood clots to form in the deep veins of your body. These clots can travel to your lungs and block blood flow (a condition called pulmonary embolism). Blood-thinning medicines and other treatments, such as compression stocking (stockings that create gentle pressure up the leg), are used to prevent blood clots.

- Prevention of intestinal bleeding. People who receive long-term support from a ventilator are at increased risk of bleeding in the intestines. Medicines can reduce this risk.

- Fluids. You may be given fluids to improve blood flow through your body and to provide nutrition. Your doctor will make sure you get the right amount of fluids. Fluids usually are given through an IV line inserted into one of your blood vessels.

Chapter 11

Nutrition Therapy in Cancer Care

Nutrition in Cancer Care

Good nutrition is important for cancer patients. Nutrition is a process in which food is taken in and used by the body for growth, to keep the body healthy, and to replace tissue. Good nutrition is important for good health. Eating the right kinds of foods before, during, and after cancer treatment can help the patient feel better and stay stronger. A healthy diet includes eating and drinking enough of the foods and liquids that have the important nutrients (vitamins, minerals, protein, carbohydrates, fat, and water) the body needs. When the body does not get or cannot absorb the nutrients needed for health, it causes a condition called malnutrition or malnourishment.

Healthy eating habits are important during cancer treatment. Nutrition therapy is used to help cancer patients get the nutrients they need to keep up their body weight and strength, keep body tissue healthy, and fight infection. Eating habits that are good for cancer patients can be very different from the usual healthy eating guidelines.

Healthy eating habits and good nutrition can help patients deal with the effects of cancer and its treatment. Some cancer treatments work better when the patient is well nourished and gets enough calories

This chapter includes text excerpted from "Nutrition in Cancer Care (PDQ®)—Patient Version," National Cancer Institute (NCI), January 8, 2016.

and protein in the diet. Patients who are well nourished may have a better prognosis (chance of recovery) and quality of life.

Cancer can change the way the body uses food. Some tumors make chemicals that change the way the body uses certain nutrients. The body's use of protein, carbohydrates, and fat may be affected, especially by tumors of the stomach or intestines. A patient may seem to be eating enough, but the body may not be able to absorb all the nutrients from the food.

Cancer and cancer treatments may affect taste, smell, appetite, and the ability to eat enough food or absorb the nutrients from food. This can cause malnutrition (a condition caused by a lack of key nutrients). Malnutrition can cause the patient to be weak, tired, and unable to fight infections or get through cancer treatment. Malnutrition may be made worse if the cancer grows or spreads. Eating too little protein and calories is a very common problem for cancer patients. Having enough protein and calories is important for healing, fighting infection, and having enough energy.

Anorexia and cachexia are common causes of malnutrition in cancer patients. Anorexia (the loss of appetite or desire to eat) is a common symptom in people with cancer. Anorexia may occur early in the disease or later, if the cancer grows or spreads. Some patients already have anorexia when they are diagnosed with cancer. Almost all patients who have advanced cancer will have anorexia. Anorexia is the most common cause of malnutrition in cancer patients.

Cachexia is a condition marked by a loss of appetite, weight loss, muscle loss, and general weakness. It is common in patients with tumors of the lung, pancreas, and upper gastrointestinal tract. It is important to watch for and treat cachexia early in cancer treatment because it is hard to correct.

Cancer patients may have anorexia and cachexia at the same time. Weight loss can be caused by eating fewer calories, using more calories, or both.

It is important to treat weight loss caused by cancer and its treatment. It is important that cancer symptoms and side effects that affect eating and cause weight loss are treated early. Both nutrition therapy and medicine can help the patient stay at a healthy weight. Medicine may be used for the following:

- to help increase appetite

- to help digest food

- to help the muscles of the stomach and intestines contract (to keep food moving along)

- to prevent or treat nausea and vomiting

- to prevent or treat diarrhea

- to prevent or treat constipation

- to prevent and treat mouth problems (such as dry mouth, infection, pain, and sores)

- to prevent and treat pain

Nutrition Therapy in Cancer Care

Screening and assessment are done before cancer treatment begins, and assessment continues during treatment. Screening is used to look for nutrition risks in a patient who has no symptoms. This can help find out if the patient is likely to become malnourished, so that steps can be taken to prevent it.

Assessment checks the nutritional health of the patient and helps to decide if nutrition therapy is needed to correct a problem.

Screening and assessment may include questions about the following:

- Weight changes over the past year.

- Changes in the amount and type of food eaten compared to what is usual for the patient.

- Problems that have affected eating, such as loss of appetite, nausea, vomiting, diarrhea, constipation, mouth sores, dry mouth, changes in taste and smell, or pain.

- Ability to walk and do other activities of daily living (dressing, getting into or out of a bed or chair, taking a bath or shower, and using the toilet).

A physical exam is also done to check the body for general health and signs of disease. The doctor will look for loss of weight, fat, and muscle, and for fluid buildup in the body.

Finding and treating nutrition problems early may improve the patient's prognosis (chance of recovery). Early nutrition screening and assessment help find problems that may affect how well the patient's body can deal with the effects of cancer treatment. Patients who are underweight or malnourished may not be able to get through treatment as well as a well-nourished patient. Finding and treating nutrition problems early can help the patient gain weight or prevent weight loss, decrease problems with the treatment, and help recovery.

A nutrition support team will check the patient's nutritional health often during cancer treatment and recovery. The team may include the following specialists:

- Physician

- Nurse

- Registered dietitian

- Social worker

- Psychologist

A patient whose religion doesn't allow eating certain foods may want to talk with a religious advisor about allowing those foods during cancer treatment and recovery.

There are three main goals of nutrition therapy for cancer patients in active treatment and recovery. The main goals of nutrition therapy for patients in active treatment and recovery are to provide nutrients that are missing, maintain nutritional health, and prevent problems. The healthcare team will use nutrition therapy to do the following:

- Prevent or treat nutrition problems, including preventing muscle and bone loss.

- Decrease side effects of cancer treatment and problems that affect nutrition.

- Keep up the patient's strength and energy.

- Help the immune system fight infection.

- Help the body recover and heal.

- Keep up or improve the patient's quality of life.

Good nutrition continues to be important for patients who are in remission or whose cancer has been cured. The goal of nutrition therapy for patients who have advanced cancer is to help with the patient's quality of life. The goals of nutrition therapy for patients who have advanced cancer include the following:

- Control side effects

- Lower the risk of infection

- Keep up strength and energy

- Improve or maintain quality of life

Types of Nutrition Care

Nutrition support gives nutrition to patients who cannot eat or digest normally. It is best to take in food by mouth whenever possible. Some patients may not be able to take in enough food by mouth because of problems from cancer or cancer treatment. Medicine to increase appetite may be used.

Nutrition support for patients who cannot eat can be given in different ways. A patient who is not able to take in enough food by mouth may be fed using enteral nutrition (through a tube inserted into the stomach or intestines) or parenteral nutrition (infused into the bloodstream). The nutrients are given in liquid formulas that have water, protein, fats, carbohydrates, vitamins, and/or minerals.

Nutrition support can improve a patient's quality of life during cancer treatment, but there are harms that should be considered before making the decision to use it. The patient and healthcare providers should discuss the harms and benefits of each type of nutrition support.

Enteral Nutrition

Enteral nutrition is also called tube feeding. Enteral nutrition is giving the patient nutrients in liquid form (formula) through a tube that is placed into the stomach or small intestine. The following types of feeding tubes may be used:

- A nasogastric tube is inserted through the nose and down the throat into the stomach or small intestine. This kind of tube is used when enteral nutrition is only needed for a few weeks.

- A gastrostomy tube is inserted into the stomach or a jejunostomy tube is inserted into the small intestine through an opening made on the outside of the abdomen. This kind of tube is usually used for long-term enteral feeding or for patients who cannot use a tube in the nose and throat.

The type of formula used is based on the specific needs of the patient. There are formulas for patients who have special health conditions, such as diabetes. Formula may be given through the tube as a constant drip (continuous feeding) or 1 to 2 cups of formula can be given 3 to 6 times a day (bolus feeding).

Enteral nutrition is sometimes used when the patient is able to eat small amounts by mouth, but cannot eat enough for health. Nutrients given through a tube feeding add the calories and nutrients needed for health.

Enteral nutrition may continue after the patient leaves the hospital. If enteral nutrition is to be part of the patient's care after leaving the hospital, the patient and caregiver will be trained to do the nutrition support care at home.

Parenteral Nutrition

Parenteral nutrition carries nutrients directly into the blood stream. Parenteral nutrition is used when the patient cannot take food by mouth or by enteral feeding. Parenteral feeding does not use the stomach or intestines to digest food. Nutrients are given to the patient directly into the blood, through a catheter (thin tube) inserted into a vein. These nutrients include proteins, fats, vitamins, and minerals. Parenteral nutrition is used only in patients who need nutrition support for five days or more.

A central venous catheter is placed beneath the skin and into a large vein in the upper chest. The catheter is put in place by a surgeon. This type of catheter is used for long-term parenteral feeding.

A peripheral venous catheter is placed into a vein in the arm. A peripheral venous catheter is put in place by trained medical staff. This type of catheter is usually used for short-term parenteral feeding.

The patient is checked often for infection or bleeding at the place where the catheter enters the body.

Parenteral nutrition support may continue after the patient leaves the hospital. If parenteral nutrition is to be part of the patient's care after leaving the hospital, the patient and caregiver will be trained to do the nutrition support care at home.

Ending parenteral nutrition support must be done under medical supervision. Going off parenteral nutrition support needs to be done slowly and is supervised by a medical team. The parenteral feedings are decreased by small amounts over time until they can be stopped, or as the patient is changed over to enteral or oral feeding.

Chapter 12

Delirium

Chapter Contents

Section 12.1

What Is Delirium?

This section includes text excerpted from "Delirium or
Sudden Confusion in Elderly Adults," U.S. Department of
Veterans Affairs (VA), August 9, 2016.

For elderly adults who have dementia, feeling confused may be expected. But when the confusion comes on suddenly, or the older adult becomes difficult to arouse, this could be a condition called delirium. This type of sudden confusion may be the first sign that the person has another illness and needs medical help right away.

One myth we often hear about aging is that it's not unusual to be confused when you're old. It's true that we can expect many changes as part of normal aging. But a sudden change in cognitive function—or the way we think and process information—is not one of them. Even if there has simply been a change in the elder's thinking or behavior, most caregivers and family members will know that something is not right. It's important to contact a doctor as soon as possible so that he or she can find the cause of the delirium and treat the underlying problem.

When Is Sudden Confusion an Emergency?

If you notice that an elderly adult has become suddenly confused or is not acting like him/herself, you may need to get help. Signs to watch for include:

- They can't focus attention or make eye contact.

- You can't fully wake them up.

- They are mumbling or their speech doesn't make sense.

- They are seeing or hearing things that aren't there.

- They have become agitated without any obvious cause.

Behavior like this may be the first sign of a medical emergency called sudden confusion or delirium.

- Elderly adults who have any of these symptoms should see their primary care doctor right away.

- If you notice any of these symptoms in the hospital, tell a staff member immediately.

It's important to remember that sudden confusion is different than other common changes in thinking that can happen as we age, such as dementia. With dementia, confusion happens slowly over time. With sudden confusion that needs medical treatment, the older adult's thinking abilities change quickly, often with no warning.

What Should I Do?

Sudden confusion in seniors can be very scary—both for the person who experiences it and the loved ones who witness it. Get medical help as soon as possible, then focus on keeping the older adult safe while they are confused.

People with sudden confusion may focus inward, showing a lack of interest in or attention to the things around them. Or they may become restless and agitated, reacting strongly to things they see, hear, or feel. It is important to remember that feeling confused can be frightening. Do your best to remain calm as you try to figure out the cause of their distress.

Some people with sudden confusion may punch, yell, kick, or act aggressively. That's why it's important to focus on keeping the confused person safe until you find out what's causing their distress. If possible, try to help them walk or change position since this may help ease discomfort.

You may try to gently reorient the person to reality, but remember that their confusion may cause them to see reality in a different way. It will help comfort them to meet them in their world until the confusion is resolved.

Can Delirium Be Prevented?

You can take a few simple steps to avoid—or help your loved ones avoid—sudden confusion.

Knowing the risk factors for sudden confusion is the first step. These include:

- Old age

- Dementia

- Sudden confusion in the past
- Multiple medications
- Problems seeing or hearing
- Not getting enough to eat or drink
- Chronic physical illness
- Alcohol or drug use
- Depression
- Problems in the brain or nervous system
- Functional disability

Important steps you can take to counter these risk factors include:

- Making sure the elderly adult gets enough calories and fluids.
- Correcting vision or hearing problems with glasses, hearing aids, or other devices.
- Helping ensure the elderly adult has good sleep habits and does not become overly tired or nap excessively during the day.
- Trying to involve the elderly adult in activities that challenge the brain, like puzzles, reading, talking about current events, or sharing memories of the past.
- Reviewing medications and dosages carefully at each doctor visit and asking questions to help make sure they aren't given any longer than necessary.

Having one or more risk factors makes an elderly adult more likely to develop sudden confusion. But a sudden event such as a severe illness, infection, or fracture is often what disrupts the brain and causes sudden confusion. This type of confusion is a medical emergency. It's important to identify the cause quickly and to start treatment as soon as possible.

Section 12.2

Delirium among Cancer Patients

This section includes text excerpted from "Delirium (PDQ®)—Patient Version," National Cancer Institute (NCI), March 9, 2016.

General Information about Delirium

Delirium is a confused mental state that can occur in patients who have cancer. Delirium is a confused mental state that can occur in patients who have cancer, especially advanced cancer. Patients with delirium have problems with the following:

- Attention
- Thinking
- Awareness
- Behavior
- Emotions
- Judgement
- Memory
- Muscle control
- Sleeping and waking

There are three types of delirium:

- **Hypoactive**. The patient is not active and seems sleepy, tired, or depressed.
- **Hyperactive**. The patient is restless or agitated.
- **Mixed**. The patient changes back and forth between being hypoactive and hyperactive.

Delirium may come and go during the day. The symptoms of delirium usually occur suddenly. They often occur within hours or days and may come and go. Delirium is often temporary and can be treated.

However, in the last 24 to 48 hours of life, delirium may be permanent because of problems like organ failure. Most advanced cancer patients have delirium that occurs in the last hours to days before death.

Causes of Delirium in Cancer Patients

Delirium may be caused by cancer, cancer treatment, or other medical conditions. There is often more than one cause of delirium in a cancer patient, especially when the cancer is advanced and the patient has many medical conditions. Causes of delirium include the following:

- Organ failure, such as liver or kidney failure.

- Electrolyte imbalances: Electrolytes are important minerals (including salt, potassium, calcium, and phosphorous) in blood and body fluids. These electrolytes are needed to keep the heart, kidneys, nerves, and muscles working the way they should.

- Infections.

- Paraneoplastic syndromes: Symptoms that occur when cancer-fighting antibodies or white blood cells attack normal cells in the nervous system by mistake.

- Side effects of medicines and treatments: Patients with cancer may take medicines with side effects that include delirium and confusion. The effects usually go away after the medicine is stopped.

- Withdrawal from medicines that depress (slow down) the central nervous system (brain and spinal cord).

It is important to know the risk factors for delirium. Patients with cancer are likely to have more than one risk factor for delirium. Identifying risk factors early may help prevent delirium or decrease the time it takes to treat it. Risk factors include the following:

- Serious illness

- Having more than one disease

- Old age

- Dementia

- Low level of albumin (protein) in the blood, which is often caused by liver problems

- Infection

- High level of nitrogen waste products in the blood, which is often caused by kidney problems
- Taking medicines that affect the mind or behavior
- Taking high doses of pain medicines, such as opioids

The risk increases when the patient has more than one risk factor. Older patients with advanced cancer who are hospitalized often have more than one risk factor for delirium.

Effects of Delirium on the Patient, Family, and Healthcare Providers

Delirium causes changes in the patient that can upset the family and caregivers. Delirium may be dangerous to the patient if his or her judgment is affected. Delirium can cause the patient to behave in unusual ways. Even a quiet or calm patient can have a sudden change in mood or become agitated and need more care.

Delirium can be upsetting to the family and caregivers. When the patient becomes agitated, family members often think the patient is in pain, but this may not be the case. Learning about differences between the symptoms of delirium and pain may help the family and caregivers understand how much pain medicine is needed. Healthcare providers can help the family and caregivers learn about these differences.

Delirium may affect physical health and communication. Patients with delirium are:

- More likely to fall.
- Sometimes unable to control bladder and/or bowels.
- More likely to become dehydrated (drink too little water to stay healthy).

They often need a longer hospital stay than patients without delirium.

The confused mental state of these patients may make them:

- Unable to talk with family members and caregivers about their needs and feelings.
- Unable to make decisions about care.

This makes it harder for healthcare providers to assess the patient's symptoms. The family may need to make decisions for the patient.

Diagnosing Delirium in Cancer Patients

Possible signs of delirium include sudden personality changes, problems thinking, and unusual anxiety or depression. When the following symptoms occur suddenly, they may be signs of delirium:

- Agitation
- Not cooperating
- Changes in personality or behavior
- Problems thinking
- Problems paying attention
- Unusual anxiety or depression

The symptoms of delirium are a lot like symptoms of depression and dementia. Early symptoms of delirium are like symptoms of depression and dementia. Delirium that causes the patient to be inactive may appear to be depression. Delirium and dementia both cause problems with memory, thinking, and judgment. Dementia may be caused by a number of medical conditions, including Alzheimer disease. Differences in the symptoms of delirium and dementia include the following:

- Patients with delirium often show changes in how alert or aware they are. Patients who have dementia usually stay alert and aware until the dementia becomes very advanced.

- Delirium occurs suddenly (within hours or days). Dementia appears gradually (over months to years) and gets worse over time.

Older patients with cancer may have both dementia and delirium. This can make it hard for the doctor to diagnose the problem. If treatment for delirium is given and the symptoms continue, then the diagnosis is more likely dementia. Checking the patient's health and symptoms over time can help diagnose delirium and dementia.

Physical exams and other laboratory tests are used to diagnose the causes of delirium. Doctors will try to find the causes of delirium.

- **Physical exam and history:** An exam of the body to check general signs of health, including checking for signs of disease, such as lumps or anything else that seems unusual. A history of the patient's health habits, past illnesses including depression, and treatments will also be taken. A physical exam can help rule out a physical condition that may be causing symptoms.

- **Laboratory tests:** Medical procedures that test samples of tissue, blood, urine, or other substances in the body. These tests help to diagnose disease, plan and check treatment, or monitor the disease over time.

Treatment of Delirium for Cancer Patients

Treatment includes looking at the causes and symptoms of delirium. Both the causes and the symptoms of delirium may be treated. Treatment depends on the following:

- Where the patient is living, such as home, hospital, or nursing home.
- How advanced the cancer is.
- How the delirium symptoms are affecting the patient.
- The wishes of the patient and family.

Treating the causes of delirium usually includes the following:

- Stopping or lowering the dose of medicines that cause delirium.
- Giving fluids to treat dehydration.
- Giving drugs to treat hypercalcemia (too much calcium in the blood).
- Giving antibiotics for infections.

In a terminally ill patient with delirium, the doctor may treat just the symptoms. The doctor will continue to watch the patient closely during treatment.

Sedation may be used for delirium at the end of life or when delirium does not get better with treatment. When the symptoms of delirium are not relieved with standard treatments and the patient is near death, in pain, or has trouble breathing, other treatment may be needed. Sometimes medicines that will sedate (calm) the patient will be used. The family and the healthcare team will make this decision together.

The decision to use sedation for delirium may be guided by the following:

- The patient will have repeated assessments by experts before the delirium is considered to be refractory (doesn't respond to treatment).

- The decision to sedate the patient is reviewed by a team of healthcare professionals and not made by one doctor.

- Temporary sedation, for short periods of time such as overnight, is considered before continuous sedation is used.

- The team of healthcare professionals will work with the family to make sure the team understands the family's views and that the family understands palliative sedation.

Part Three

Medical Decisions Surrounding the End of Life

Chapter 13

Understanding Healthcare Decisions

Issues You May Face

Maybe you are now faced with making end-of-life choices for some-one close to you. You've thought about that person's values and opin-ions, and you've asked the healthcare team to explain the treatment plan and what you can expect to happen.

But, there are other issues that are important to understand in case they arise. What if the dying person starts to have trouble breathing and a doctor says a ventilator might be needed? Maybe one family member wants the healthcare team to do everything possible to keep this relative alive. What does that involve? Or, what if family members can't agree on end-of-life care or they disagree with the doctor? What happens then?

Here are some other common end-of-life issues. They will give you a general understanding and may help your conversations with the doctors.

If We Say Do Everything Possible, What Does That Mean?

This means that if someone is dying, all measures that might keep vital organs working will be tried—for example, using a ventilator to

This chapter includes text excerpted from "End of Life: Helping with Comfort and Care," National Institute on Aging (NIA), National Institutes of Health (NIH), July 2016.

support breathing or starting dialysis for failing kidneys. Such life support can sometimes be a temporary measure that allows the body to heal itself and begin to work normally again. It is not intended to be used indefinitely in someone who is dying.

What Can Be Done If Someone's Heart Stops Beating (Cardiac Arrest)?

CPR (cardiopulmonary resuscitation) can sometimes restart a stopped heart. It is most effective in people who were generally healthy before their heart stopped. During CPR, the doctor repeatedly pushes on the chest with great force and periodically puts air into the lungs. Electric shocks (called defibrillation) may also be used to correct an abnormal heart rhythm, and some medicines might also be given. Although not usually shown on television, the force required for CPR can cause broken ribs or a collapsed lung. Often, CPR does not succeed in older adults who have multiple chronic illnesses or who are already frail.

What If Someone Needs Help Breathing or Completely Stops Breathing (Respiratory Arrest)?

If a patient has very severe breathing problems or has stopped breathing, a ventilator may be needed. A ventilator forces the lungs to work. Initially, this involves intubation, putting a tube attached to a ventilator down the throat into the trachea or windpipe. Because this tube can be quite uncomfortable, people are often sedated with very strong intravenous medicines. Restraints may be used to prevent them from pulling out the tube. If the person needs ventilator support for more than a few days, the doctor might suggest a tracheotomy, sometimes called a "trach" (rhymes with "make"). This tube is then attached to the ventilator. This is more comfortable than a tube down the throat and may not require sedation. Inserting the tube into the trachea is a bedside surgery. A tracheotomy can carry risks, including a collapsed lung, a plugged tracheotomy tube, or bleeding.

How Can I Be Sure the Medical Staff Knows That We Don't Want Efforts to Restore a Heartbeat or Breathing?

Tell the doctor in charge as soon as the patient or person making healthcare decisions decides that CPR or other life-support procedures should not be performed. The doctor will then write this on the patient's chart using terms such as DNR (Do Not Resuscitate),

DNAR (Do Not Attempt to Resuscitate), AND (Allow Natural Death), or DNI (Do Not Intubate). DNR forms vary by State and are usually available online.

If end-of-life care is given at home, a special non-hospital DNR, signed by a doctor, is needed. This ensures that if emergency medical technicians (EMTs) are called to the house, they will respect your wishes. Make sure it is kept in a prominent place so EMTs can see it. Without a non-hospital DNR, in many States EMTs are required to perform CPR and similar techniques. Hospice staff can help determine whether a medical condition is part of the normal dying process or something that needs the attention of EMTs.

DNR orders do not stop all treatment. They only mean that CPR and a ventilator will not be used. These orders are not permanent— they can be changed if the situation changes.

What about Pacemakers (or Similar Devices)—Should They Be Turned Off?

A pacemaker is a device implanted under the skin on the chest that keeps a heartbeat regular. It will not keep a dying person alive. Some people have an implantable cardioverter defibrillator (ICD) under the skin. An ICD shocks the heart back into regular rhythm when needed. The ICD should be turned off at the point when life support is no longer wanted. This can be done at the bedside without surgery.

What If the Doctor Suggests a Feeding Tube?

If a patient can't or won't eat or drink, the doctor might suggest a feeding tube. While a patient recovers from an illness, getting nutrition temporarily through a feeding tube can be helpful. But, at the end of life, a feeding tube might cause more discomfort than not eating. For people with dementia, tube feeding does not prolong life or prevent aspiration.

As death approaches, loss of appetite is common. Body systems start shutting down, and fluids and food are not needed as before. Some experts believe that at this point few nutrients are absorbed from any type of nutrition, including those received through a feeding tube. Further, after a feeding tube is inserted, the family might need to make a difficult decision about when, or if, to remove it.

If tube feeding will be tried, there are two methods that could be used. In the first, a feeding tube, known as a nasogastric or NG tube, is threaded through the nose down to the stomach to give nutrition for a short time. Sometimes, the tube is uncomfortable. Someone with an NG tube might try to remove it. This usually means the person has to be restrained, which could mean binding his or her hands to the bed.

If tube feeding is required for an extended time, then a gastric or G tube is put directly into the stomach through an opening made in the side or abdomen. This second method is sometimes called a PEG (percutaneous endoscopic gastrostomy) tube. It carries risks of infection, pneumonia, and nausea.

Hand feeding (sometimes called assisted oral feeding) is an alternative to tube feeding. This approach may have fewer risks, especially for people with dementia.

Should Someone Who Is Dying Be Sedated?

Sometimes, for patients very near the end of life, the doctor might suggest sedation to manage symptoms that are not responding to other treatments and are still making the patient uncomfortable. This means using medicines to put the patient in a sleep-like state. Many doctors suggest continuing to use comfort care measures like pain medicine even if the dying person is sedated. Sedatives can be stopped at any time. A person who is sedated may still be able to hear what you are saying—so try to keep speaking directly to, not about, him or her. Do not say things you would not want the patient to hear.

What about Antibiotics?

Antibiotics are medicines that fight infections caused by bacteria. Lower respiratory infections (such as pneumonia) and urinary tract infections are often caused by bacteria and are common in older people who are dying. Many antibiotics have side effects, so the value of trying to treat an infection in a dying person should be weighed against any unpleasant side effects. If someone is already dying when the infection began, giving antibiotics is probably not going to prevent death but might make the person feel more comfortable.

Questions to Ask about Healthcare Decisions

Here are some questions you might want to ask the medical staff:

- What is the care plan? What are the benefits and risks?

- How often should we reassess the care plan?

- If we try using the ventilator to help with breathing and decide to stop, how will that be done?

- If my family member is dying, why does he or she have to be connected to all those tubes and machines? Why do we need more tests?

- What is the best way for our family to work with the care staff?

- How can I make sure I get a daily update on my family member's condition?

- Will you call me if there is a change in his or her condition?

Thoughts to Share

Make sure the healthcare team knows what is important to your family surrounding the end of life. You might say:

- In my religion, we . . . (then describe your religious traditions regarding death).

- Where we come from . . . (tell what customs are important to you at the time of death).

- In our family when someone is dying, we prefer . . . (describe what you hope to have happen).

Chapter 14

Preferences for Care at the End of Life

What Is Advance Care Planning?

Advance care planning involves learning about the types of decisions that might need to be made, considering those decisions ahead of time, and then letting others know about your preferences, often by putting them into an advance directive. An advance directive is a legal document that goes into effect only if you are incapacitated and unable to speak for yourself. This could be the result of disease or severe injury—no matter how old you are. It helps others know what type of medical care you want. It also allows you to express your values and desires related to end-of-life care. You might think of an advance directive as a living document—one that you can adjust as your situation changes because of new information or a change in your health.

Decisions That Could Come up near Death

Sometimes when doctors believe a cure is no longer possible and you are dying, decisions must be made about the use of emergency treatments to keep you alive. Doctors can use several artificial or

This chapter includes text excerpted from "Advance Care Planning," National Institute on Aging (NIA), National Institutes of Health (NIH), March 2014.

mechanical ways to try to do this. Decisions that might come up at this time relate to:

- CPR (cardiopulmonary resuscitation)

- Ventilator use

- Artificial nutrition (tube feeding) or artificial hydration (intravenous fluids)

- Comfort care

CPR. CPR (cardiopulmonary resuscitation) might restore your heartbeat if your heart stops or is in a life-threatening abnormal rhythm. The heart of a young, otherwise healthy person might resume beating normally after CPR. An otherwise healthy older person, whose heart is beating erratically or not beating at all, might also be helped by CPR. CPR is less likely to work for an older person who is ill, can't be successfully treated, and is already close to death. It involves repeatedly pushing on the chest with force, while putting air into the lungs. This force has to be quite strong, and sometimes ribs are broken or a lung collapses. Electric shocks known as defibrillation and medicines might also be used as part of the process.

Ventilator use. Ventilators are machines that help you breathe. A tube connected to the ventilator is put through the throat into the trachea (windpipe) so the machine can force air into the lungs. Putting the tube down the throat is called intubation. Because the tube is uncomfortable, medicines are used to keep you sedated (unconscious) while on a ventilator. If you can't breathe on your own after a few days, a doctor may perform a tracheotomy or "trach" (rhymes with "make"). During this bedside surgery, the tube is inserted directly into the trachea through a hole in the neck. For long-term help with breathing, a trach is more comfortable, and sedation is not needed. People using such a breathing tube aren't able to speak without special help because exhaled air goes out of the trach rather than past their vocal cords.

Artificial nutrition or artificial hydration. A feeding tube and/or intravenous (IV) liquids are sometimes used to provide nutrition when a person is not able to eat or drink. These measures can be helpful if you are recovering from an illness. However, if you are near death, these could actually make you more uncomfortable. For example, IV liquids, which are given through a plastic tube put into a vein, can increase the burden on failing kidneys. Or if the body is shutting down near death, it is not able to digest food properly, even when provided through a feeding tube. At first, the feeding tube is threaded through the nose down to the stomach. In time, if tube feeding is still needed, the tube is surgically inserted into the stomach.

Comfort care. Comfort care is anything that can be done to soothe you and relieve suffering while staying in line with your wishes. Comfort care includes managing shortness of breath; offering ice chips for dry mouth; limiting medical testing; providing spiritual and emotional counseling; and giving medication for pain, anxiety, nausea, or constipation. Often this is done through hospice, which may be offered in the home, in a hospice facility, in a skilled nursing facility, or in a hospital. With hospice, a team of healthcare providers works together to provide the best possible quality of life in a patient's final days, weeks, or months. After death, the hospice team continues to offer support to the family. Learn more about providing comfort at the end of life.

Getting Started

Start by thinking about what kind of treatment you do or do not want in a medical emergency. It might help to talk with your doctor about how your present health conditions might influence your health in the future. For example, what decisions would you or your family face if your high blood pressure leads to a stroke?

If you don't have any medical issues now, your family medical history might be a clue to thinking about the future. Talk to your doctor about decisions that might come up if you develop health problems similar to those of other family members.

In considering treatment decisions, your personal values are key. Is your main desire to have the most days of life, or to have the most life in your days? What if an illness leaves you paralyzed or in a permanent coma and you need to be on a ventilator? Would you want that?

What makes life meaningful to you? You might want doctors to try CPR if your heart stops or to try using a ventilator for a short time if you've had trouble breathing, if that means that, in the future, you could be well enough to spend time with your family. Even if the emergency leaves you simply able to spend your days listening to books on tape or gazing out the window watching the birds and squirrels compete for seeds in the bird feeder, you might be content with that.

But, there are many other scenarios. Here are a few. What would you decide?

- If a stroke leaves you paralyzed and then your heart stops, would you want CPR? What if you were also mentally impaired by a stroke—does your decision change?

- What if you develop dementia, don't recognize family and friends, and, in time, cannot feed yourself? Would you want a feeding tube used to give you nutrition?

- What if you are permanently unconscious and then develop pneumonia? Would you want antibiotics and a ventilator used?

For some people, staying alive as long as medically possible is the most important thing. An advance directive can help make sure that happens.

Your decisions about how to handle any of these situations could be different at age 40 than at age 85. Or they could be different if you have an incurable condition as opposed to being generally healthy. An advance directive allows you to provide instructions for these types of situations and then to change the instructions as you get older or if your viewpoint changes.

Making Your Wishes Known

There are two elements in an advance directive—a living will and a durable power of attorney for healthcare. There are also other documents that can supplement your advance directive or stand alone. You can choose which documents to create, depending on how you want decisions to be made. These documents include:

- Living will

- Durable power of attorney for healthcare

- Other documents discussing DNR (do not resuscitate) orders, organ and tissue donation, dialysis, and blood transfusions

Living will. A living will is a written document that helps you tell doctors how you want to be treated if you are dying or permanently unconscious and cannot make decisions about emergency treatment. In a living will, you can say which of the procedures described above you would want, which ones you wouldn't want, and under which conditions each of your choices applies.

Durable power of attorney for healthcare. A durable power of attorney for healthcare is a legal document naming a healthcare proxy, someone to make medical decisions for you at times when you might not be able to do so. Your proxy, also known as a surrogate or agent, should be familiar with your values and wishes. This means that he or she will be able to decide as you would when treatment decisions need to be made. A proxy can be chosen in addition to or instead of a living will. Having a healthcare proxy helps you plan for situations that cannot be foreseen, like a serious auto accident.

A durable power of attorney for healthcare enables you to be more specific about your medical treatment than a living will.

Some people are reluctant to put specific health decisions in writing. For them, naming a healthcare agent might be a good approach, especially if there is someone they feel comfortable talking with about their values and preferences.

Other advance care planning documents. You might also want to prepare separate documents to express your wishes about a single medical issue or something not already covered in your advance directive. A living will usually covers only the specific life-sustaining treatments discussed earlier. You might want to give your healthcare proxy specific instructions about other issues, such as blood transfusion or kidney dialysis. This is especially important if your doctor suggests that, given your health condition, such treatments might be needed in the future.

Two medical issues that might arise at the end of life are DNR (do not resuscitate) orders and organ and tissue donation.

A DNR (do not resuscitate) order tells medical staff in a hospital or nursing facility that you do not want them to try to return your heart to a normal rhythm if it stops or is beating unevenly. Even though a living will might say CPR is not wanted, it is helpful to have a DNR order as part of your medical file if you go to a hospital. Posting a DNR next to your bed might avoid confusion in an emergency situation. Without a DNR order, medical staff will make every effort to restore the normal rhythm of your heart. A non-hospital DNR will alert emergency medical personnel to your wishes regarding CPR and other measures to restore your heartbeat if you are not in the hospital. A similar document that is less familiar is called a DNI (do not intubate) order. A DNI tells medical staff in a hospital or nursing facility that you do not want to be put on a breathing machine.

Organ and tissue donation allows organs or body parts from a generally healthy person who has died to be transplanted into people who need them. Commonly, the heart, lungs, pancreas, kidneys, corneas, liver, and skin are donated. There is no age limit for organ and tissue donation. You can carry a donation card in your wallet. Some states allow you to add this decision to your driver's license. Some people also include organ donation in their advance care planning documents. At the time of death, family may be asked about organ donation. If those close to you, especially your proxy, know how you feel about organ donation, they will be ready to respond.

Selecting Your Healthcare Proxy

If you decide to choose a proxy, think about people you know who share your views and values about life and medical decisions. Your proxy might be a family member, a friend, your lawyer, or someone with whom you worship. It's a good idea to also name an alternate proxy. It is especially important to have a detailed living will if you choose not to name a proxy.

You can decide how much authority your proxy has over your medical care—whether he or she is entitled to make a wide range of decisions or only a few specific ones. Try not to include guidelines that make it impossible for the proxy to fulfill his or her duties. For example, it's probably not unusual for someone to say in conversation, "I don't want to go to a nursing home," but think carefully about whether you want a restriction like that in your advance directive. Sometimes, for financial or medical reasons, that may be the best choice for you.

Of course, check with those you choose as your healthcare proxy and alternate before you name them officially. Make sure they are comfortable with this responsibility.

Making It Official

Once you have talked with your doctor and have an idea of the types of decisions that could come up in the future and whom you would like as a proxy, if you want one at all, the next step is to fill out the legal forms detailing your wishes. A lawyer can help but is not required. If you decide to use a lawyer, don't depend on him or her to help you understand different medical treatments. That's why you should start the planning process by talking with your doctor.

Many states have their own advance directive forms. Your local Area Agency on Aging can help you locate the right forms. You can find your area agency phone number by calling the Eldercare Locator toll-free at 1-800-677-1116.

Some states want your advance directive to be witnessed; some want your signature notarized. A notary is a person licensed by the state to witness signatures. You might find a notary at your bank, post office, or local library, or call your insurance agent. Some notaries charge a fee.

Some people spend a lot of time in more than one state—for example, visiting children and grandchildren. If that's your situation also, you might consider preparing an advance directive using forms for each state—and keep a copy in each place, too.

After You Set up Your Advance Directive

There are key people who should be told that you have an advance directive. Give copies to your healthcare proxy and alternate proxy. Give your doctor a copy for your medical records. Tell key family members and friends where you keep a copy. If you have to go to the hospital, give staff there a copy to include in your records. Because you might change your advance directive in the future, it's a good idea to keep track of who receives a copy.

Review your advance care planning decisions from time to time—for example, every 10 years, if not more often. You might want to revise your preferences for care if your situation or your health changes. Or, you might want to make adjustments if you receive a serious diagnosis; if you get married, separated, or divorced; if your spouse dies; or if something happens to your proxy or alternate. If your preferences change, you will want to make sure your doctor, proxy, and family know about them.

Still Not Sure?

What happens if you have no advance directive or have made no plans and you become unable to speak for yourself? In such cases, the state where you live will assign someone to make medical decisions on your behalf. This will probably be your spouse, your parents if they are available, or your children if they are adults. If you have no family members, the state will choose someone to represent your best interests.

Always remember, an advance directive is only used if you are in danger of dying and need certain emergency or special measures to keep you alive but are not able to make those decisions on your own. An advance directive allows you to continue to make your wishes about medical treatment known.

Looking toward the Future

Nobody can predict the future. You may never face a medical situation where you are unable to speak for yourself and make your wishes known. But having an advance directive may give you and those close to you some peace of mind.

Chapter 15

Alzheimer Disease and End-of-Life Issues

Alzheimer: An Incurable Disease

Despite our best research efforts, Alzheimer disease (AD) remains incurable. Researchers are using sophisticated technologies to pinpoint how Alzheimer Disease progressively steals memories and destroys personality; and yet, AD remains irreversible. Although one does not die of Alzheimer disease, during the course of the disease, the body's defense mechanisms ultimately weaken, increasing susceptibility to catastrophic infection and other causes of death related to frailty. At some point after the mind has been lost to this devastating disease, the body will be lost as well.

Families and caregivers of people with AD face many challenges as they cope with the steady loss of their loved one's mental and physical skills. As the disease moves to its end stages, certain steps can provide measures of comfort-both to the caregiver and to the person with AD. Healthcare professionals can help caregivers fill the last days with love and tenderness even through the wrenching turmoil of letting go.

Many caregivers are unaware that resources and healthcare professionals are available to provide comfort and help each AD patient

This chapter includes text excerpted from "Alzheimer Disease and End-of-Life Issues," National Institute on Aging (NIA), National Institutes of Health (NIH), February 26, 2015.

end life with dignity. They face emotional conflict and unnecessary guilt.

"A lot of what we think about death and dying is based on the cancer model," says Dr. Stephen Post, professor in the department of bio-ethics at Case Western University School of Medicine. "Alzheimer is a complicated and difficult disease." Late-stage AD is characterized by the inability to communicate by speech or recognize family members, the inability to move about without assistance, incontinence, loss of appetite, and loss of the ability to swallow, with death usually resulting from aspiration pneumonia, infection, or coronary arrest. On the average, the advanced stage of AD lasts 1.5 to 2 years, according to Dr. Post, though 20–30% of patients will "linger" 4, 5, 6, or even as long as 10 years, he says.

Doctors, nurses, social workers, and other healthcare professionals can help caregivers understand the dying process and the role of palliative care for the AD patient. This is the purpose of palliative care-to provide comfort and symptom relief, without the use of aggressive treatments, such as tube feeding, mechanical respiration, dialysis, and cardiopulmonary resuscitation, which often only prolong the suffering of the patient. Community programs, such as hospice, can be of great service to family members and healthcare professionals by assisting with medications, patient physical care, and counseling. The objective in managing the advanced stages of Alzheimer disease should be to maximize comfort while preserving patient dignity and respect.

The Palliative Course

Experts agree that palliative care is the most appropriate course of action for advanced Alzheimer disease. Use of aggressive medical interventions in the advanced stage, such as Cardiopulmonary resuscitation (CPR), feeding tubes, intravenous antibiotics, even dialysis, is considered by experts to be of little benefit, and may impose a further burden of suffering on the patient. "The Alzheimer's Association firmly recommends palliative care and hospice approach in the advanced stages of the disease," says Dr. Post. "Family members should never be made to feel guilty in making a decision to allow a person with AD to die naturally."

"Healthcare professionals are duty-bound to do more than simply present technological options like items on a laundry list, without clarifying the burdens that these technologies create for people with advanced dementia," Dr. Post says. Healthcare teams in these circumstances must be nonjudgmental and listen attentively to family wishes, while providing accurate facts on the adverse implications of prolonging end-of-life treatments.

Artificial Feeding and Hydration

Family members should be warned about the potential medical problems associated with artificial feeding and hydration. These include, in the case of nasograstric tubes, pain and discomfort related to the forceful introduction of physical devices in the esophagus, needed sedation, and infections often resulting from the procedure. "Many family members are not aware that no longer eating and drinking is part of the dying process, and it is normal," says Dr. Post.

"Our modern culture tends to treat dying as unnatural. Our technology allows us to forestall death, yet cannot prevent it. Family members need to be informed, with great compassion, sensitivity, and patience, about the dying process and how natural and inevitable it truly is. The body is shutting down. The natural process of dying means that the body no longer wants or needs food or fluids. This is often viewed as unnatural by caregivers, and even some healthcare professionals. However, we need to explore our own feelings and attitudes toward death and dying before we can help families through this transitional process, this time of loss and change," comments Darby Morhardt, MSW, Social Worker, Northwestern University Alzheimer's Disease Center.

Cessation of food intake results in the release of endorphins, which reduce pain. Feeding tubes and hydration block the release of endorphins and can result in weeks of "unnecessary suffering" Dr. Post said, with patients "uremic and bloated and unable to clear mucus from their lungs." Percutaneous endoscopic gastronomy (PEG) feeding can result in back-up to the esophagus, increasing the risk of aspiration pneumonia, while lack of ambulation-PEG feeding often requires physical restraint to prevent patients from pulling out their feeding tubes-increases the risk for bed ulcers and skin infections.

Artificial feeding also deprives a patient of taste, says Dr. Ladislav Volicer, clinical director of the Geriatric Research, Education and Clinical Center (GRECC) at the E.N.R.M. Veterans Hospital in Bedford, Massachusetts. "Alzheimer's patients love sweets," Dr. Volicer says, "even in the later stages-things like milk shakes and ice cream." Artificial feeding also deprives patients and caregivers of personal contact, which is a meaningful activity.

"We haven't had any tube feeding in the last 10 years," says Dr. Volicer, who often converts patients back to assisted feeding on arrival.

"They can always eat to some degree," he says, "except during the actual dying process." Patients in the dying phase do not experience hunger and thirst, he adds.

Problems with choking can be addressed by substituting thick liquids, such as yogurt instead of milk, and by using commercial thickeners. "What we are trying to do is switch the emphasis of care from high tech to high touch," he says. "That also includes very aggressive management of pain. We use a lot of narcotics in the management of late-stage dementia."

Antibiotics may be useful for urinary tract infections, but they are not reliable against chest infections, because of increasing resistance, says Dr. Post. Some physicians prefer to recommend acetaminophen (like Tylenol) for fever.

Hospital transfers should also be discouraged. "There is published evidence," says Dr. Volicer, "that the 3-month mortality rate is lower if patients are treated in a nursing home than if they are transferred to the hospital."

The End Draws Near

It's difficult to predict when an AD patient is going to die. "The average clinicians are not as good at this as they would be for cancer," says Dr. Jason Karlawish, of the University of Pennsylvania's Institute of Aging, "because there is a lack of clear understanding of this stage of AD." Dying for the Alzheimer patient is marked by little if any verbal output, complete dependency in all aspects of daily living, and the complications of brain failure, which include episodes of aspiration, urinary tract infections, fevers, skin breakdowns, and more than 10% loss of body weight. "This is the typical profile of a patient who I would expect could die within a year," says Dr. Karlawish.

Working with Family Members

In the absence of advance directives, the healthcare team should work with family members to arrive at a consensus of care and abide by final decisions. There are often conflicts over the use of heroic efforts to prolong life. At odds are everything from the philosophies of individual providers and institutional caregivers to issues of patient competence in the absence of legal instruments.

The solution: arrival at a plan by way of a narrative consensus. Healthcare workers can guide this effort by creating an environment of "equal standing," Dr. Karlawish says, in which all family members are encouraged to discuss how they perceive the patient's illness and arrive at a consensus that will provide the patient with the most comfort and the highest quality of remaining life. "You should be hearing yourself talking about half the time in the beginning," Dr. Karlawish says, "but if you've done it right, the caregiver should wind up doing most of the talking." Physicians should not be hesitant to recommend hospice as an option, he says.

Sparing a Lifetime of Guilt

Doctors can educate themselves to make knowledgeable recommendations. "Nothing should be left to surrogate decision-making without clear data and recommendations," Dr. Post says. "Family members need to be spared a lifetime of guilt."

Social workers make good moderators at consensus meetings. Clergy can also play an important role for both family and the patient, says Dr. Post, who views the AD patient as still having an emotional, recreational, and symbolic self. "Pastoral care involves symbols," he says. "Oftentimes, we underestimate the importance of pastoral care for reconnecting these people with some aspect of themselves that is otherwise ignored."

Healthcare professionals also can help families understand that all feelings—anger, sadness, guilt, relief, conflict, fear-are normal as they witness the patient going through the dying process.

A Healing Death

If there is a kind point in the progression of AD, Dr. Post suggests, it is the point at which the patient begins to forget what they have forgotten, where they no longer have insight into their behavior. But for family members with memories intact, there is no such kind point. There is only a series of losses at each stage of the disease, as their loved one slips away. "So many of the healing aspects of death and dying are lost with Alzheimer's disease," says Dr. Post.

Much of the understanding family members have of the dying process is what the healthcare team brings to them. In the absence of advanced directives, the healthcare team must provide the means by which family members can arrive at a consensus that will preserve patient dignity and quality of life, and the best chance for healing for those left behind.

Chapter 16

Advanced Cancer and End-of-Life Issues

End-of-Life Care in Advanced Cancer

When you learn you have advanced cancer, you're faced with many decisions about your end-of-life care. Talking about these decisions early can make it easier on you and your family later. The following are some questions you may want to think about:

- What's important to you during this time?

- Is it most important that you be as comfortable and alert as possible during the last stages of cancer?

- Is it most important to continue with treatments that may help you live longer but make you uncomfortable?

Some patients choose to receive all possible treatments. Others choose to receive only some treatments or no treatment at all. Some choose to receive only care that will keep them comfortable. Having information about your options will help you make these choices. Together, you, your family, and your doctor can decide on a plan for your care during the advanced stages of cancer.

This chapter includes text excerpted from "Planning the Transition to End-of-Life Care in Advanced Cancer (PDQ®)—Patient Version," National Cancer Institute (NCI), November 24, 2015.

Quality Care at the End of Life

Your care continues even after all treatments have stopped. End-of-life care is more than what happens moments before dying. Care is needed in the days, weeks, and sometimes even months before death. During this time, many patients feel it's important to:

- Have their pain and symptoms controlled.
- Avoid a long process of dying.
- Feel a sense of control over what is happening to them.
- Cause less emotional and financial burden on the family.
- Become closer with loved ones.

Your doctors and family need to know the kind of end-of-life care you want.

Make End-of-Life Care Decisions Early

You may be able to think about your options more clearly if you talk about them before the decisions need to be made. It's a good idea to let your doctors, family, and caregivers know your wishes before there is an emergency.

End-of-Life Care Decisions to Be Made

Care decisions for the last stages of cancer can be about treatments and procedures, pain control, place of care, and spiritual issues.

Chemotherapy

Some patients choose to begin new chemotherapy treatment in the end stages of cancer. Others wish to let the disease take its course when a cure is not expected. In the end stages of cancer, chemotherapy usually doesn't help you live longer and it may lower the quality of the time that remains. Each person and each cancer is different. Talking with your doctor about the effects of treatment and your quality of life can help you make a decision. You can ask if the treatment will make you comfortable or if it will help you live longer.

Pain and Symptom Control

Controlling pain and other symptoms can help you have a better quality of life in the end stages of cancer. Pain and symptom control can be part of your care in any place of care, such as the hospital, home, and hospice.

Cardiopulmonary Resuscitation (CPR)

It's important to decide if you will want to have cardiopulmonary resuscitation (CPR). CPR is a procedure used to try to restart the heart and breathing when it stops. In advanced cancer, the heart, lungs, and other organs begin to fail and it's harder to restart them with CPR. Your doctor can help you understand how CPR works and talk with you about whether CPR is likely to work for you.

People who are near the end of life may choose not to have CPR done. Your decision about having CPR is personal. Your own spiritual or religious views about death and dying may help you decide. If you decide you don't want CPR, you can ask your doctor to write a do-not-resuscitate (DNR) order. This tells other healthcare professionals not to perform CPR if your heart or breathing stops. You can remove the DNR order at any time.

Talk with your doctors and other caregivers about CPR as early as possible (for example, when being admitted to the hospital), in case you're not able to make the decision later. If you do choose to have your doctor write a DNR, it's important to tell all your family members and caregivers about it.

In the United States, if there is no DNR order, you will be given CPR to keep you alive.

Ventilator Use

A ventilator is a machine used to help you breathe and keep you alive after normal breathing stops. It doesn't treat a disease or condition. It's used only for life support. You can tell doctors whether you would want to be put on a ventilator if your lungs stop working or if you cannot breathe on your own after CPR. If your goal of care is to live longer, you may choose to have a ventilator used. Or you may choose to have a ventilator for only a certain length of time. It's important to tell your family and healthcare providers what you want before you have trouble breathing.

Religious and Spiritual Support

Your religious or spiritual beliefs may help you with end-of-life decisions. Clergy and chaplains can give counseling. You can also talk with a member of your church, a social worker, or even other people who have cancer.

Talking with Your Doctor about End-of-Life Care

Some doctors don't ask patients about end-of-life issues. If you want to make choices about these issues, talk with your doctors so that your wishes can be carried out. Open communication can help you and your doctors make decisions together and create a plan of care that meets your goals and wishes. If your doctor is not comfortable talking about end-of-life plans, you can talk to other specialists for help.

Understand Your Prognosis

Having a good understanding of your prognosis is important when making decisions about your care and treatment during advanced cancer. You will probably want to know how long you have to live. That's a hard question for doctors to answer. It can be different for each person and depends on the type of cancer, where it has spread, and whether you have other illnesses. Treatments can work differently for each person. Your doctor can talk about the treatment options with you and your family and explain the effects they may have on your cancer and your quality of life. Knowing the benefits and risks of available treatments can help you decide on your goals of care for the last stages of the cancer.

Decide on Your Care Goals

Your care goals for advanced cancer depend in part on whether quality of life or length of life is more important to you. Your goals of care may change as your condition changes or if new treatments become available. Tell your doctor what your goals of care are, even if you aren't asked. It's important that you and your doctor are working toward the same goals.

Take Part in Making Decisions

Do you want to take part in making the decisions about your care? Or would you rather have your family and your doctors make those decisions? This is a personal choice and your family and doctors need to know what you want.

Early communication with your doctors can help you feel more prepared for end-of-life issues.

Many patients who start talking with their doctors early about end-of-life issues report feeling better prepared. Better communication with your doctors may make it easier to deal with concerns about being older, living alone, relieving symptoms, spiritual well-being, and how your family will cope in the future.

There are ways to improve communication with your doctors.

Tell your doctor how you and your family wish to receive information and the type of information you want. Also ask how you can get information at times when you can't meet face-to-face.

Remembering what your doctor said and even remembering what you want to ask can be hard to do. Some of the following may help communication and help you remember what was said:

- Have a family member go with you when you meet with your doctor.

- Make a list of the questions you want to ask the doctor during your visit.

- Get the information in writing.

- Record the discussion with tape recorders, smart phones, or on video.

- Ask if your doctor or clinic offers any of the following:

- A cancer consultation preparation package, which includes aids such as a question idea sheet, booklets on decision making and patient rights, and information about the clinic.

- A talk with a psychologist about advance planning and end-of-life issues.

- An end-of-life preference interview, which includes a list of questions that can help you explain your wishes about the end of life.

Supportive Care, Palliative Care, and Hospice

Even when treatments can no longer cure the cancer, medical care is still needed. Some of the end-of-life care options are supportive care, palliative care, and hospice.

Supportive Care

Supportive care is given to prevent or treat, as early as possible, the symptoms of the cancer, side effects caused by treatments, and psychological, social, and spiritual problems related to the cancer or its treatment. During active treatment to cure the cancer, supportive care helps you stay healthy and comfortable enough to continue receiving the cancer treatments. In the last stages of cancer, when a cure is no longer the goal, supportive care is used for side effects that continue.

Palliative Care

Palliative care is specialized medical care for people with serious or life-threatening illnesses. The focus of palliative care is relief from pain and other symptoms, both during active treatment and when treatment has been stopped. Palliative care is offered in some hospitals, outpatient centers, and in the home.

Palliative care helps to improve your quality of life by preventing and relieving suffering. When you're more comfortable, your family's quality of life may also be better. Palliative care includes treating physical symptoms such as pain, and helping you and your family with emotional, social, and spiritual concerns. When palliative treatment is given at the end of life, the focus is on relieving symptoms and distress caused by the process of dying and to make sure your goals of care are followed.

Hospice Care

When treatment is no longer helping, you may choose hospice. Hospice is a program that gives care to people who are near the end of life and have stopped treatment to cure or control their cancer. Hospice care focuses on quality of life rather than length of life. The hospice team offers physical, emotional, and spiritual support for patients who are expected to live no longer than six months. The goal of hospice is to help patients live each day to the fullest by making them comfortable and relieving their symptoms. This may include supportive and palliative care to control pain and other symptoms so you can be as alert and comfortable as possible. Services to help with the emotional, social, and spiritual needs of you and your family are also an important part of hospice care.

Hospice programs are designed to keep the patient at home with family and friends, but hospice care may also be given in hospice centers and in some hospitals and nursing homes. The hospice team includes doctors, nurses, spiritual advisors, social workers, nutritionists, and volunteers. Team members are specially trained on issues that occur at the end of life. The hospice program continues to give help, including grief counseling, to the family after their loved one dies. Ask your doctor for information if you wish to receive hospice care.

Advance Planning

Making end-of-life care decisions early can ease your mind and decrease stress on your family. There may come a time when you can't tell the healthcare team what you want. When that happens, would you prefer to have your doctor and family make decisions? Or would you rather make decisions early, so your wishes will be known and can be followed when the time comes? If not planned far ahead of time, the end-of-life decisions must be made by someone other than you.

Planning ahead for end-of-life care helps with the following:

- Makes sure your doctors and family know what your wishes are.

- Allows you to refuse the use of treatments.

- Decreases the emotional stress on your family, who would have to make decisions if you aren't able to.

- Reduces the cost of care, if you choose not to receive life-saving procedures.

- Eases your mind to have these decisions already made.

You can make your wishes known with an advance directive.

Advance directive is the general term for different types of documents that state what your wishes are for certain medical treatments when you can no longer tell those wishes to your caregivers. In addition to decisions about relieving symptoms at the end of life, it is also helpful to decide if and when you want certain treatments to stop. Advance directives make sure your wishes about treatments and life-saving procedures to keep you alive are known ahead of time. Without knowing your wishes, doctors will do everything medically possible to keep you alive, such as cardiopulmonary resuscitation (CPR) and the use of a ventilator (breathing machine).

Each state has its own laws for advance directives. Make sure your advance directives follow the laws of the state where you live and are being treated.

The following are types of documents that communicate your wishes in advance:

- **Living will:** A legal document that states whether you want certain life-saving medical treatments to be used or not used under certain circumstances. Some of the treatments covered by a living will include CPR, use of a ventilator (breathing machine), and tube-feeding.

- **Healthcare proxy (HCP):** A document in which you choose a person (called a proxy) to make medical decisions if you become unable to do so. It's important that your proxy knows your values and wishes, so that he or she can make the decisions you would make if you were able. You do not have to state specific decisions about individual treatments in the document, just state that the proxy will make medical decisions for you. HCP is also known as durable power of attorney for healthcare (DPOAHC) or medical power of attorney (MPOA).

- **Do-Not-Resuscitate (DNR) order:** A document that tells medical staff in the hospital not to do cardiopulmonary resuscitation (CPR) if your heart or breathing stops. A DNR order is a decision only about CPR. It does not affect other treatments that may be used to keep you alive, such as medicine or food.

- **Out-of-hospital DNR order:** A document that tells emergency medical workers outside of a hospital that you do not wish to have CPR or other types of resuscitation. Each state has its own rules for a legal out-of-hospital DNR order, but it is usually signed by the patient, a witness, and the doctor. It's best to have several copies so one can quickly be given to emergency medical workers when needed.

- **Do-Not-Intubate (DNI) order:** A document that tells medical staff in a hospital or nursing facility that you do not wish to have a breathing tube inserted and to be put on a ventilator (breathing machine).

- **Physician Orders for Life-Sustaining Treatment (POLST):** A form that states what kind of medical treatment you want toward the end of your life. It is signed by you and your doctor.

- **Medical Orders for Life-Sustaining Treatment (MOLST):** A form that states the care you would like to receive if you are not able to communicate. This care includes CPR, intubation (breathing tubes), and other life-saving procedures. Under current law, the information in a MOLST form must be followed both in the home and hospital by all medical staff, including emergency medical workers.

Give copies of your advance directives to your doctors, caregivers, and family members. Advance directives need to move with you. If your doctors or your place of care changes, copies of your advance directives need to be given to your new caregivers. This will make sure that your wishes are known through all cancer stages and places of care. You can change or cancel an advance directive at any time.

The Transition to End-of-Life Care

The word transition can mean a passage from one place to another. The transition or change from looking toward recovery to receiving end-of-life care is not an easy one and there are important decisions to be made. If you become too sick before you have made your wishes known, others will make care and treatment decisions for you, without knowing what you would have wanted. It may be less stressful for everyone if you, your family, and your healthcare providers have planned ahead for this time.

The goal of end-of-life care is to prevent suffering and relieve symptoms. The right time to transition to end-of-life care is when this supports your changing condition and changing goals of care.

There are certain times when you may think about stopping treatment and transitioning to comfort care. These include:

- Finding out that the cancer is not responding to treatment and that more treatment is not likely to help.

- Having poor quality of life due to the side effects or complications of treatment.

- Being unable to carry out daily activities when the disease progresses.

Together with your doctor, you and your family members can share an understanding about treatment choices and when transition to end-of-life care is the best choice. When you make the decisions and plans, doctors and family members can be sure they are doing what you want.

Chapter 17

Human Immunodeficiency Virus/Acquired Immune Deficiency Syndrome (HIV/ AIDS) and End-of-Life Issues

HIV/AIDS Basics

HIV stands for human immunodeficiency virus. It is the virus that can lead to acquired immunodeficiency syndrome or AIDS if not treated. Unlike some other viruses, the human body can't get rid of HIV completely, even with treatment. So once you get HIV, you have it for life.

HIV attacks the body's immune system, specifically the CD4 cells (T cells), which help the immune system fight off infections. Untreated,

This chapter contains text excerpted from the following sources: Text under the heading "HIV/AIDS Basics" is excerpted from "About HIV/AIDS," Centers for Disease Control and Prevention (CDC), September 21, 2016; Text beginning with the heading "Hospitalization and HIV" is excerpted from "Hospitalization and Palliative Care," AIDS*info*, U.S. Department of Health and Human Services (HHS), June 1, 2012. Reviewed October 2016; Text beginning with the heading "Initiating Antiretroviral Therapy in the Older HIV Patient" is excerpted from "HIV and the Older Patient," AIDS*info*, U.S. Department of Health and Human Services (HHS), January 28, 2016.

HIV reduces the number of CD4 cells (T cells) in the body, making the person more likely to get other infections or infection-related cancers. Over time, HIV can destroy so many of these cells that the body can't fight off infections and disease. These opportunistic infections or cancers take advantage of a very weak immune system and signal that the person has Acquired Immune Deficiency Syndrome (AIDS), the last stage of HIV infection.

No effective cure currently exists, but with proper medical care, HIV can be controlled. The medicine used to treat HIV is called antiretroviral therapy or ART. If taken the right way, every day, this medicine can dramatically prolong the lives of many people infected with HIV, keep them healthy, and greatly lower their chance of infecting others. Before the introduction of ART in the mid-1990s, people with HIV could progress to AIDS in just a few years. Today, someone diagnosed with HIV and treated before the disease is far advanced can live nearly as long as someone who does not have HIV.

Hospitalization and HIV

There are a number of HIV-related reasons you might have to be admitted to the hospital. Acute respiratory failure is a major one—it accounts for approximately 25–50% of intensive care unit (ICU) admissions for people with HIV disease. Respiratory failure is usually a product of infection, with Pneumocystis jiroveci pneumonia (PCP) and bacterial pneumonia being the most common culprits. Other common indications for ICU admission include central nervous system infections (like cryptococcal meningitis or encephalitis) and sepsis.

Surgery with HIV

There is good news if you're HIV-positive and need or want to have surgery. Studies have found that there isn't much difference in the rate of complications between HIV-positive and HIV-negative patients. So simply having HIV should not keep you from having either elective or emergency surgery.

If you are scheduling a surgical procedure, you need to make sure your healthcare provider has the most up-to-date information on your medical history—including your CD4 count, viral load, and a list of your current medications. You should talk to your provider in detail about potential complications, recovery time, and any special instructions or tests you may need before your surgery.

Palliative Care

Palliative care is medical care that focuses on relieving pain and suffering for people with advanced illness and their families. Palliative care does not aim to cure you of an illness, but to improve your quality of life by managing symptoms and complications. You can have palliative care at any point in your illness, and at the same time as treatment that is meant to cure you.

If you are receiving end-of-life care, palliative care may cover psychosocial and spiritual support, as well as pain and symptom management. Your palliative caregivers may talk with you about your goals and values around end-of-life care, and they may refer you to hospice care when appropriate.

Initiating Antiretroviral Therapy (ART) in the Older HIV Patient

Antiretroviral therapy (ART) is recommended for all HIV-infected individuals. Early treatment may be particularly important in older adults in part because of decreased immune recovery and increased risk of serious non-AIDS events in this population. In a modeling study based on data from an observational cohort, the beneficial effects of early ART were projected to be greatest in the oldest age group (patients between ages 45 and 65 years). No data support a preference for any one of the Panel's recommended initial ART regimens on the basis of patient age. The choice of regimen should instead be informed by a comprehensive review of the patient's other medical conditions and medications. The What to Start section of these guidelines provides guidance on selecting an antiretroviral regimen based on an older patient's characteristics and specific clinical conditions (e.g., kidney disease, elevated risk for cardiovascular disease, osteoporosis). In older patients with reduced renal function, dosage adjustment of nucleoside reverse transcriptase inhibitors (NRTIs) may be necessary. In addition, ARV regimen selection may be influenced by potential interaction of antiretroviral medications with drugs used concomitantly to manage co-morbidities. Adults age >50 years should be monitored for ART effectiveness and safety similarly to other HIV-infected populations; however, in older patients, special attention should be paid to the greater potential for adverse effects of ART on renal, liver, cardiovascular, metabolic, and bone health.

HIV, Aging, and Antiretroviral Therapy

The efficacy, PKs, adverse effects, and drug interaction potentials of ART in the older adult have not been studied systematically. There is no evidence that the virologic response to ART differs in older and younger patients. In a recent observational study, a higher rate of viral suppression was seen in patients >55 years old than in younger patients. However, ART-associated CD4 cell recovery in older patients is generally slower and lower in magnitude than in younger patients. This observation suggests that starting ART at a younger age may result in better immunologic response and possibly clinical outcomes.

Hepatic metabolism and renal elimination are the major routes of drug clearance, including the clearance of ARV drugs. Both liver and kidney functions decrease with age and may result in impaired drug elimination and increased drug exposure. Most clinical trials have included only a small proportion of participants over 50 years of age, and current ARV dosing recommendations are based on PK and pharmacodynamic data derived from participants with normal organ function. Whether drug accumulation in the older patient may lead to greater incidence and severity of adverse effects than seen in younger patients is unknown.

HIV-infected patients with aging-associated comorbidities may require additional pharmacologic interventions that can complicate therapeutic management. In addition to taking medications to manage HIV infection and comorbid conditions, many older HIV-infected patients also are taking medications to relieve discomfort (e.g., pain medications, sedatives) or to manage adverse effects of medications (e.g., anti-emetics). They also may self-medicate with over-the-counter medicines or supplements. In HIV-negative older patients, polypharmacy is a major cause of iatrogenic complications. Some of these complications may be caused by medication errors (by prescribers or patients), medication non-adherence, additive drug toxicities, and drug-drug interactions. Older HIV-infected patients are probably at an even greater risk of polypharmacy-related adverse consequences than younger HIV-infected or similarly aged HIV-uninfected patients. When evaluating any new clinical complaint or laboratory abnormality in HIV-infected patients, especially in older patients, clinicians should always consider the possible role of adverse drug reactions from both ARV drugs and other concomitantly administered medications.

Drug-drug interactions are common with ART and can be easily overlooked by prescribers. The available drug interaction information on ARV agents is derived primarily from PK studies performed in small numbers of relatively young, HIV-uninfected participants with normal organ function. Data from these studies provide clinicians with a basis to assess whether a significant interaction may exist. However, the magnitude of the interaction may be greater in older HIV-infected patients than in younger HIV-infected patients.

Nonadherence is the most common cause of treatment failure. Complex dosing requirements, high pill burden, inability to access medications because of cost or availability, limited health literacy including misunderstanding of instructions, depression, and neurocognitive impairment are among the key reasons for nonadherence. Although many of these factors associated with non-adherence may be more prevalent in older patients, some studies have shown that older HIV-infected patients may actually be more adherent to ART than younger patients. Clinicians should regularly assess older patients to identify any factors, such as neurocognitive deficits, that may decrease adherence. To facilitate medication adherence, it may be useful to discontinue unnecessary medications, simplify regimens, and recommend evidence-based behavioral approaches including the use of adherence aids such as pillboxes or daily calendars, and support from family members.

Switching, Interrupting, and Discontinuing Antiretroviral Therapy in Older Patients

Given the greater incidence of co-morbidities, non-AIDS complications and frailty among older HIV-infected patients, switching one or more ARVs in an HIV regimen may be necessary to minimize toxicities and drug-drug interactions. For example, expert guidance now recommends bone density monitoring in men aged ≥50 years and postmenopausal women, and suggests switching from tenofovir disoproxil fumarate or boosted protease inhibitors to other ARVs in older patients at high risk for fragility fractures.

Few data exist on the use of ART in severely debilitated patients with chronic, severe, or non-AIDS terminal conditions. Withdrawal of ART usually results in rebound viremia and a decline in CD4 cell count. Acute retroviral syndrome after abrupt discontinuation of ART has been reported. In severely debilitated patients, if there are no significant adverse reactions to ART, most clinicians would continue therapy. In cases where ART negatively affects quality of life, the decision to continue therapy should be made together with the patient and/or family members after a discussion on the risks and benefits of continuing or withdrawing ART.

End-of-Life Issues

Important issues to discuss with aging HIV-infected patients are living wills, advance directives, and long-term care planning, including related financial concerns. Out-of-pocket healthcare expenses (e.g., copayments, deductibles), loss of employment, and other financial-related factors can cause temporary interruptions in treatment, including ART, which should be avoided whenever possible. The increased life expectancy and the higher prevalence of chronic complications in aging HIV populations can place greater demands upon HIV services. Facilitating a patient's continued access to insurance can minimize treatment interruptions and reduce the need for other services to manage concomitant chronic disorders.

Conclusion

HIV disease can be overlooked in aging adults who tend to present with more advanced disease and experience accelerated CD4 loss. HIV induces immune-phenotypic changes that have been compared to accelerated aging. Effective ART has prolonged the life expectancy of HIV infected patients, increasing the number of patients >50 years of age living with HIV. However, unique challenges in this population include greater incidence of complications and co-morbidities, and some of these complications may be exacerbated or accelerated by long term use of some ARV drugs. Providing comprehensive multidisciplinary medical and psychosocial support to patients and their families (the "Medical Home" concept) is of paramount importance in the aging population. Continued involvement of HIV experts, geriatricians, and other specialists in the care of older HIV-infected patients is warranted.

Chapter 18

Ethics and Legal Issues in Palliative Care

The life expectancy of the American people has reached an all-time high, but along with the increased life expectancy is an increase in the number of people living with, and dying from, chronic debilitating diseases such as heart disease, cancer, stroke and chronic obstructive pulmonary disease While the elderly with chronic illnesses comprise a group one might associate with end-of-life issues, there are other groups for whom these concerns are important.

Examples extend across the life span including neonates in intensive care units, children with AIDS, teens with cancer, and young adults with degenerative diseases. Coupled with this spectrum of individuals is the increased availability of technologies and treatments that can be used to prolong life and, in some cases, death. Defining when these technologies and treatments shift from life saving interventions to burdensome and futile procedures that negatively impact quality of life has proved elusive. When these technologies and treatments become futile, the individuals' families and significant others may be involved in a difficult period of decision-making about how

This chapter contains text excerpted from the following sources: Text in this chapter begins with excerpts from "Quality of Life for Individuals at the End-of-Life," National Institutes of Health (NIH), August 2, 2000. Reviewed October 2016; Text under the heading "Ethics" is excerpted from "Ethical Practices in End-of-Life Care," U.S. Department of Veterans Affairs (VA), December 9, 2013.

much aggressive treatment to try and when to stop. Conversely there is widespread fear that the only alternative to aggressive treatment is abandonment and suffering.

For many Americans, end-of-life care is fragmented, painful, and emotionally distressing, with unnecessary transitions between health-care institutions, community-based organizations and home care settings. There are many national initiatives underway to improve care of the dying. Significant efforts are being made to better train health professionals and to encourage public awareness of the issues. Yet important gaps in knowledge limit our ability to help individuals who are dying achieve the highest possible quality of life. "From the cellular to the social level, much remains to be learned about how people die and how reliably excellent and compassionate care can be achieved" (IOM, 1997).

Research is needed to better define what is meant by end-of-life, to identify aspects of an optimal death experience within the cultural and ethnic context of the individual so better palliative care can be provided, to facilitate communication and ethical decision-making among those involved in end-of-life decisions, and to support the development of a well-integrated healthcare system that includes the family and the multidisciplinary team.

More needs to be understood about the physical, emotional, social, cultural and spiritual experiences of people who are dying and about the environmental context which influences the quality of the life remaining. Issues related to research methods are important to consider with inquiry into dying. There are pressing needs to better define key concepts, identify and test appropriate measures, develop strategies to minimize subject burden, and devise methods for complex data analysis. Advances in understanding how to help individuals who are dying to attain the highest quality of life possible can be advanced with innovative, science-based research.

Ethics

Historically, end-of-life care was shaped by a presumption in favor of curative medical interventions. Any decision not directed specifically at maximizing survival was understood negatively as "withdrawing," "withholding," or "refusing" treatment. With the evolution of hospice and palliative care, care-giving goals of comfort, relief of suffering, and a dignified death have come to be recognized as positive and appropriate for patients with advanced illness. To honor the range of end-of-life options available to patients, palliative care emphasizes shared decision making that is based on explicitly identifying achievable and desired goals of care.

Your responsibility to provide respectful and clinically appropriate care at the end of life is based on four ethical obligations:

1. Your obligation to respect the patient's right to self-determination. This right, sometimes referred to as autonomy, is well established in law and ethics, and best summarized in the words of Justice Benjamin Cardozo in the 1914 court case that gave legal recognition to the concept of informed consent:"Every human being of adult years and sound mind has a right to determine what shall be done with his own body."

2. Your obligation to prevent or remove harm and to promote the patient's good. This is also known as beneficence.

3. Your obligation to refrain from causing harm or imposing unnecessary risk. This is also known as nonmaleficence.

4. Your obligation to not abandon the patient. The healing relationship is distinguished by the vulnerability of the patient, the imbalance of knowledge and power between the healthcare provider and patient, and the expectation that healthcare providers will use their knowledge and skill to help the patient. Patients have a legitimate expectation that their welfare will be paramount and that they will not be abandoned by their healthcare providers.

Chapter 19

Life Support Choices

Life-Sustaining Treatments in the Last Days of Life

In the last days of life, patients and family members are faced with making decisions about treatments to keep the patient alive. Decisions about whether to use life-sustaining treatments that may extend life in the final weeks or days cause a great deal of confusion and anxiety. Some of these treatments are ventilator use, parenteral nutrition, and dialysis.

Patients may be guided by their oncologist, but have the right to make their own choices about life-sustaining treatments. The following are some of the questions to discuss:

- What are the patient's goals of care?

- How would the possible benefits of life-sustaining treatments help reach the patient's goals of care, and how likely would this be?

- How would the possible harms of life-sustaining treatments affect the patient's goals of care? Is the possible benefit worth the possible harm?

- Besides possible benefits and harms of life-sustaining treatments, what else can affect the decision?

This chapter includes text excerpted from "Last Days of Life (PDQ®)—Patient Version," National Cancer Institute (NCI), April 8, 2016.

- Are there other professionals, such as a chaplain or medical ethicist, who could help the patient or family decide about life-sustaining treatments?

Choices about care and treatment at the end of life should be made while the patient is able to make them. A patient may wish to receive all possible treatments, only some treatments, or no treatment at all in the last days of life. These decisions may be written down ahead of time in an advance directive, such as a living will. Advance directive is the general term for different types of legal documents that describe the treatment or care a patient wishes to receive or not receive when he or she is no longer able to speak their wishes.

Studies have shown that cancer patients who have end-of-life discussions with their doctors choose to have fewer procedures, such as resuscitation or the use of a ventilator. They are also less likely to be in intensive care, and the cost of their healthcare is lower during their final week of life. Reports from their caregivers show that these patients live as long as patients who choose to have more procedures and that they have a better quality of life in their last days.

Care that supports a patient's spiritual health may improve quality of life. A spiritual assessment is a method or tool used by doctors to understand the role that religious and spiritual beliefs have in the patient's life. This may help the doctor understand how these beliefs affect the way the patient copes with cancer and makes decisions about cancer treatment.

Serious illnesses like cancer may cause patients or family caregivers to have doubts about their beliefs or religious values and cause spiritual distress. Some studies show that patients with cancer may feel anger at God or may have a loss of faith after being diagnosed. Other patients may have feelings of spiritual distress when coping with cancer. Spiritual distress may affect end-of-life decisions and increase depression.

Doctors and nurses, together with social workers and psychologists, may be able to offer care that supports a patient's spiritual health. They may encourage patients to meet with their spiritual or religious leaders or join a spiritual support group. This may improve patients' quality of life and ability to cope. When patients with advanced cancer receive spiritual support from the medical team, they are more likely to choose hospice care and less aggressive treatment at the end of life.

Fluids

The goals of giving fluids at the end of life should be discussed by patient, family, and doctors. Fluids may be given when the patient can no longer eat or drink normally. Fluids may be given with an intravenous (IV) catheter or through a needle under the skin. Decisions about giving fluids should be based on the patient's goals of care. Giving fluids has not been shown to help patients live longer or to improve quality of life. However, the harms are minor and the family may feel there are benefits if the patient is less fatigued and more alert. The family may also be able to give the patient sips of water or ice chips, or swab the mouth and lips to keep them moist.

Nutrition Support

The goals of nutrition support for patients in the last days of life are different from the goals during cancer treatment. Nutrition support can improve health and boost healing during cancer treatment. The goals of nutrition therapy for patients during the last days of life are different from the goals for patients in active cancer treatment and recovery. In the final days of life, patients often lose the desire to eat or drink and may not want food or fluids that are offered to them. Also, procedures used to put in feeding tubes may be hard on a patient.

Making plans for nutrition support in the last days is helpful. The goal of end-of-life care is to prevent suffering and relieve symptoms. If nutrition support causes the patient more discomfort than help, then nutrition support near the end of life may be stopped. The needs and best interests of each patient guide the decision to give nutrition support. When decisions and plans about nutrition support are made by the patient, doctors and family members can be sure they are doing what the patient wants.

Two types of nutrition support are commonly used. If the patient cannot swallow, two types of nutrition support are commonly used:

- Enteral nutrition uses a tube inserted into the stomach or intestine.

- Parenteral nutrition uses an intravenous (IV) catheter inserted into a vein.

Each type of nutrition support has benefits and risks.

Antibiotics

The benefits of using antibiotics in the last days of life are unclear. The use of antibiotics and other treatments for infection is common in patients in the last days of life, but it is hard to tell how well they work. It is also hard to tell if there are any benefits of using antibiotics at the end of life.

Overall, doctors want to make the patient comfortable in the last days of life rather than give treatments that may not help them live longer.

Transfusions

The decision to use blood transfusions in advanced cancer depends on goals of care and other factors.

Many patients with advanced cancer have anemia. Patients with advanced blood cancers may have thrombocytopenia (a condition in which there is a lower-than-normal number of platelets in the blood). Deciding whether to use blood transfusions for these conditions is based on the following:

- Goals of care.

- How long the patient is expected to live.

- The benefits and risks of the transfusion.

The decision is hard to make since patients usually need to receive transfusions in a medical setting rather than at home. Many patients are used to receiving blood transfusions during active treatment or supportive care, and may want to continue transfusions to feel better. However, studies have not shown that transfusions are safe and effective at the end of life.

Resuscitation

Patients should decide whether or not they want cardiopulmonary resuscitation (CPR). An important decision for the patient to make is whether to have cardiopulmonary resuscitation (CPR) (trying to restart the heart and breathing when it stops). It is best if patients talk with their family, doctors, and caregivers about their wishes for CPR as early as possible (for example, when being admitted to the hospital or when active cancer treatment is stopped). A do-not-resuscitate (DNR) order is written by a doctor to tell other health professionals not to perform CPR at the moment of death, so that the natural process of dying occurs. If the patient wishes, he or she can ask the doctor to write a DNR order. The patient can ask that the DNR order be changed or removed at any time.

Chapter 20

Termination of Life-Sustaining Treatment

Last Days in the Hospital or Intensive Care Unit

Choices about whether to use intensive care should be discussed. Near the end of life, patients with advanced cancer may be admitted to a hospital or intensive care unit (ICU) if they have not made other choices for their care. In the ICU, patients or family members have to make hard decisions about whether to start, continue, or stop aggressive treatments that may make the patient live longer, but do not improve the patient's quality of life. Families may be unsure of their feelings or have trouble deciding whether to limit or avoid treatments.

Sometimes, treatments like dialysis or blood transfusions may be tried for a short time. However, at any time, patients or families may talk with doctors about whether they want to continue with ICU care. They may choose instead to change over to comfort care in the final days.

Ventilator use may keep the patient alive after normal breathing stops. A ventilator is a machine that helps patients breathe. Sometimes, using a ventilator will not improve the patient's condition, but will keep the patient alive longer. If the goal of care is to help the patient live longer, a ventilator may be used, according to the patient's

This chapter includes text excerpted from "Last Days of Life (PDQ®)—Patient Version," National Cancer Institute (NCI), April 8, 2016.

wishes. If ventilator support stops helping the patient or is no longer what the patient wants, the patient, family, and healthcare team may decide to turn the ventilator off.

Before a ventilator is turned off. Family members will be given information about how the patient may respond when the ventilator is removed and about pain relief or sedation to keep the patient comfortable. Family members will be given time to contact other loved ones who wish to be there. Chaplains or social workers may be called to give help and support to the family.

Suffering and Palliative Sedation at the End of Life

The emotions of patients and caregivers are closely connected. Patients and caregivers share the distress of cancer, with the caregiver's distress sometimes being greater than the patient's. Since caregiver suffering can affect the patient's well-being and the caregiver's adjustment to loss, early and constant support of the caregiver is very important.

Palliative sedation lowers the level of consciousness and relieves extreme pain and suffering. Palliative sedation uses special drugs called sedatives to relieve extreme suffering by making a patient calm and unaware.

The decision whether to sedate a patient at the end-of-life is a hard one. Sedation may be considered for a patient's comfort or for a physical condition such as uncontrolled pain. Palliative sedation may be temporary. A patient's thoughts and feelings about end-of-life sedation may depend greatly on his or her own culture and beliefs. Some patients who become anxious facing the end of life may want to be sedated. Some patients and their families may wish to have a level of sedation that allows them to communicate with each other. Other patients may wish to have no procedures, including sedation, just before death.

Studies have not shown that palliative sedation shortens life when used in the last days. It is important for the patient to tell family members and healthcare providers of his or her wishes about sedation at the end of life. When patients make their wishes about sedation known ahead of time, doctors and family members can be sure they are doing what the patient would want. Families may need support from the healthcare team and mental health counselors while palliative sedation is used.

Chapter 21

Organ Donation and Transplantation

What Is Organ Donation and Transplantation?

Organ transplantation is the surgical removal of an organ or tissues from one person (the donor) and placing it in another person (the recipient). Organ donation is when you allow your organs or tissues to be removed and given to someone else. Most donated organs and tissues are from people who have died. But, a living person can donate some organs. Blood, stem cells, and platelets can also be donated.

What Is the Status of Organ Donation and Transplantation in the United States?

Currently there are 119,929 candidates for transplant on the U.S. national waiting list. Nearly 2 out of every 3 people on the waiting

This chapter contains text excerpted from the following sources: Text under heading "What Is Organ Donation and Transplantation?" is excerpted from "Organ Donation and Transplantation Fact Sheet," Office on Women's Health (OWH), U.S. Department of Health and Human Services (HHS), July 16, 2012. Reviewed October 2016; text under heading "What Is the Status of Organ Donation and Transplantation in the United States?" is excerpted from "Organ Donation Statistics," Organdonor.gov, U.S. Department of Health and Human Services (HHS), March 22, 2016; text under heading "Organ Donation FAQs" is excerpted from "Organ Donation FAQs," Organdonor.gov, U.S. Department of Health and Human Services (HHS), March 22, 2016.

list are over the age of 50. Almost 2,000 children under 18 are on the waiting list. Almost 70,000 people (58%) on the list are ethnic minorities.

Frequently Asked Questions on Organ Donation

Who Can Become an Organ Donor?

All adults in the U.S. and in some states people under the age of 18 can indicate their commitment to donation by signing up to be an organ donor. Whether someone is suitable for donation is determined at the time of death. Authorization by a parent or guardian is generally necessary for individuals under 18 who have died to become an actual donor.

Are There Age Limits for Donating Your Organs?

There are no age limitations on who can donate. Newborns as well as senior citizens have been organ donors. Whether or not you can donate depends on your physical condition and the condition of your organs, not age.

Can Non-Residents Donate and Receive Organs in the United States?

Non-resident aliens—people who don't live in the United States or aren't citizens—can donate and receive organs in the United States. Organs are given to patients according to medical need, not citizenship.

However, only about 1 in 100 people who receive transplants are non U.S. residents.

If I Have a Medical Condition, Can I Still Donate?

Don't rule yourself out from being an organ donor because you have a health condition. You're always encouraged to register. There are very few conditions that would prevent someone from being an organ, eye, or tissue donor—such as HIV infection, active cancer, or a systemic infection. Even with an illness, you may be able to donate your organs or tissues.

The transplant team will determine what can be used at the time of your death based on a clinical evaluation, medical history and other factors. Even if there's only one organ or tissue that can be used, that's one life saved or improved.

Can I Be an Organ and Tissue Donor, and Also Donate My Body to Medical Science?

Total body donation generally is not an option if you choose to be an organ and tissue donor. However eye donors still may be accepted. There are also a few medical schools and research organizations that may accept an organ donor for research.

If you wish to donate your entire body, you should contact the medical organization of your choice directly and make arrangements. Medical schools, research facilities, and other agencies study bodies to understand how disease affects human beings. This research is vital to saving and improving lives.

Can I Register as an Organ Donor?

Anyone over the age of 18 is eligible to sign up, and in many states, people younger than 18 can register as well. There are several ways to sign up.

You can register online in your state.

You can also sign up when you visit your state motor vehicle office.

Either way, be sure to tell your family about your decision. If the time comes, they won't be surprised and they can help carry out your wishes. They may be asked to provide information to the transplant team.

What Am I Signing up for When I Register?

When you register as an organ donor in your state, you're authorizing donation of your organs if you die in circumstances that make donation possible. Generally, that means dying in a hospital and on artificial support. You can read more about the deceased donation process here. You will remain on your state's registry unless you opt out.

I Have an Organ Donor Card. Is That Enough?

No. There's no way of knowing if the card would be with you or if it would be examined in the event of your death. If you wish to be a donor, sign up in your state registry.

I Have My Organ Donor Status on My Driver's License. Is That Enough?

That's an important step, but it's also important to share your wishes with your family. Most families want to carry out the wishes of their loved one, so please be sure to tell them how you feel.

Can I Specify What I Want to Donate?

When registering online, most states give you the option to choose which organs and tissues you donate, or to donate everything that can be used. Check with your state registry to learn more.

Can I Remove Myself from the Registered Donors List?

Yes, you can change your donor status at any time. Look for an option such as "updating your status" on your state's site.

If you have a donor designation on your driver's license, removing yourself from the registry will not change that. So, unless your state uses a removable sticker on the license to identify donors, you will likely need to change your license at your local motor vehicle office.

If I Register as a Donor, Will My Wishes Be Carried Out?

If you signed up as a deceased donor in your state registry and you are over 18, then you have legally authorized your donation and no one can overrule your consent. Signing a card isn't enough. If you are under 18, your parents or legal guardian must authorize donation.

What Organs and Tissues Can Be Donated?

- Eight vital organs can be donated: heart, kidneys (2), pancreas, lungs (2), liver, and intestines. Hands and faces have also recently been added to the list.

- Tissue: cornea, skin, heart valves, bone, blood vessels, and connective tissue

- Bone marrow and stem cells, umbilical cord blood, peripheral blood stem cells (PBSC)

If I'm a Registered Donor, Will It Affect the Medical Care I Receive at the Hospital?

No! The medical team trying to save your life is separate from the transplant team. Every effort is made to save your life before donation becomes a possibility.

Will Donation Disfigure My Body? Can There Be an Open Casket Funeral?

Donation does not interfere with having an open casket service. Surgical techniques are used to retrieve organs and tissues, and all incisions are closed.

Are There Any Costs to My Family for Donation?

No. Your family pays for your medical care and funeral costs, but not for organ donation. Costs related to donation are paid by the recipient, usually through insurance, Medicare, or Medicaid.

Can I Sell My Organs?

No! The National Organ Transplant Act (Public Law 98–507) makes it illegal to sell human organs and tissues in the United States. Violators are subject to fines and imprisonment.

One reason Congress made this law was to make sure the wealthy do not have an unfair advantage for obtaining donated organs and tissues.

Can People of Different Races and Ethnicities Match Each Other?

Yes. People of different ethnicities frequently match each other.

How Are Donated Organs Distributed?

Organs are matched to patients based on a number of factors, including blood and tissue typing, medical need, time on the waiting list, and geographical location.

I'd Like to Donate a Kidney to Someone. How Can I Be Tested to See If I Am a Match?

Within the United States, living donations of a kidney can be made to a family member, friend, or anyone on the waiting list. Living donations are arranged through many kidney transplant centers throughout the United States. They will test to see if you are a match and if you are healthy enough to safely undergo surgery.

Remember that there is a lot to do before you can be considered a living donor.

How Many People Are Currently Waiting for Organs?

The number of patients waiting for organs varies every day, but on average, the number is well over 120,000 and climbing. Every 10 minutes, another person is added to the waiting list.

The number of patients now on the waiting list and other data are available on the Organ Procurement and Transplantation Network website. The number of people requiring a lifesaving transplant continues to rise faster than the number of available donors. Approximately 300 new transplant candidates are added to the waiting list each month.

Why Do Minorities Have a Higher Need for Transplants?

More than half of all people on the transplant waiting list are from a racial or ethnic minority group. That is because some diseases that cause end-stage organ failure are more common in these populations than in the general population.

For example, African Americans, Asians, Native Hawaiians and Pacific Islanders, and Hispanics/Latinos are 3 times more likely than Whites to suffer from end-stage renal (kidney) disease, often as the result of high blood pressure.

Native Americans are 4 times more likely than Whites to suffer from diabetes. An organ transplant is sometimes the best—or only— option for saving a life.

Chapter 22

Physician-Assisted Suicide

Requests to End Suffering

Suffering has always been a part of human existence. Requests to end suffering by means of death through both physician-assisted suicide and euthanasia have likely occurred since the beginning of medicine. Patient requests for assistance in suicide are relatively common. A national survey of physicians who care for terminally ill patients found that over 18% had been asked by a patient at least once to assist in suicide and over 11% had been asked to give a lethal injection. Cancer specialists are especially likely to encounter these issues. In a 1996 survey, more than half of responding oncologists reported having received a request for assisted suicide or euthanasia.

Physical pain, dependency, and depression are all associated with consideration of euthanasia or physician-assisted suicide. While concerns about pain are common among people who are seriously ill, published studies have found pain not to be a dominant factor motivating people to seek or commit assisted suicide. Clinical depression and hopelessness have both been associated with the desire for a hastened death among cancer patients. Issues of dependence on others and loss of autonomy have contributed to the suicides of terminally ill cancer patients receiving palliative care. A desire to control the circumstances of death was an important factor in patients' decisions in a survey of Oregon nurses and social workers who cared for hospice patients who

This chapter includes text excerpted from "Physician-Assisted Suicide," National Cancer Institute (NCI), September 15, 2016.

died by legally prescribed medication. Similarly, loss of control, being dependent on others, and being a burden were the most frequently perceived causes of patients' requests for assistance with suicide in a survey of Washington physicians.

Physical symptoms such as pain, dyspnea, and fatigue are common in patients with cancer and become more prevalent in advanced stages of disease. The same is true for the syndrome of depression. These sources of suffering do more than erode the quality of people's lives. Pain, fatigue, depression, and self-rated assessments of health have all been shown to correlate with shorter survival.

Despite its prevalence among patients with serious illness, clinical depression is often unrecognized. Because many of the constitutional symptoms of depression, such as loss of appetite, fatigue, disturbance of sleep, and diminished libido, are all attributable to cancer or its treatment, the diagnosis may be obscured. Oncologists more readily diagnose depression when patients exhibit outward manifestations, such as crying and sad affect. The response to a single question, "Are you depressed?" has been shown to correlate well with longer survey tools in diagnosing depression. Inquiring about whether a patient feels a sense of hopelessness is also an effective screening tool for depression.

Patients with advanced, incurable illness may experience total pain that has physical, emotional, social, and spiritual dimensions. The nature of suffering entails a sense of impending disintegration of the person and a felt loss of meaning and purpose in life. Social suffering can derive from a sense of being a burden to one's family or society. While unrelieved physical suffering may have been widespread in the past, modern medicine now has more knowledge and skills to relieve suffering than ever before.

Today, specialists in palliative care believe that if all patients had access to careful assessment and optimal symptom control and supportive care, the suffering of most patients with life-threatening illnesses could be reduced sufficiently to eliminate their desire for hastened death. Even when the desire persists, avenues other than physician-assisted suicide or euthanasia are available to remedy suffering and still avoid prolonging life against the patient's wishes.

This chapter presents an approach for responding compassionately and competently to such requests. The focus is not on the debate to legalize PAS or euthanasia, but rather on the practical steps that a physician can take to assess the patient's request, begin to address its root causes, and ensure optimum quality of the patient's end-of-life.

Why Patients Ask for Physician-Assisted Suicide

Requests by a patient for assistance in suicide can be startling and understandably are often emotionally difficult for physicians. It is with empathy that a physician feels suffering when a patient is suffering enough to seek early death. To a physician, a patient's expression of a wish to die can sound like a condemnation of the care he or she is receiving. However hard for the physician to hear, it is essential for such requests to be understood as invitations for communication and opportunities for therapeutic intervention. The courage it takes for an ill and vulnerable person to make such a request of his or her physician is, in itself, evidence of the patient's trust and opens the door to deeper conversation.

Advocates of legalizing physician-assisted suicide assert that patients may feel abandoned if their doctor declines to write a lethal prescription. A countervailing concern is that agreeing to a request could curtail rather than open communication and that by even considering assisting a patient in suicide, a physician risks reinforcing the sense of helplessness, hopelessness, and worthlessness that may underlie the patient's despair. Given the risk that either approach may worsen the suffering, start instead by listening and exploring the patient's motivations.

Patients ask physicians about physician-assisted suicide (PAS) for a variety of reasons. It is a rare patient with a life-threatening illness who doesn't think about suicide, if only in passing. Some patients may approach the physician about PAS with the intent of "thinking out loud" about their current and future condition. Others may raise the question based on lifelong values. For some, a request for PAS is a sign that unmet needs have built to an intolerable level. In any case, the request for PAS should prompt the physician to assess the underlying cause for the request. Patients make requests for many different reasons that may arise from physical, psychological, social, or spiritual suffering, or practical concerns. Each person will have a unique set of needs and reasons why he or she would like to hasten death. In many surveys of patients' reasons, unrelieved psychosocial and mental suffering is the most common stimulus for requests. Studies have documented that patients who are depressed are more likely to have made serious inquiries about PAS or euthanasia. Fear of future suffering, loss of control, indignity, or being a burden are also prominent reasons for requests.

Physical suffering, including pain, is a less-frequent motivator than many think. In one above-noted study, pain alone was a motivator in

3% of requests; pain was one of several motivators in 46% of requests; and in the remaining 51% of requests pain was not cited as a factor at all. Nonetheless, the contribution of physical suffering is important because it is often treatable.

The fear of being a burden and losing independence are the most important correlates of a desire for hastened death, and are more distressing for many patients than physical symptoms. It remains crucial to address physical symptoms in cases of requests for hastened death, but in relative terms, the psychosocial aspect is more important. The key point for physicians is that phrases such as "we can control your symptoms, even if we have to sedate you" or "we can keep you comfortable" may not be reassuring to the majority of patients. Rather, exploring and addressing psychosocial concerns will be most fruitful.

The Legal and Ethical Debate

The debate about legalizing active steps to intentionally end life as a means to end suffering remains controversial. Because of the added risk of misunderstanding or overriding the patient's wishes, there is currently less support for euthanasia than for physician-assisted suicide. Nonetheless, both requests do occur and physicians need to know how to respond to either type of request.

In any discussion of physician-assisted suicide or euthanasia, it is important that the terminology be clear. Euthanasia is defined as the act of bringing about the death of a hopelessly ill and suffering person in a relatively quick and painless way for reasons of mercy. Physician-assisted suicide is defined as the act of a physician in providing the means for a patient to hasten his or her death. Although they may have similar goals, physician-assisted suicide and euthanasia differ in whether or not the physician participates in the action that finally ends life.

In physician-assisted suicide, the physician provides the necessary means or information and the patient performs the act.

In euthanasia, the physician performs the intervention.

In the current debate, there are two principles on which virtually all agree. First, physicians have an obligation to relieve pain and suffering and promote the dignity of dying patients in their care. Second, the principle of patient bodily integrity requires that physicians respect patients' competent decisions to forgo life-sustaining treatment.

An important event in the present debate occurred in 1997, when the United States Supreme Court recognized that there is no federal constitutional right to physician assisted suicide but did affirm that state legislatures may choose to legalize it. As of early 1999, Oregon is the only state that has voted to legalize PAS. In contrast to the PAS debate, the right to palliative care is uniformly acknowledged. The same U.S. Supreme Court Justices' concurring opinions supported the right of all Americans to receive quality palliative care.

Part Four

End-of-Life Care Facilities

Chapter 23

Hospice Care

What Is Hospice, and How Is It Used in Cancer Care?

Hospice is a special type of care in which medical, psychological, and spiritual support are provided to patients and their loved ones when cancer therapies are no longer controlling the disease. Hospice care focuses on controlling pain and other symptoms of illness so patients can remain as comfortable as possible near the end of life. Hospice focuses on caring, not curing. The goal is to neither hasten nor postpone death. If the patient's condition improves or the cancer goes into remission, hospice care can be discontinued and active treatment may resume. Choosing hospice care doesn't mean giving up. It just means that the goal of treatment has changed.

The hospice team usually includes doctors, nurses, home health aides, social workers, clergy or other counselors, and trained volunteers. The team may also include speech, physical, and occupational therapists, if needed. A hospice team member is on-call 24 hours a day, 7 days a week to provide support. The hospice team will work with the patient on the patient's goals for end-of-life care, not a predetermined plan or scenario. Hospice care is very individualized.

Hospice services may include doctor or nursing care, medical supplies and equipment, home health aide services, short-term respite (relief) services for caregivers, drugs to help manage cancer-related symptoms, spiritual support and counseling, and social work services.

This chapter includes text excerpted from "Hospice Care," National Cancer Institute (NCI), October 25, 2012. Reviewed October 2016.

Patients' families are also an important focus of hospice care, and services are designed to give them assistance and support. Hospice care most often takes place at home. However, hospice care can also be delivered in special in-patient facilities, hospitals, and nursing homes.

Who Is Eligible for Hospice Care?

Under most insurance plans in the United States, including Medicare, acceptance into hospice care requires a statement by a doctor and the hospice medical director that the patient has a life expectancy of 6 months or less if the disease runs its normal course. The patient also signs a statement saying that he or she is choosing hospice care. (Hospice care can be continued if the patient lives longer than 6 months, as long as the hospice medical director or other hospice doctor recertifies the patient's condition.)

The hospice team or insurance provider can answer questions about whether specific care decisions, such as getting a second opinion or participating in a clinical trial while in hospice care, would affect eligibility for hospice services.

How Can People Get Help Paying for Hospice Services?

Medicare and most Medicaid and private insurance plans cover hospice services. Medicare is a government health insurance program for the elderly and disabled that is administered by the Centers for Medicare and Medicaid Services (CMS). The Medicare hotline can answer general questions about Medicare benefits and refer people to their regional home health intermediary for information about Medicare-certified hospice programs. The hotline number is 1–800–MEDICARE (1–800–633–4227); callers with TTY equipment can call 1–877–486–2048. The booklet Medicare Hospice Benefits is available on the Medicare website. The Hospice and Respite Care page, also on the Medicare website, has answers to frequently asked questions about Medicare coverage for hospice and respite care.

Medicaid, a federal-state partnership program that is part of CMS and is administered by each state, is designed for people who need financial assistance for medical expenses. Information about coverage is available from local state welfare offices, state public health departments, state social services agencies, or the state Medicaid office. Information about specific state locations can also be found online.

Information about the types of costs covered by a particular private policy is available from a hospital business office or hospice social worker, or directly from the insurance company. Local civic, charitable, or religious organizations may also be able to help patients and their families with hospice expenses.

What Is the Difference between Hospice and Palliative Care?

Although hospice and palliative care share the same principles of providing comfort and support for patients, palliative care is available throughout a patient's experience with cancer, whereas hospice is offered only toward the end of life. A person's cancer treatment continues to be administered and assessed while he or she is receiving palliative care, but with hospice care the focus has shifted to just relieving symptoms and providing support.

Chapter 24

Types of Long-Term Care

What Is Long-Term Care?

Long-term care involves a variety of services designed to meet a person's health or personal care needs during a short or long period of time. These services help people live as independently and safely as possible when they can no longer perform everyday activities on their own.

Most Care Provided at Home

Long-term care is provided in different places by different caregivers, depending on a person's needs. Most long-term care is provided at home by unpaid family members and friends. It can also be given in a facility such as a nursing home or in the community, for example, in an adult day care center.

The most common type of long-term care is personal care—help with everyday activities, also called "activities of daily living." These activities include bathing, dressing, grooming, using the toilet, eating, and moving around—for example, getting out of bed and into a chair.

This chapter contains text excerpted from the following sources: Text under the heading "What Is Long-Term Care?" is excerpted from "Long-Term Care," NIHSeniorHealth, National Institute on Aging (NIA), May 2015; text under the heading "What Are My Other Long-Term Care Choices?" is excerpted from "What Are My Other Long-Term Care Choices?" Medicare.gov, Centers for Medicare and Medicaid Services (CMS), September 7, 2012. Reviewed October 2016.

Long-term care also includes community services such as meals, adult day care, and transportation services. These services may be provided free or for a fee.

Health Drives the Need for Care

People often need long-term care when they have a serious, ongoing health condition or disability. The need for long-term care can arise suddenly, such as after a heart attack or stroke. Most often, however, it develops gradually, as people get older and frailer or as an illness or disability gets worse.

How Long Does Care Last?

Long-term care can last a short time or a long time. Short-term care lasts several weeks or a few months while someone is recovering from a sudden illness or injury. For example, a person may get short-term rehabilitation therapy at a nursing facility after hip surgery, then go home.

Long-term care can be ongoing, as with someone who is severely disabled from a stroke or who has Alzheimer disease. Many people can remain at home if they have help from family and friends or paid services. But some people move permanently to a nursing home or other type of facility if their needs can no longer be met at home.

About 70 percent of people over age 65 need some type of long-term care during their lifetime. More than 40 percent need care in a nursing home for some period of time.

Who Will Need Long-Term Care?

It is difficult to predict how much or what type of long-term care a person might need. Several things increase the risk of needing long-term care.

- **Age**. The risk generally increases as people get older.

- **Gender**. Women are at higher risk than men, primarily because they often live longer.

- **Marital status**. Single people are more likely than married people to need care from a paid provider.

- **Lifestyle**. Poor diet and exercise habits can increase a person's risk.

- **Health and family history**. These factors also affect risk.

What Are My Other Long-Term Care Choices?

A nursing home may not be your only choice. Before you make any decisions about long term care, talk to your family, your doctor or other healthcare provider, a person-centered counselor, or a social worker to understand more about other long-term care services and supports like the ones listed below.

Community Services

There are a variety of community services that might help you with your personal care and activities, as well as home modification and equipment to support you staying at home. Some services, like volunteer groups that help with shopping or transportation, may be low cost or the group may ask for a voluntary donation. Some services may be available at varied costs depending on where you live and the services you need. These home services and programs may be available in your community:

Adult Day Care

- Adult day healthcare, which offers nursing and therapy
- Meal programs (like Meals-on-Wheels)
- Senior centers
- Friendly visitor programs
- Help with shopping and transportation
- Help with legal questions, bill paying, or other financial matters

Home Care

Depending on your needs, you may be able to get help with your personal activities (like laundry, shopping, cooking, and cleaning) at home from family members, friends, or volunteer groups. Home care agencies are also available to help with personal care, like help walking or bathing.

If you think you need home care, talk to your family to see if they can help with your care or help arrange for other care providers. There are also some home healthcare agencies that can help with nursing or attendant care in your home. Medicare will only pay for these if you meet certain conditions.

Home Healthcare

There are also some home healthcare agencies that can help with nursing care in your home. Home healthcare agencies may also provide other services, like physical therapy, occupational therapy, and help bathing. Medicare only covers short-term home healthcare if you meet certain limited conditions.

Accessory Dwelling Unit (ADU)

If you or a loved one owns a single-family home, adding an accessory dwelling unit (ADU) may help you keep your independence. An ADU (also called an "in-law" or "accessory" apartment, or a "second unit") is a second living space within a home or on a lot. It has a separate living and sleeping area, a place to cook, and a bathroom. Sometimes people turn an upper floor, basement, attic, or space over a garage into an ADU, and sometimes people build somewhere else on the property.

Check with your local zoning office to be sure ADUs are allowed in your area and find out if there are special rules. The cost for an ADU can vary widely depending on the size and cost of building materials and workers.

Subsidized Senior Housing

There are federal and state programs that help pay for housing for some older people with low to moderate incomes. Some of these housing programs also offer help with meals and other activities, like housekeeping, shopping, and doing the laundry. People usually live in their own apartments in the complex and pay rent that's a percentage of their income.

Residential Care Facilities

Residential care facilities include board and care homes (sometimes called "group homes" or "personal care homes"), and assisted living. Board and care homes and assisted living communities are group living arrangements that provide help with some activities of daily living. Whether they provide nursing services or help with medications varies among states. In some states, board and care homes and assisted living mean the same thing.

The term "assisted living" may mean different things in different facilities within the same state. Not all assisted living facilities provide the same services. It's important to contact the facility and make sure they can meet your needs. In assisted living, people often live in their own room or apartment within a building or group of buildings and have some or all of their meals together with other residents. Social and recreational activities are usually provided. Some of these facilities have health services on site.

In most cases, board and care home and assisted living residents pay a regular monthly rent and pay additional fees for the services they get. Medicare doesn't pay for assisted living facilities.

Assisted Living Facilities

These facilities provide help with activities of daily living. Some help with care most people can do themselves (like taking medicine, using eye drops, getting to appointments, or preparing meals). Residents often live in their own room or apartment within a building or group of buildings and have some or all of their meals together. Social and recreational activities are usually provided. Some of these facilities have health services on site.

Not all assisted living facilities provide the same services. In most cases, assisted living residents pay a regular monthly rent, and then pay additional fees for the services they get.

Continuing Care Retirement Communities (CCRC)

Continuing Care Retirement Communities (CCRCs) are retirement communities that offer more than one kind of housing and different levels of care. In the same community, there may be individual homes or apartments for people who still live on their own, an assisted living facility for people who need some help with daily care, and a nursing home for those who require higher levels of care. Residents move from one level to another based on their needs, but usually stay within the CCRC. If you're considering a CCRC, be sure to check the quality of the nursing home.

Your CCRC contract usually requires you to use the CCRC's nursing home if you need nursing home care. Some CCRC's will only admit people into their nursing home if they've previously lived in another section of the retirement community, like their assisted living or an independent area. Many CCRCs generally require a large payment before you move in (called an "entry fee") and charge monthly fees.

Hospice and Respite Care

Hospice is a program of care and support for people who are terminally ill. Hospice helps people who are terminally ill live comfortably.

The focus is on comfort, not on curing an illness. Respite care is a very short inpatient stay given to a hospice patient so that their usual caregiver can rest.

Pace (Program of All-Inclusive Care for the Elderly)

PACE (Program of All-inclusive Care for the Elderly) is a Medicare/Medicaid program that helps people meet healthcare needs in community.

Home and Community-Based Waiver Programs

If you're already eligible for Medicaid (or would be eligible for Medicaid coverage in a nursing home), you may be able to get help with the costs of some home- and community-based services, like homemaker services, personal care, and respite care. States have home- and community-based waiver programs to help people keep their independence while getting the care they need outside of an inpatient facility.

Chapter 25

Long-Term Care:
Making the Right Decisions

Planning for Long-Term Care

You can never know for sure if you will need long-term care. Maybe you will never need it. But an unexpected accident, illness, or injury can change your needs, sometimes suddenly. The best time to think about long-term care is before you need it.

Planning for the possibility of long-term care gives you time to learn about services in your community and what they cost. It also allows you to make important decisions while you are still able. You will need to make:

- housing decisions

- health decisions

- legal decisions

- financial decisions

People with Alzheimer disease or other cognitive impairment should begin planning for long-term care as soon as possible.

This chapter includes text excerpted from "Long-Term Care: Planning for Long-Term Care," NIHSeniorHealth, National Institute on Aging (NIA), May 2015.

Housing Decisions: Staying in Your Home

In thinking about long-term care, it is important to consider where you will live as you age and how your place of residence can best support your needs if you can no longer fully care for yourself.

Most people prefer to stay in their own home for as long as possible. When planning to receive long-term care in your home, there are many things to consider including:

- the condition of your home

- whether it can be modified, if necessary, to accommodate a wheelchair or other devices/equipment

- the availability of long-term care services in your area, such as adult day care or nearby medical facilities

- how "age-friendly" your community is. Does it offer public transportation, home delivered meals and other needed services?

- tax and legal issues

Housing Decisions: Housing with Services

If it becomes necessary, several types of housing come with support services. Primarily, these are:

- Public Housing for low-to-moderate income elderly and persons with disabilities. Typically assistance with services is provided by a staff person called a Service Coordinator

- Assisted Living or "board and care" homes are group living settings that offer housing in addition to assistance with personal care and other services, such as meals. Generally, they do not provide medical care

- Continuing Care Retirement Communities (CCRCs) provide a range of housing options, including independent living units, assisted living and nursing homes, all on the same campus. Nursing facilities, or nursing homes, are the most service-intensive housing option, providing skilled nursing services and therapies as needed.

Decisions about Your Health

Begin by thinking about what would happen if you became seriously ill or disabled. Talk with your family and friends about who would provide care if you needed help for a long time. You might delay or prevent the need for long-term care by staying healthy and independent. Talk to your doctor about your medical and family history and lifestyle. He or she may suggest actions you can take to improve your health.

Healthy eating, regular physical activity, not smoking, and limited drinking of alcohol can help you stay healthy. So can an active social life, a safe home, and regular healthcare.

Legal Decisions

Planning for long-term care includes legal planning. That means creating official documents—often called "advance directives"—that state your wishes for medical care in an emergency and at the end of life. You can also decide who will make healthcare decisions for you if you cannot make them yourself. It is important to consider what you want before you need long-term care. Discuss the options with family members, a lawyer, and others. These discussions can be hard, but telling others your wishes ahead of time answers questions they might have later and takes the burden off your family.

Experts recommend creating three types of legal documents, or advance directives. These are:

- a healthcare power of attorney
- a living will
- a do-not-resuscitate order, if desired.

Healthcare Power of Attorney

A healthcare power of attorney, also called a durable power of attorney for healthcare, is a legal document that names the person who will make medical decisions for you if you cannot make them yourself. This healthcare "agent" or "proxy" is your substitute decision maker. The person you choose should understand and respect your values and beliefs about healthcare. Talk with that person to make sure he or she is comfortable with this role.

Living Will

A living will, also called a healthcare directive, is a legal document that records your wishes for medical treatment near the end of life. It spells out what life-sustaining treatment you do or do not want if you are terminally ill, permanently unconscious, or in the final stage

171

of a fatal illness. For example, the document can state whether or not you want to receive artificial breathing if you can no longer breathe on your own.

Do-Not-Resuscitate (DNR) Order

A do-not-resuscitate (DNR) order tells healthcare providers not to perform cardiopulmonary resuscitation (CPR) or other life-support procedures if your heart stops or if you stop breathing. A DNR order is signed by a healthcare provider and put in your medical chart. Hospitals and long-term care facilities have DNR forms that a staff member can help you fill out. You do not have to have a DNR order.

Getting Expert Advice

Lawyers and other professionals can help you create legal documents to ensure that your healthcare wishes are expressed. These experts understand state laws and how changes, such as a divorce, move from your home, or death in the family, affect the way documents are prepared and maintained.

Be sure to discuss your preferences and give copies of your legal documents to family members, your healthcare proxy, and your doctor. It's important to review documents regularly and update them as needed.

Financial Decisions

Financial planning is another important part of long-term care planning. Government health insurance programs, including Medicare and Medicaid, pay for some long-term care services but not others. Most people do not have enough money to pay for all of their long-term care needs, especially if those needs are extensive or last a long time.

Reviewing Your Resources

Think about your financial resources and how you feel about using them to pay for long-term care. These resources may include:

- Social Security
- a pension or other retirement fund
- personal savings
- income from stocks and bonds

Your home is another type of asset that could be used if needed. It's a good idea to review your insurance coverage, too. Many health insurance plans provide little, if any, coverage for long-term care. Review any private health insurance, Medicare, and Medigap policies to learn exactly what is covered and what is not.

Other Options

Consider other possible ways to pay for long-term care. An increasing number of private payment options are available. Two of the more common options are long-term care insurance and reverse mortgages.

Chapter 26

Paying for Long-Term Care

Long-term care involves a variety of services provided at home, in the community, and in facilities. These services include:

- home-based care such as home health aides
- community-based care such as adult day care
- facility-based care such as assisted living and nursing homes.

Costs Can Be High

Long-term care can be expensive. Americans spend billions of dollars a year on various services. How people pay for long-term care depends on their financial situation and the kinds of services they use. Often, they rely on a variety of payment sources, including;

- personal funds
- government health insurance programs, such as Medicare and Medicaid
- private financing options, such as long-term care insurance.

Personal Funds

At first, many people pay for long-term care services with their own money. They may use personal savings, a pension or other retirement

This chapter includes text excerpted from "Long-Term Care: Paying for Long-Term Care," NIHSeniorHealth, National Institute on Aging (NIA), May 2015.

fund, income from stocks and bonds, or proceeds from the sale of a home.

Much home-based care is paid for using personal funds ("out of pocket"). Initially, family and friends often provide personal care and other services, such as transportation, for free. But as a person's needs increase, paid services may be needed.

Many older adults also pay out-of-pocket to participate in adult day service programs, meals, and other community-based services provided by local governments and nonprofit groups, which help them remain in their homes.

Professional care given in assisted living facilities and continuing care retirement communities is almost always paid for out of pocket, though in some states Medicaid may pay some costs for people who meet financial and health requirements.

Medicare and Medicaid

Another source of funds for long-term care are government insurance programs like Medicare and Medicaid. Medicare is Federal health insurance for people age 65 and older, younger people with certain disabilities, and all people with late-stage kidney failure. Medicaid is a Federal and State health insurance program for people with limited income and resources. These programs have rules limiting who is eligible and what services are covered.

Medicare Coverage Is Limited

Contrary to what many people think, Medicare does not cover most long-term care costs. It does pay for some part-time services for people who are homebound and for short-term skilled nursing care, but it does not cover ongoing personal care at home, like help with bathing. It may cover part of the first 100 days in a nursing home.

"Medigap" policies, which supplement Medicare, are not designed to meet long-term care needs. But some policies cover co-payments for nursing home stays that qualify for Medicare coverage.

Medicaid Coverage Is Broader

Medicaid pays for healthcare services for people with limited income, and it is an important source of payment for long-term care services. Personal care, home healthcare, adult day care, and nursing home care are examples of the types of Medicaid-covered services used by older adults. However, Medicaid is not available for everyone. To be eligible, you must meet certain financial and health requirements. People with financial resources above a certain limit will most likely not qualify unless they first use up their own resources to pay for care, which is called "spending down." Who is eligible and what services are covered vary from state to state.

Paying for Nursing Home Care

Nursing homes and 24-hour skilled care at home are the most expensive types of long-term care. Because nursing homes cost so much—thousands of dollars a month—most people who live in them for more than 6 months cannot pay the entire bill on their own. At first, many residents pay with their own money. They "spend down" their resources until they qualify for Medicaid. There are rules for spending down resources. Long-term care in facilities generally costs more than home-based care unless you need extensive services at home.

Veterans' Benefits

Veterans' benefits are another source of government funds, and they may help veterans with disabilities and their spouses pay for personal care and homemaker services provided at home. Disabled or aging veterans with long-term care needs may be able to get help from the U.S. Department of Veterans Affairs (VA). Its benefits pay for care in VA nursing homes and certain services at home.

Older Americans Act Programs

The Older Americans Act is a Federal program designed to organize, coordinate, and provide home- and community-based services to older adults and their families. A broad array of programs help older adults remain in the community as independently as possible.

Services under the Older Americans Act are provided by state and local agencies and other organizations. They include in-home personal care and homemaker services for frail older adults, meals in the community and for homebound elderly, local transportation services, respite care, and services for older Native Americans.

You do not have to have a certain income to use these programs, but they are targeted at low-income, frail, or disabled seniors over age 60; minority older adults; and older adults living in rural areas.

Private Financing Options

Most people don't have enough money to pay for all long-term care costs on their own, especially ongoing or expensive services like a nursing home. By planning ahead, they can use other private payment options, including:

- long-term care insurance
- reverse mortgages
- certain life insurance policies
- annuities
- trusts

Which private financing option is best for a person depends on many factors. These factors include the person's age, health status, personal finances, and risk of needing long-term care.

Long-Term Care Insurance

Long-term care insurance pays for many types of long-term care. The exact coverage depends on the type of policy you buy and what services are covered. You can purchase nursing home—only coverage or a comprehensive policy that includes both home care and facility care. Many companies sell long-term care insurance. It is a good idea to shop around and compare policies.

Buying long-term care insurance can be a good choice for younger, relatively healthy people at low risk of needing long-term care. Costs go up for people who are older, have health problems, or want more benefits.

Reverse Mortgages

A reverse mortgage is a special type of home loan that lets a homeowner convert part of the ownership value in his or her home into cash. Unlike a traditional home loan, no repayment is required until the borrower sells the home, no longer uses it as a main residence, or dies.

There are no income or medical requirements to get a reverse mortgage. The loan amount is tax-free and can be used for any expense, including long-term care. If long-term care costs are higher than the amount you borrow, selling your home is not required, but doing so may provide enough funds to repay the loan.

Life Settlements

Some life insurance policies can help pay for long-term care. Policies with an "accelerated death benefit" provide cash advances while you are still alive. The advance is subtracted from the amount your beneficiaries (the people who get the insurance proceeds) will receive when you die.

You can get an accelerated death benefit if you live permanently in a nursing home, need long-term care for an extended time, are terminally ill, or have a life-threatening diagnosis such as acquired immune deficiency syndrome (AIDS). Check your life insurance policy to see exactly what it covers.

You may be able to raise cash by selling your life insurance policy for its current value. This option, known as a "life settlement," is usually available only to people age 70 and older. The proceeds are taxable and can be used for any reason, including paying for long-term care.

A similar arrangement, called a "viatical settlement," allows a terminally ill person to sell his or her life insurance policy to an insurance company. This option is typically used by people who are expected to live 2 years or less. A viatical settlement provides immediate cash, but it can be hard to get.

Annuities

You may choose to enter into an annuity contract with an insurance company to help pay for long-term care services. In exchange for a single payment or a series of payments, the insurance company will send you an annuity, which is a series of regular payments over a specified and defined period of time. There are two types of annuities: immediate annuities and deferred long-term care annuities.

- If you have an immediate long-term care annuity, the insurance company will send you a specified monthly income in return for a single premium payment.

- Deferred long-term care annuities are available to people up to age 85. Similar to other annuities, in exchange for a single premium payment, you receive a stream of monthly income for a specified period of time.

Trusts

A trust is a legal entity that allows a person (the trustor) to transfer assets to another person (the trustee). Once the trustor establishes the trust, the trustee manages and controls the assets for the trustor or for another beneficiary.

You may choose to use a trust to provide flexible control of assets for the benefit of minor children. Another common use of a trust is to provide flexible control of assets for an older adult or a person with a disability, which could include yourself or your spouse. Two types of trusts can help pay for long-term care services: charitable remainder trusts and Medicaid disability trusts.

Chapter 27

Nursing Home Care

What Is a Nursing Home?

A nursing home, also known as a skilled nursing facility, is a place for people who don't need to be in a hospital but can no longer be cared for at home. This can include people with critical injuries or serious illnesses, or those needing care after surgery. Most nursing homes have aides and skilled nurses on hand 24 hours a day. Talk to your healthcare provider to find out if a nursing home is the best choice for you or a member of your family.

Nursing homes can be:

Hospital-like. This type of nursing home is often set up like a hospital. Members of the staff give medical care, as well as physical, speech, and occupational therapy. There can be a nurses' station on each floor. As a rule, one or two people live in a room. A number of nursing homes will let couples live together. Things that make a room special, like family photos, are often welcome.

Household-like. These facilities are designed to be more like homes, and the day-to-day routine is not fixed. Teams of staff and residents try to create a relaxed feeling. Kitchens are often open to residents, decorations give a sense of home, and the staff is encouraged to develop relationships with residents.

This chapter includes text excerpted from "Nursing Homes: Making the Right Choice," National Institute on Aging (NIA), National Institutes of Health (NIH), September 2012. Reviewed October 2016.

Combination. Some nursing homes have a combination of hospital-like and household-like units.

Many nursing homes have visiting doctors who see their patients on site. Other nursing homes have patients visit the doctor's office. Nursing homes sometimes have separate areas called "Special Care Units" for people with serious memory problems, like dementia.

Tips to Keep in Mind

If you need to go to a nursing home after a hospital stay, the hospital staff can help you find one that will provide the kind of care that's best for you. Most hospitals have social workers who can help you with these decisions. If you are looking for a nursing home, ask your doctor's office for some recommendations. Once you know what choices you have, it's a good idea to:

Consider. What is important to you—nursing care, meals, physical therapy, a religious connection, hospice care, or Special Care Units for dementia patients? Do you want a place close to family and friends so they can easily visit?

Ask. Talk with friends, relatives, social workers, and religious groups to find out what places they suggest. Check with healthcare providers about which nursing homes they feel provide good care. Use their suggestions to make a list of homes that offer the types of services you want.

Call. Get in touch with each place on your list. Ask questions about how many people live there and what it costs. Find out about waiting lists.

Visit. Make plans to meet with the director and the nursing director. The Medicare Nursing Home Checklist at https://www.medicare.gov/nursinghomecompare/search.html has some good ideas to consider when visiting. For example, look for:

- Medicare and Medicaid certification
- Handicap access
- Residents who look well cared for
- Warm interaction between staff and residents

Talk. Don't be afraid to ask questions. For example, you can ask the staff to explain any strong odors. Bad smells might indicate a problem; good ones might hide a problem. You might want to find out how long the director and heads of nursing, food, and social services departments have worked at the nursing home. If key members of the staff change often, that could mean there's something wrong.

Visit again. Make a second visit without calling ahead. Try another day of the week or time of day so you will meet other staff members and see different activities. Stop by at mealtime. Is the dining room attractive and clean? Does the food look tempting?

Understand. Once you select a nursing home, carefully read the contract. Question the director or assistant director about anything you don't understand. Ask a good friend or family member to read over the contract before you sign it.

Do Nursing Homes Have to Meet Standards?

The Centers for Medicare and Medicaid Services (CMS) requires each State to inspect any nursing home that gets money from the government. Homes that don't pass inspection are not certified. Ask to see the current inspection report and certification of any nursing home you are considering.

Paying for Nursing Home Care

It's important to check with Medicare, Medicaid, and any private insurance provider you have to find out their current rules about covering the costs of long-term care. You can pay for nursing home care in several ways. Here are some examples:

Medicare. For someone who needs special care, Medicare, a Federal program, will cover part of the cost in a skilled nursing home approved by Medicare. Check with Medicare for details.

Medicaid. Medicaid is a State/Federal program that provides health benefits to some people with low incomes. Contact your county family services department to see if you qualify.

Private pay. Some people pay for long-term care with their own savings for as long as possible. When that is no longer possible, they may apply for help from Medicaid. If you think you may need to apply for Medicaid at some point, make sure the nursing home you're interested in accepts Medicaid payments. Not all do.

Long-term care insurance. Some people buy private long-term care insurance. It can pay part of the costs for a nursing home or other long-term care for the length of time stated in your policy. This type of insurance is sold by many different companies and benefits vary widely. Look carefully at several policies before making a choice.

When thinking about nursing home costs, keep in mind that you can have extra out-of-pocket charges for some supplies or personal care, for instance, hair appointments, laundry, and services that are outside routine care.

Chapter 28

Home Care for Critically Ill Patients

Chapter Contents

Section 28.1

Home Healthcare

This section includes text excerpted from "There's No
Place Like Home—for Growing Old," National Institute
on Aging (NIA), National Institutes of Health (NIH),
March 2012. Reviewed October 2016.

What Do I Do First?

Planning ahead is hard because you never know how your needs
might change. But, the first step is to think about the kinds of help
you might want in the near future. Maybe you live alone, so there is
no one living in your home who is available to help you. Maybe you
don't need help right now, but you live with a husband or wife who
does. Everyone has a different situation, but one way to begin planning is to look at any illnesses like diabetes or emphysema that you or
your spouse might have. Talk to your doctor about how these health
problems could make it hard for someone to get around or take care
of him- or herself in the future. Help getting dressed in the morning,
fixing a meal, or remembering to take medicine may be all you need
to stay in your own home.

What Kinds of Help Can I Get?

You can get almost any type of help you want in your home—often
for a cost. The following list includes some common things people need.
You can get more information on many of these services from your
local Area Agency on Aging, local and State offices on aging or social
services, tribal organization, or nearby senior center.

Personal care. Is bathing, washing your hair, or dressing getting
harder to do? Maybe a relative or friend could help. Or, you could hire
a trained aide for a short time each day.

Homemaking. Do you need help with chores like housecleaning,
yard work, grocery shopping, or laundry? Some grocery stores and drug
stores will take your order over the phone and bring the items to your

home. There are cleaning services you can hire, or maybe someone you know has a housekeeper to suggest. Some housekeepers will help with laundry. Some dry cleaners will pick up and deliver your clothes.

Meals. Worried that you might not be eating nutritious meals or tired of eating alone? Sometimes you could share cooking with a friend or have a potluck dinner with a group of friends. Find out if meals are served at a nearby senior center, church, or synagogue. Eating out may give you a chance to visit with others. Is it hard for you to get out? Ask someone to bring you a healthy meal a few times a week. Also, meal delivery programs bring hot meals into your home.

Money management. Do you worry about paying bills late or not at all? Are health insurance claim forms confusing? Maybe you can get help with these tasks. Ask a trusted relative to lend a hand. Volunteers, financial counselors, or geriatric care managers can also help. Just make sure you get the referral from a trustworthy source, like your local Area Agency on Aging. If you are familiar with computers, you could pay your bills online. Check with someone at your bank about this option. Some people have their regular bills, like utilities and rent or mortgage, paid automatically from their checking account.

When you sign up for Federal benefits for the first time, you must choose either electronic direct deposit to your bank or a special debit card.

Be careful to avoid money scams. Never give your Social Security number, credit card account numbers, or bank account numbers to someone on the phone (unless you placed the call) or in response to an email you receive on your computer. Always check all bills, including utility bills, for charges you do not recognize.

Even though you might not need it now, think about giving someone you trust permission to discuss your bills with creditors or your Social Security or Medicare benefits with those agencies. Or, you could give overall permission to handle a variety of legal matters for you in the form of a durable power of attorney. "Durable" means the permission remains in effect if you cannot make decisions yourself, but you can change the power of attorney or cancel it at any time.

Healthcare. Do you forget to take your medicine? There are devices available to remind you when it is time for your next dose. Special pill boxes allow you or someone else to set out your pills for an entire week. Have you just gotten out of the hospital and still need nursing care at home for a short time? The hospital discharge planner can help you make arrangements, and Medicare might pay for a home health aide to come to your home.

If you can't remember what the doctor told you to do, try to have someone go to your doctor visits with you. Ask them to write down everything you are supposed to do, or if you are by yourself, ask the doctor to put all recommendations in writing.

Products to Make Life Easier

Is it getting harder to turn a door knob or put on your socks? Devices are available to make daily activities easier. The Department of Education's website, has information on more than 30,000 assistive-technology products designed to make it easier for people to do things for themselves. If you can't use a computer, you can call 1-800-227-0216.

Getting around—at home and in town. Are you having trouble walking? Perhaps a walker would help. If you need more, think about getting an electric chair or scooter. These are sometimes covered by Medicare. Do you need someone to go with you to the doctor or shopping? Volunteer escort services may be available. If you are no longer driving a car, check if there are free or low-cost public transportation and taxis in your area. Maybe a relative, friend, or neighbor would take you along when they go on errands or do yours for you.

Activities and friends. Are you bored staying at home? Your local senior center offers a variety of activities. You might see friends there and meet new people too. Is it hard for you to leave your home? Maybe you would enjoy visits from someone. Volunteers, called "Friendly Visitors," "Senior Volunteers," or "Senior Companions," are sometimes available to stop by or call once a week. They can just keep you company, or you can talk about any problems you are having. Call your local Area Agency on Aging to see if they are available near you.

Safety. Are you worried about crime in your neighborhood, physical abuse, or losing money as a result of a scam? Talk to the staff at your local Area Agency on Aging. Do you live alone, and are you afraid of becoming sick with no one around to help? You might want to get an emergency alert system. You just push a special button that you wear, and emergency medical personnel are called. A monthly fee is charged.

Housing. Would a few changes make your home easier and safer to live in? Think about things like a ramp at the front door, grab bars in the tub or shower, nonskid floors, more comfortable handles on doors or faucets, and better insulation. Sound expensive? You might be able to get help paying for these changes. Check with your local or State Area Agency on Aging, State housing finance agency, welfare department, community development groups, or the Federal Government.

Where Can I Look For Help?

Here are some resources to start with:

People you know. Family, friends, and neighbors are the biggest source of help for many older people. Talk with those close to you about the best way to get what you need. If you are physically able, think about trading services with a friend or neighbor. One could do the grocery shopping, and the other could cook dinner, for example.

Community and local government resources. Learn about the services found in your community. Healthcare providers and social workers may have suggestions. The local Area Agency on Aging, local and State offices on aging or social services, and your tribal organization may have lists of services of services. Look in the phone book under "Government." If you belong to a religious group, talk to the clergy, or check with its local offices about any senior services they offer.

Geriatric care managers. These specially trained professionals can help find resources to make your daily life easier. They will work with you to form a long-term care plan and find the services you need. They will charge for this help, and their fees probably won't be covered by any insurance plan. Geriatric care managers can be very helpful when family members live far apart. If asked, they will check in with you from time to time to make sure your needs haven't changed.

Federal Government sources. There are many resources from the Federal Government where you can start looking for information. Some are only available on the Internet. If you don't have Internet access, you might be able to use a computer with Internet access in your local library or senior center. Perhaps your son or daughter, grandchild, niece, nephew, or a friend or neighbor could look on the Internet for you.

How Much Will This Cost?

An important part of planning is thinking about how you are going to pay for the help you need. Some things you want may cost a lot.

Others may be free. Some might be covered by Medicare, private "Medigap" policies or other private health insurance, Medicaid, or long- term care insurance. Some may not. Check with your insurance provider(s). There is a chance that paying for just a few services out of pocket could cost less in the long run than moving into an independent living, assisted living, or long-term care facility. And you will have your wish of still living on your own.

Are you eligible for veterans benefits from the U.S. Department of Veterans Affairs? The VA sometimes provides medical care in your home. In some areas they also offer homemaker/ home health aide services, adult day healthcare, and hospice.

Section 28.2

Assistive Technology: Help for Patients with Chronic Conditions

This section includes text excerpted from "Assistive Technology," Eldercare Locator, U.S. Department of Health and Human Services (HHS), October 15, 2015.

Assistive Technology (AT)

Assistive technology (AT) is any service or tool that helps older adults or persons with disabilities perform activities that might otherwise be difficult or impossible.

For older adults, such technology may be a walker to improve mobility or an amplification device to make sounds easier to hear. It could also include a magnifying glass for someone who has poor vision or a scooter that makes it possible for someone to travel over distances that are too far to walk. In short, AT is anything that aids continued participation in daily activities.

AT allows many people to live independently without long-term nursing or home healthcare. For some, it is critical to the ability to perform simple activities of daily living, such as bathing.

Choosing AT

Older adults should carefully evaluate their needs before purchasing AT. Using AT may change the mix of services that they require or affect the way that those services are provided. Needs assessment and planning are very important.

Usually, a needs assessment is most effective when done by a team working with the older adult in a place where the AT will be used. For example, someone who has trouble communicating or hearing might consult his or her doctor, an audiology specialist, a speech-language therapist, and family and friends. Together, they can identify precise challenges and help select the most effective devices available at the lowest cost. A professional member of the team, such as the audiology specialist, can also arrange for any training needed to use the equipment.

When considering AT, it is useful to consider high-tech and low-tech solutions. Older adults should also think about how their needs might change over time. High-tech devices tend to be more expensive but may address many different needs. Low-tech equipment is usually less expensive but also less adaptable.

Paying for AT

Right now, no single private insurance plan or public program will pay for all types of AT under any circumstances. However, Medicare Part B will cover up to 80% of the cost, if the items are durable medical equipment—devices that are "primarily and customarily used to serve a medical purpose, and generally are not useful to a person in the absence of illness or injury." Contact Medicare to determine whether a particular type of AT is covered.

Depending on where you live, the state-run Medicaid program may pay for some AT. Keep in mind that when Medicaid covers part of the cost, the benefits do not usually provide the total amount needed to buy an expensive piece of equipment, such as a power wheelchair.

Older adults who are eligible for veteran benefits may be eligible for assistance from the U.S. Department of Veterans Affairs (VA), which has a model structure in place to pay for the large volume of equipment that it buys. The VA also invests in training people to use assistive devices.

Subsidy programs provide some types of AT at a reduced cost or for free. Many businesses and nonprofit groups offer discounts, grants, or rebates to get consumers to try a specific product. Older adults should be cautious about participating in subsidy programs run by businesses with commercial interests in the product or service because of the potential for fraud.

Local Resources

Most states have at least one agency that deals specifically with AT issues. The Assistive Technology Act (Tech Act) provides funds for the development of statewide consumer information and training programs.

Some Area Agencies on Aging (AAA) have programs or link to services that assist older people obtain low-cost assistive technology. To locate your AAA, call the Eldercare Locator at 1-800-677-1116.

Local civic, faith-based, and veterans' organizations as well as senior centers may also be able to refer you to AT resources.

Section 28.3

Home Care for Cancer Patients

This section contains text excerpted from the following sources:
Text beginning with the heading "Home Care Services" is
excerpted from "Finding Health Care Services," National Cancer
Institute (NCI), March 10, 2015; Text beginning with heading "Who
Are Caregivers, and How Do They Support Cancer Survivors?" is
excerpted from "Basic Information for Cancer Survivors' Family,
Friends, and Caregivers," Centers for Disease Control and
Prevention (CDC), March 8, 2016.

Home Care Services

Sometimes cancer patients want to be cared for at home so they can be in familiar surroundings with family and friends. Home care services can help the patients stay at home by using a team approach with doctors, nurses, social workers, physical therapists, and others.

If the cancer patient qualifies for home care services, such services may include:

- Managing symptoms and monitoring care

- Delivery of medications

- Physical therapy

- Emotional and spiritual care

- Help with preparing meals and personal hygiene

- Providing medical equipment

For many patients and families, home care can be both rewarding and demanding. It can change relationships and require families to cope with all aspects of patient care. New issues may also arise that families need to address such as the logistics of having home care providers coming into the home at regular intervals. To prepare for these changes, patients and caregivers should ask questions and get as much information as possible from the home care team or organization. A doctor, nurse, or social worker can provide information about a patient's specific needs, the availability of services, and the local home care agencies.

Getting Financial Assistance for Home Care

Help with paying for home care services may be available from public or private sources. Private health insurance may cover some home care services, but benefits vary from plan to plan.

Some public resources to help pay for home care are:

- Centers for Medicare and Medicaid Services (CMS): A government agency responsible for the administration of several key federal healthcare programs. Two of these are

- Medicare: A government health insurance program for the elderly or disabled.

- Medicaid: A joint federal and state health insurance program for those who need help with medical expenses. Coverage varies by state.

Both Medicare and Medicaid may cover home care services for the cancer patients who qualify, but some rules apply. Talk to a social worker and other members of the healthcare team to find out more about home care providers and agencies.

- Eldercare Locator: Run by the U.S. Administration on Aging (AOA), it provides information about local Area Agencies on Aging and other assistance for older people. These agencies may provide funds for home care. Eldercare Locator can be reached at 1-800-677-1116 for more information.

- The U.S. Department of Veterans Affairs (VA) Veterans who are disabled as a result of military service can receive home care services from the U.S. Department of Veterans Affairs (VA). However, only home care services provided by VA hospitals may be used. More information about these benefits can be found on their website or by calling 1–877–222–8387 (1–877–222–VETS).

Who Are Caregivers, and How Do They Support Cancer Survivors?

A caregiver is a person who provides help and care to someone who has been diagnosed with cancer. Cancer survivors may get help from caregivers with regular day-to-day tasks, such as household chores, as well as tasks related to their cancer, such as coordinating treatment and follow-up care with healthcare providers. Caregiving relationships can be formal or informal.

Formal caregivers are trained and paid to provide care, such as nurses, therapists, social workers, and home health aides. Formal caregivers may work for home care agencies, community or social service agencies, or for-profit providers.

Informal caregivers provide unpaid care out of love, respect, or friendship. Some examples of informal caregiving relationships are:

- Adult children caring for parents.

- Parents or grandparents caring for a child with cancer.

- A spouse or partner caring for his or her spouse or partner.

- A neighbor or close friend caring for the cancer survivor.

The types of care that informal caregivers provide ranges from simple, occasional tasks, like driving the cancer patient to the doctor, to full-time care. The demands on caregivers often change over time. Some of the types of help caregivers provide include:

- Cooking, cleaning, and other household chores.

- Running errands such as buying groceries and getting prescriptions filled.

- Helping the cancer patient bathe, get dressed, use the bathroom, eat, and take medicine.

- Paying bills and filing insurance claims.

- Providing encouragement and support to the survivor, and helping him or her stay in touch with friends and family members.

- Telling the doctor if the survivor gets worse or has side effects from treatment.

Researchers are studying the roles caregivers play in supporting survivors, and the challenges and benefits associated with caregiving, so they can suggest ways in which caregivers can be supported.

Part Five

End-of-Life Caregiving

Chapter 29

Communications among Patients, Families, and Providers

Chapter Contents

Section 29.1

Effective Communication for Effective Care

This section includes text excerpted from "Communication
in Cancer Care (PDQ®)—Patient Version," National Cancer
Institute (NCI), March 27, 2015.

Good communication between patients, family caregivers, and the healthcare team is very important. Good communication between patients with cancer, family caregivers, and the healthcare team helps improve patients' well-being and quality of life. Communicating about concerns and decision making is important during all phases of treatment and supportive care.

The goals of good communication in cancer care are to:

- Build a trusting relationship between the patient, family caregivers, and the healthcare team.

- Help the patient, family caregivers, and healthcare team share information with each other.

- Help the patient and family talk about feelings and concerns.

Patients, their families, and their healthcare team face many issues when cancer is diagnosed. Cancer is a life-threatening illness, even though advances in treatments have increased the chances of a cure or remission. A patient who is diagnosed with cancer may feel fear and anxiety about treatments that are often difficult, expensive, and complicated. Decisions about the patient's care can be very hard to make. Good communication can help patients, families, and doctors make these decisions together and improve the patient's well-being and quality of life.

Studies show that when patients and doctors communicate well during cancer care, there are many positive results. Patients are usually:

- More satisfied with care and feel more in control.

- More likely to follow through with treatment.

- More informed.

- More likely to take part in a clinical trial.

- Better able to make the change from care that is given to treat the cancer to palliative care.

Some patients and families want a lot of information and choose to make decisions about care. Patients and their families should let the healthcare team know how much information they want about the cancer and its treatment. Some patients and families want a lot of detailed information. Others want less detail. Also, the need for information may change as the patient moves through diagnosis and treatment. Some patients with advanced disease want less information about their condition.

There may be differences in how involved patients and families want to be in making decisions about cancer care. Some patients and families may want to be very involved and make their own decisions about cancer care. Others may want to leave decisions to the doctor.

Communication is important throughout cancer care, but especially when important decisions are to be made. These important decision times include:

- When the patient is first diagnosed.

- Any time new decisions about treatment need to be made.

- After treatment, when discussing how well it worked.

- Whenever the goal of care changes.

- When the patient makes his or her wishes known about advance directives, such as a living will.

End-of life discussions with the healthcare team may lead to fewer procedures and better quality of life. Studies have shown that cancer patients who have end-of-life discussions with their doctors choose to have fewer procedures, such as resuscitation or the use of a ventilator. They are also less likely to be in intensive care, and the cost of their healthcare is lower during their final week of life. Reports from their caregivers show that these patients live as long as patients who choose to have more procedures and that they have a better quality of life in their last days.

The Role of Family Caregivers

Family caregivers are partners in communication. Families can help patients make better decisions about their cancer care. Patients and their family members can join together as partners to communicate with the doctor and healthcare team. When possible, patients should decide how much help they want from family members when making decisions. Communication between family caregivers and the healthcare team should continue throughout cancer care. It should include information about the goals of treatment, plans for the patient's care, and what to expect over time.

Communication with the doctor helps caregivers as well as patients. Communication that includes the patient and family is called family-centered communication. Family-centered communication with the doctor helps the family understand its role in caregiving. Family caregivers who get specific and practical direction from the healthcare team are more confident about giving care. When caregivers receive this help, they can give the patient better care.

Language and culture can affect communication. Communication can be more difficult if the doctor does not speak the same language as the patient and family, or if there are cultural differences. Every patient with cancer has the right to get clear information about the diagnosis and treatment so he or she can take full part in making decisions. Most medical centers have trained interpreters or have other ways to help with language differences.

If cultural beliefs will affect decisions about treatment and care, the healthcare team should be told about these beliefs. For example, a common Western belief is that an informed patient should make the final decision about cancer care.

There may be problems with communication. There are many things that can block communication between the patient and doctor. This can happen if:

- The patient does not fully understand all the facts about treatment.

- The medical information is not given in a way the patient can understand.

- The patient believes the doctor will tell them the important facts about treatment and doesn't ask questions.

- The patient is afraid to ask too many questions.

- The patient is afraid to take too much of the doctor's time and doesn't ask questions.

Family caregivers can sometimes help when communication problems come up.

The Role of Parents

Children with cancer need information that is right for their age. Studies show that children with cancer want to know about their illness and how it will be treated. The amount of information a child wants depends in part on his or her age. Most children worry about how their illness and treatment will affect their daily lives and the people around them. Studies also show that children have less doubt and fear when they are given information about their illness, even if it is bad news.

There are many ways for parents to communicate with their child.

When a child is seriously ill, parents may find that communication is better when they:

- Talk with the doctor at the beginning of cancer care about open communication with their child and other family members. Parents should discuss how the family feels about sharing medical information with their child, and talk about any concerns they have.

- Talk with their child and share information throughout the course of the illness.

- Find out what their child already knows and wants to know about the illness. This will help clear up any confusion their child may have about the medical facts.

- Explain medical information according to what is right for their child's age and needs.

- Are sensitive to their child's emotions and reactions.

- Encourage their child by promising they will be there to listen to and protect him or her.

Talking with the Healthcare Team

Patients and family caregivers can get ready for medical appointments. It is helpful for patients and caregivers to plan ahead for doctor visits. The following may help you get the most out of these visits:

- Keep a file or notebook of the patient's medical information that includes test and procedure dates, test results, and other records. Bring this file with you to the medical appointment.

- Keep a list of names and doses of medicines and how often they are taken. Bring this list with you.

- Use only trusted sources, such as government and national organizations, if you do research about the medical condition. Bring this research with you to discuss with the doctor.

- Make a list of questions and concerns. List your most important questions first.

- If you have a lot to discuss with the doctor, ask if you can:

  - Schedule a longer appointment.

  - Ask questions by phone or email.

  - Talk with a nurse or other member of the healthcare team. Nurses are an important part of the healthcare team and can share information with you and your doctor.

- Bring a tape recorder or take notes so that later on you can listen to or review what you discussed.

- Bring a family caregiver or friend to the doctor visit so they can help you remember important information after the visit.

- Patients and family caregivers should talk before the appointment to help get ready for possible bad news or information that is different than expected.

Patients and caregivers can make a checklist of specific questions about treatment. When talking with the doctor, ask specific questions about any concerns you have. If an answer is not clear to you, ask the doctor to explain it in a way that you can understand. Include the following questions about the patient's treatment:

- What medical records should the patient bring to treatment?

- What can the patient do ahead of time to get ready for treatment?

- How long will the treatment take?

- Can the patient go to and from treatment alone? Should someone else go along?

- Can a family member be with the patient during treatment?

- What can be done to help the patient feel more comfortable during treatment?

- What are the side effects of treatment?

- After treatment, what problems should be watched for? When should a doctor be called?

- Who can help with questions about filing insurance claims?

Section 29.2

Talk about End-of-Life Wishes

This section includes text excerpted from "Planning for End-of-Life Care Decisions," National Institute on Aging (NIA), National Institutes of Health (NIH), July 2016.

The simplest, but not always the easiest, way is to talk about end-of-life care before an illness. Discussing your thoughts, values, and desires about end-of-life care before you become sick will help people who are close to you to know what care you want. You could discuss how you feel about using life-prolonging measures (for example, CPR or a ventilator) or where you would like to be cared for (for example, home or nursing home). Doctors should be told about these wishes as well.

For some people, it makes sense to bring this up at a small family gathering. Some may find that telling their family they have made a will (or updated an existing one) provides an opportunity to bring up this subject with other family members. As hard as it might be to talk about your end-of-life wishes, knowing your preferences ahead of time can make decision-making easier for your family. You may also have some comfort knowing that your family can choose what you want.

On the other hand, if your parents (or another close relative or friend) are aging and you are unsure about what they want, you might introduce the subject. You can try to explain that having this conversation will help you care for them and do what they want. You might start by talking about what you think their values are, instead of talking about specific treatments. Try saying something like, "When Uncle Isaiah had a stroke, I thought you seemed upset that his kids wanted to put him on a respirator." Or, "I've always wondered why Grandpa didn't die at home. Do you know?"

Encourage your parents to share the type of care they would choose to have at the end of life, rather than what they don't want. There is no right or wrong plan, only what they would like. If they are reluctant to have this conversation, don't force it, but try to bring it up again at a later time.

Prepare Advance Directives and Other Documents

Written instructions letting others know the type of care you want if you are seriously ill or dying are called advance directives. These include a living will and healthcare power of attorney. A living will records your end-of-life care wishes in case you are no longer able to speak or make decisions for yourself.

You might want to talk with your doctor or other healthcare provider before preparing a living will. This will help you have a better understanding of what types of decisions might need to be made. Make sure your doctor and family have seen your living will and understand your instructions.

Because a living will cannot give guidance for every possible situation, you probably want to name someone to make care decisions for you if you are unable to do so for yourself. You might choose a family member, friend, lawyer, or someone in your religious community. Of course, you should make sure the person you have named (and alternates) understand your views about end-of-life care and are willing to make those decisions on your behalf. You can do this either in the advance directives or through a durable power of attorney for healthcare that names a healthcare proxy, who is also called a representative, surrogate, agent, or attorney-in-fact.

Durable means it remains in effect even if you are unable to make decisions. A durable power of attorney for healthcare is a useful document if you don't want to be specific—if you'd rather let a proxy evaluate each situation or treatment option independently. This document is particularly important if your healthcare proxy—the person you want to make choices for you—is not a legal member of your family.

If you don't name someone, the State you live in probably has an order of priority based on family relationships to determine who decides for you. Don't confuse a durable power of attorney for healthcare with a durable power of attorney. The first is limited to decisions related to healthcare, while the latter covers decisions regarding property or financial matters.

A lawyer can prepare these papers, or you can do them yourself. Forms are available from your local or State government, from private groups, or on the Internet. Often, these forms need to be witnessed. That means that people who are not related to you watch as you sign and date the paperwork and then sign and date it themselves as proof that the signature is indeed yours.

Make sure you give copies to your primary doctor and your healthcare proxy. Have copies in your files as well. Hospitals might ask for a copy when you are admitted, even if you are not seriously ill. You should also give permission to your doctors and insurance companies to share your personal information with your healthcare proxy. This lets your proxy discuss your case with the doctor and handle insurance issues that may come up.

Sometimes, people change their minds as they get older or after they become ill. Review the decisions in your advance directives from time to time, and make changes if your views or your health needs have changed. Be sure to discuss these changes with your healthcare proxy and your doctor. Replace all copies of the older version with the updated ones, witnessed and signed if appropriate.

Do you live in one State, but spend a lot of time in another? Maybe you live in the north and spend winter months in a southern State. Or, perhaps your children and grandchildren live in a different State and you visit them often. Because States' rules and regulations may differ, make sure your forms are legal in both your home State and the State you travel to often. If not, make an advance directive with copies for that State, too, and be sure your family there has a copy.

Chapter 30

Long-Distance Caregiving

What Is a Long-Distance Caregiver?

If you live an hour or more away from a person who needs care, you can think of yourself as a long-distance caregiver. This kind of care can take many forms—from helping with finances or money management to arranging for in-home care, from providing respite care for a primary caregiver to creating a plan in case of emergencies.

Many long-distance caregivers act as information coordinators, helping aging parents understand the confusing maze of new needs, including home health aides, insurance benefits and claims, and durable medical equipment.

Caregiving, no matter where the caregiver lives, is often long-lasting and ever-expanding. For the long-distance caregiver, what may start out as an occasional social phone call to share family news can eventually turn into regular phone calls about managing household bills, getting medical information, and arranging for grocery deliveries. What begins as a monthly trip to check on Mom may become a larger project to move her to a new home or nursing facility closer to where you live.

Anyone, anywhere can be a long-distance caregiver. Gender, income, age, social status, employment—none of these prevents you

This chapter includes text excerpted from "Long-Distance Caregiving: Twenty Questions and Answers," National Institute on Aging (NIA), National Institutes of Health (NIH), June 2016.

from taking on at least some caregiving responsibilities and possibly feeling some of the satisfaction.

How Will I Know If My Aging Relative or Friend Needs Help?

Uncle Simon sounds fine on the phone, but I don't know if he really is okay. Sometimes, your relative will ask for help. Or, the sudden start of a severe illness will make it clear that assistance is needed. But, when you live far away, some detective work might be necessary to uncover possible signs that support or help is needed.

A phone call is not always the best way to tell whether or not an older person needs help handling daily activities. Uncle Simon might not want to worry his nephew, Brad, who lives a few hours away, or he might not want to admit that he's often too tired to cook an entire meal. But how can Brad know this? If he calls at dinnertime and asks "what's cooking," Brad might get a sense that dinner is a bowl of cereal. If so, he might want to talk with his uncle and offer some help.

With Simon's permission, Brad might contact people who see his uncle regularly—neighbors, friends, doctors, or local relatives, for example—and ask them to call Brad if they have concerns about Simon. Brad might also ask if he could check in with them periodically. When Brad spends a weekend with his uncle, he can look around for possible trouble areas—it's easier to disguise problems during a short phone call than during a longer visit.

Brad can make the most of his visit if he takes some time in advance to develop a list of possible problem areas he wants to check out while visiting his uncle. That's a good idea for anyone in this type of situation. Of course, it may not be possible to do everything in one trip—but make sure that any potentially dangerous situations are taken care of as soon as possible. If you can't correct everything on your list, see if you can arrange for someone else to finish up.

In addition to safety issues and the overall condition of the home, try to determine the older person's mood and general health status. Sometimes people confuse depression in older people with normal aging. A depressed older person might brighten up for a phone call or short visit, but it's harder to hide serious mood problems during an extended visit.

How Can I Really Help from Far Away?

My sister lives close to our parents and has gradually been doing more and more for them. I'm halfway across the country. I'd like to help them and my sister, but I don't feel comfortable just jumping in.

Many long-distance caregivers provide emotional support and occasional respite to a primary caregiver. Staying in contact with your parents by phone or email might also take some pressure off your sister. Long-distance caregivers can play a part in arranging for professional caregivers, hiring home health and nursing aides, or locating care in an assisted living facility or nursing home (also known as a skilled nursing facility). Some long-distance caregivers find they can be helpful by handling things online—for example, researching health problems or medicines, paying bills, or keeping family and friends updated. Some long-distance caregivers help a parent pay for care, while others step in to manage finances.

Caregiving is not easy for anyone—not for the caregiver and not for the care recipient. There are sacrifices and adjustments for everyone. When you don't live where the care is needed, it may be especially hard to feel that what you are doing is enough and that what you are doing is important. It often is.

How Can My Family Decide about Sharing Responsibilities?

My brother lives closest to our grandmother, but he's uncomfortable coordinating her medical care. This is a question that many families have to work out. You could start by setting up a family meeting and, if your grandmother is capable, include her in the discussion. This is best done when there is not an emergency. A calm conversation about what kind of care is needed in the present and might be called for in the future can avoid a lot of confusion. Ask your grandmother what she wants. Use her wishes as the basis for a plan. Decide who will be responsible for each task. Many families find the best first step is to name a primary caregiver, even if one is not needed immediately. That way the primary caregiver can step in if there is a crisis.

Think about your schedules and how to adapt them to give respite to a primary caregiver or to coordinate holiday and vacation times. One family found that it worked to have the long-distance caregiver come to town while the primary caregiver was away. Many families report that offering appreciation, reassurance, and positive feedback to the primary caregiver is an important, but sometimes forgotten, contribution.

What Is a Geriatric Care Manager, and How Can I Find One?

A friend of mine suggested that having a professional on the scene to help my dad would take some of the pressure off me. Professional care managers are usually licensed nurses or social workers who specialize in geriatrics. Some families hire a geriatric care manager to evaluate and assess a parent's needs and to coordinate care through community resources. The cost of an initial evaluation varies and may be expensive, but depending on your family circumstances, geriatric care managers might offer a useful service.

A geriatric care manager is a sort of "professional relative" who can help you and your family to identify needs and find ways to meet your needs. These professionals can also help by leading family discussions about sensitive subjects.

When interviewing a geriatric care manager, you might want to ask:

- Are you a licensed geriatric care manager?

- How long have you been providing care management services?

- Are you available for emergencies around the clock?

- Does your company also provide home care services?

- How will you communicate information to me?

- What are your fees? Will you provide information on fees in writing prior to starting services?

- Can you provide references?

There are organizations that can help you find a care manager near your family member's community. You can also call or write to the Eldercare Locator for recommendations. In some cases, support groups for diseases related to aging may be able to recommend geriatric care managers who have assisted other families.

How Can I Lighten the Load for My Mother?

Over the years, Dad's condition has worsened, and now when we talk, Mom sounds exhausted. Your mother may be hesitant to ask for help or to say that she needs a break. Be sure to acknowledge how important her care has been for your father. Also, discuss the physical and emotional effects caregiving can have on people. Although caregiving can be satisfying, it also can be very hard work. Offer to arrange for respite care.

Respite care will give your mother a break from her caregiving responsibilities. Respite care can be arranged for just an afternoon or for several days. Care can be provided in the family home, or your dad may spend the time in an adult day services program or at a skilled nursing facility.

The ARCH National Respite Locator Service can help you find services in your parent's community. You might suggest your mother contact the Well Spouse Association—it offers support to the wives, husbands, and partners of chronically ill or disabled people and has a nationwide listing of local groups.

Your parents may need more help from home-based care to continue to live in their own home. Some people find it hard to have paid caregivers in the house, but most also say that the assistance is invaluable. If your mother is reluctant, point out that with an in-home aide, she may have more energy to devote to your father's care and some time for herself. Suggest she try it for a short time, and then decide.

In time, your father may have to move to assisted living or a nursing home. If that happens, your mother will need your support. You can help her select a facility. She may need help adjusting to his absence or to living alone in their home. Just listening may not sound like much help, but often it is.

Should I Encourage My Parents to Get More Help?

The last time I visited, my mom seemed very confused, like she just wasn't quite there. Dad didn't seem to notice and didn't want to talk about it when I asked him.

If you do not see your parent often, changes in his or her health may seem dramatic. In contrast, the primary caregiver might not notice such changes or realize that more help, medical treatment, or supervision is needed. Or, the primary caregiver might not want to accept the fact that the health of his or her spouse or parent is failing. Sometimes a geriatric care manager or other professional is the first to notice changes.

For families dealing with Alzheimer disease or another dementia, it can be easier to cover for the patient—doing things for him or her, filling in information in conversations, and so on—than to acknowledge what is happening.

A few good conversation starters are:

- If you thought there might be a change in Aunt Joan's condition, whose opinion would you seek?

- I didn't notice Dad repeating himself so much the last time I was here. Do you remember when it started?

Some changes may not be what you think. Occasional forgetfulness does not necessarily indicate dementia. Before you raise the issue of what needs to be done, talk to your parent and the primary caregiver about your concerns.

Try not to sound critical when you raise the subject. Instead, mention your particular worry, for example, "Mom, it looks like you don't have much food in the house—are you having trouble getting to the store?" and explain why you are asking. Listen to what the primary caregiver says about the situation and whether he or she believes there are problems.

Discuss what you think could be done. For example, you could ask:

- Would you like me to arrange to have groceries delivered on a regular basis?

- Do we need to get a second opinion about the diagnosis?

- Can you follow the medication schedule?

- Would you like some help with housework?

Try to follow your suggestions with practical help, and give specific examples of what you can do. For example, you might arrange to have a personal or home health aide come in once a week. You might schedule doctors' appointments or arrange for transportation.

In some cases, you may have to be forceful, especially if you feel that the situation is unhealthy or unsafe. Do not leave a frail adult at risk. If you have to act against the wishes of your parent or the primary caregiver, be direct and explain what you are going to do. Discuss your plan, and say why you are taking action.

How Can I Help My Parents Decide If It Is Time for Them to Move from Their Home?

My mom is getting frailer, and my dad admits that keeping up with chores around their house is getting to be too much. I'm at a loss about what to do.

The decision about whether your parents should move is often tricky and emotional. Each family will have its own reasons for wanting (or not wanting) to take such a step. One family may decide a move is right because the parents can no longer manage the home. For another family, the need for hands-on care in a long-term care facility motivates a change.

In some cases, a move frees up cash so that the parent can afford a more suitable situation. For others, the desire to move to a safer location is hampered by a lack of funds to cover the cost of the new home.

In the case of long-distance caregivers, the notion of moving can seem like a solution to the problem of not being close enough to help. For some caregivers, moving a sick or aging parent to their own home or community can be a viable alternative. Some families decide to have an adult child move back to the parent's home to become the primary caregiver.

Keep in mind that leaving a home, community, and familiar medical care can be very disruptive and difficult for the older parent, especially if they are not enthusiastic about the change. You might first want to explore what services are available in your parents' community to help them in their home—including home healthcare, housekeeping, personal care, and transportation services.

Check with your parents' friends and doctors, a local social worker, senior centers, and other resources in their area and on the internet for possible sources of help.

Older adults and their families have some options when it comes to deciding where to live, but these choices can be limited by factors such as illness, ability to perform activities of daily living (for example, eating, bathing, using the toilet, dressing, walking, and moving from bed to chair), financial resources, and personal preferences.

Making a decision that is best for your parent—and making that decision with your parent—can be difficult. Try to learn as much as you can about possible housing options.

Older adults, or those with serious illness, can choose to:

- stay in their own home or move to a smaller one

- move to an assisted-living facility

- move to a long-term care facility

- move in with a family member

Some families find a conference call is a good way to talk together about the pros and cons of each option. The goal of this call is to come up with a plan that works for everyone, especially your parent. If the decision involves a move for your mom or dad, you could, even from a distance, offer to arrange tours of some places for their consideration.

Experts advise families to think carefully before moving an aging adult into an adult child's home. There are a lot of questions to consider, for example:

- Is there space in your home?

- Is someone around to help the older person during the whole day?

- What are your parents able to do for themselves?

- What personal care are you willing and able to provide—moving your parent from a chair to a bed or toilet, changing adult diapers, or using a feeding tube, for example?

- What kinds of home care services are available in your community?

- What kind of specialized medical care is available nearby?

How Do We Find a Nursing Home?

If the decision is made that your parent needs the intensive care found in a nursing home (skilled nursing facility), you could talk with his or her doctor or a social worker about which facilities would be appropriate. Once you have the names of several places, the primary caregiver could visit them and meet with staff there. Then, when you have narrowed down the list, you can compare the quality of the remaining homes at Nursing Home Compare on the Medicare website or call Medicare for help.

What Happens If Mom Gets Too Sick to Stay at Home?

My mother is terrified of ending up in an institution and has asked me to promise that I won't "put" her in a nursing home. It's hard for me to figure out what to say.

If you are over 40, chances are you've had a similar conversation with someone you love. It might come up if you see a segment about nursing homes while watching the evening news. "I never want to be in a nursing home," your mother says. This thought usually reflects what most of us want: to stay in our own homes, to maintain independence, to turn to family and friends for help.

Sometimes, however, parents want their adult children to promise that they won't go to a nursing home. Think carefully before doing so. According to the Centers for Medicare and Medicaid Services, "Quality of care means doing the right thing, at the right time, in the right way, for the right person, and having the best possible results."

Agreeing that you will not put someone in a nursing home may close the door to the right care option for your family. It requires you to know that no matter what happens you will be able to care for your parent. The fact is that for some illnesses and for some people, professional healthcare in a long-term care facility is the only reasonable choice.

When faced with a parent who is truly ill or frail, long-distance caregivers may find that some promises hamper their ability to do what is necessary, either for their own health or for their parent's well-being. Many people discover too late that promises they made, such as, "Of course you will be able to die at home," cannot be kept.

Try to focus your commitments on what you know here and now. If asked to make a promise, you could say something like, "Dad, I will make sure you have the best care we can arrange. You can count on me to try and do what's best for everyone. I can't think of a situation where I'd walk out on you."

Base your promises and decisions on a realistic assessment of the current situation or diagnosis, and realize that you might need to revisit your agreement. Your father's condition might change. Your circumstances might change. You truly do not know what will happen in the future—disease and illness can necessitate enormous adjustments. And, of course, it's not only your parent's health that changes—your own health may alter over time.

If you've already made a promise to your parent, remember you can bring the subject up again. You can modify your answer to something more specific, something you feel you can undertake. As hard as that conversation might be, it may be better than risking the guilt of a promise not kept.

Chapter 31

End-of-Life Care for People Who Have Cancer

What Does End-of-Life Care Mean for People Who Have Cancer?

When a cancer patient's healthcare team determines that the cancer can no longer be controlled, medical testing and cancer treatment often stop. But the person's care continues, with an emphasis on improving their quality of life and that of their loved ones, and making them comfortable for the following weeks or months.

Medicines and treatments people receive at the end of life can control pain and other symptoms, such as constipation, nausea, and shortness of breath. Some people remain at home while receiving these treatments, whereas others enter a hospital or other facility. Either way, services are available to help patients and their families with the medical, psychological, social, and spiritual issues around dying. Hospice programs are the most comprehensive and coordinated providers of these services.

The period at the end of life is different for each person. The signs and symptoms people have vary as their illness continues, and each person has unique needs for information and support. Questions and

This chapter includes text excerpted from "End-of-Life Care for People Who Have Cancer," National Cancer Institute (NCI), May 10, 2012. Reviewed October 2016.

concerns that family members have about the end of life should be discussed with each other, as well as with the healthcare team, as they arise.

Communication about end-of-life care and decision making during the final months of a person's life are very important. Research has shown that if a person who has advanced cancer discusses his or her options for care with a doctor early on, that person's level of stress decreases and their ability to cope with illness increases. Studies also show that patients prefer an open and honest conversation with their doctor about choices for end-of-life care early in the course of their disease, and arc more satisfied when they have this talk.

Experts strongly encourage patients to complete advance directives, which are documents stating a person's wishes for care. They also designate who the patient chooses as the decision-maker for their care when they are unable to decide. It's important for people with cancer to have these decisions made before they become too sick to make them. However, if a person does become too sick before they have completed an advance directive, it's helpful for family caregivers to know what type of care their loved one would want to receive.

How Do Doctors Know How Long a Person Will Continue to Live?

Patients and their family members often want to know how long a person who has cancer will continue to live. It's normal to want to be prepared for the future. But predicting how long someone will continue to live is a hard question to answer. A number of factors, including the type of cancer, its location, and whether the patient has other illnesses, can affect what will happen.

Although doctors may be able to estimate the amount of time someone will continue to live based on what they know about that person, they might be hesitant to do so. They may be concerned about over- or under-estimating the person's remaining life span. They also might be fearful of giving false hope or destroying a person's will to live.

When Should Someone Call for Professional Help If They're Caring for a Person Who Has Cancer at Home?

People caring for patients at home should ask them if they're comfortable, if they feel any pain, and if they're having any other physical problems.

There may be times when the caregiver needs assistance from the patient's healthcare team. A caregiver can contact the patient's doctor or nurse for help in any of the following situations:

- The patient is in pain that is not relieved by the prescribed dose of pain medication.

- The patient is experiencing onset of new symptoms, such as nausea, vomiting, increasing confusion, anxiety or restlessness.

- The patient is experiencing symptoms that were previously well controlled.

- The patient shows discomfort, such as by grimacing or moaning.

- The patient is having trouble breathing and seems upset.

- The patient is unable to urinate or empty the bowels.

- The patient has fallen.

- The patient is very depressed or talking about committing suicide.

- The caregiver has difficulty giving medicines to the patient.

- The caregiver is overwhelmed by caring for the patient, is too sad, or is afraid to be with the patient.

- The caregiver doesn't know how to handle a certain situation.

Keep in mind that palliative care experts can be called upon by the patient's physician at any point in the person's illness to help with these issues. They are increasingly available not only in the hospital, but also in the outpatient setting.

When Is the Right Time to Use Hospice Care?

Many people believe that hospice care is only appropriate in the last days or weeks of life. Yet Medicare states that it can be used as much as 6 months before death is anticipated. And those who have lost loved ones say that they wish they had called in hospice care sooner.

Research has shown that patients and families who use hospice services report a higher quality of life than those who don't. Hospice care offers many helpful services, including medical care, counseling, and respite care. People usually qualify for hospice when their doctor signs a statement saying that patients with their type and stage of disease, on average, aren't likely to survive beyond 6 months.

What Are Some Ways to Provide Emotional Support to a Person Who Is Living with and Dying of Cancer?

Everyone has different needs, but some worries are common to most dying patients. Two of these concerns are fear of abandonment and fear of being a burden. People who are dying also have concerns about loss of dignity and loss of control. Some ways caregivers can provide comfort to a person with these worries are listed below:

- Keep the person company. Talk, watch movies, read, or just be with him or her.

- Allow the person to express fears and concerns about dying, such as leaving family and friends behind. Be prepared to listen.

- Be willing to reminisce about the person's life.

- Avoid withholding difficult information. Most patients prefer to be included in discussions about issues that concern them.

- Reassure the patient that you will honor advance directives, such as living wills.

- Ask if there is anything you can do.

- Respect the person's need for privacy.

- Support the person's spirituality. Let them talk about what has meaning for them, pray with them if they'd like, and arrange visits by spiritual leaders and church members, if appropriate. Keep objects that are meaningful to the person close at hand.

What Other Issues Should Caregivers Be Aware Of?

It's just as important for caregivers to take care of their own health at this time. Family caregivers are affected by their loved one's health more than they realize. Taking care of a sick person often causes physical and emotional fatigue, stress, depression, and anxiety. Because of this, it's important for caregivers to take care of their own body, mind, and spirit. Helping themselves will give them more energy, help them cope with stress, and cause them to be better caregivers as a result.

It's also helpful if caregivers ask for support from friends and family members. Such help is important to help lessen the many tasks involved in taking care of a loved one who is sick or dying.

What Are Some Topics Patients and Family Members Can Talk About?

For many people, it's hard to know what to say to someone at the end of life. It's normal to want to be upbeat and positive, rather than talk about death. And yet, it's important to be realistic about how sick the person may be. Caregivers can encourage their loved one without giving false hope. Although it can be a time for grieving and accepting loss, the end of life can also be a time for looking for meaning and rethinking what's important.

During this period, many people tend to look back and reflect on life, legacies created, and loved ones who will be left behind. Some questions to explore with a patient at the end of life are the following:

- What are the happiest and saddest times we have shared together?
- What are the defining or most important moments of our life together?
- What are we most proud of?
- What have we taught each other?

Patients with serious, life-threatening illness have stated that being positive or adding humor remains an important outlet for them. Even at this challenging moment, laughter may still be the best medicine.

How Should Caregivers Talk to Their Children about Advanced Cancer?

Children deserve to be told the truth about a family member's prognosis so they can be prepared if their loved one dies. It's important to answer all of their questions gently and honestly so they don't imagine things that are worse than reality. They need to be reassured that they will be taken care of no matter what happens.

Caregivers need to be prepared to answer tough questions. To do this, they should know what their own feelings and thoughts are about the situation. They need to be able to show children how to hope for the best while preparing for and accepting that their loved one may die.

How Does Cancer Cause Death?

Every patient is different, and the way cancer causes death varies. The process can depend on the type of cancer, where it is in the body, and how fast it's growing.

For some people, the cancer can't be controlled anymore and spreads to healthy tissues and organs. Cancer cells take up the needed space and nutrients that the healthy organs would use. As a result, the healthy organs can no longer function. For other people, complications from treatment can cause death.

During the final stages of cancer, problems may occur in several parts of the body.

- **Digestive system:** If cancer is in the digestive system (e.g., stomach, pancreas, or colon), food or waste may not be able to pass through, causing bloating, nausea, or vomiting. If the cancer prevents food from being digested or absorbed, patients can also become malnourished.

- **Lungs:** If too little healthy lung tissue is left, or if cancer blocks off part of the lung, the person may have trouble breathing and getting enough oxygen. Or, if the lung collapses, it may become infected, which may be too hard for someone with advanced cancer to fight.

- **Bones:** If cancer is in the bones, too much calcium may go into the bloodstream, which can cause unconsciousness and death. Bones with tumors may also break and not heal.

- **Liver:** The liver removes toxins from the blood, helps digest food, and converts food into substances needed to live. If there isn't enough healthy liver tissue, the body's chemical balance is upset. The person may eventually go into a coma.

- **Bone marrow:** When cancer is in the bone marrow, the body can't make enough healthy blood cells. A lack of red blood cells will cause anemia, and the body won't have enough oxygen in the blood. A low white blood cell count will make it hard to fight infection. And a drop in platelets will prevent the blood from clotting, making it hard to control abnormal bleeding.

- **Brain:** A large tumor in the brain may cause memory problems, balance problems, bleeding in the brain, or loss of function in another body part, which may eventually lead to a coma.

In some cases, the exact cause can't be pinpointed and patients simply decline slowly, becoming weaker and weaker until they succumb to the cancer. Again, every patient is different and all processes have different stages and rates in which they advance. And some conditions have treatments that can help slow the process or make the patient more comfortable. It's very important to keep having conversations with the patient's healthcare team.

What Are the Signs That Death Is Approaching, and What Can the Caregiver Do to Make the Person Comfortable during This Time?

Certain signs and symptoms can help a caregiver anticipate when death is near. They are described below, along with suggestions for managing them. However, each person's experience at the end of life is different. What may happen to one person may not happen for another. Also, the presence of one or more of these symptoms doesn't necessarily mean that the patient is close to death. A member of the healthcare team can give family members and caregivers more information about what to expect.

Withdrawal from friends and family:

- People often focus inward during the last weeks of life. This doesn't necessarily mean that patients are angry or depressed or that they don't love their caregivers. It could be caused by decreased oxygen to the brain, decreased blood flow, and/or mental preparation for dying.

- They may lose interest in things they used to enjoy, such as favorite TV shows, friends, or pets.

- Caregivers can let the patient know they are there for support. The person may be aware and able to hear, even if they are unable to respond. Experts advise that giving them permission to "let go" may be helpful. If they do feel like talking, they may want to reminisce about joys and sorrows, or tie up loose ends.

Sleep changes:

- People may have drowsiness, increased sleep, intermittent sleep, or confusion when they first wake up.

- Worries or concerns may keep patients up at night. Caregivers can ask them if they would like to sit in the room with them while they fall asleep.

- Patients may sleep more and more as time passes. Caregivers should continue to talk to them, even if they're unconscious, for the patient may still hear them.

Hard-to-control pain:

- It may become harder to control pain as the cancer gets worse. It's important to provide pain medication regularly. Caregivers should ask to see a palliative care doctor or a pain specialist for advice on the correct medicines and doses. It may be helpful to explore other pain control methods such as massage and relaxation techniques.

Increasing weakness:

- Weakness and fatigue will increase over time. The patient may have good days and bad days, so they may need more help with daily personal care and getting around.

- Caregivers can help patients save energy for the things that are most important to them.

Appetite changes:

- As the body naturally shuts down, the person with cancer will often need and want less food. The loss of appetite is caused by the body's need to conserve energy and its decreasing ability to use food and fluids properly.

- Patients should be allowed to choose whether and when to eat or drink. Caregivers can offer small amounts of the foods the patient enjoys. Since chewing takes energy, they may prefer milkshakes, ice cream, or pudding. If the patient doesn't have trouble with swallowing, offer sips of fluids and use a flexible straw if they can't sit up. If a person can no longer swallow, offer ice chips. Keep their lips moist with lip balm and their mouth clean with a soft, damp cloth.

Awareness:

- Near the end of life, people often have episodes of confusion or waking dreams. They may get confused about time, place, and the identity of loved ones. Caregivers can gently remind patients where they are and who is with them. They should be calm and reassuring. But if the patient is agitated, they should not attempt to restrain them. Let the healthcare providers know if significant agitation occurs, as there are treatments available to help control or reverse it.

- Sometimes patients report seeing or speaking with loved ones who have died. They may talk about going on a trip, seeing lights, butterflies, or other symbols of reality we can't see. As long as these things aren't disturbing to the patient, caregivers can ask them to say more. They can let them share their visions and dreams, not trying to talk them out of what they believe they see.

The dying process:

- There may be a loss of bladder or bowel control due to the muscles relaxing in the pelvis. Caregivers should continue to provide clean, dry bedding and gentle personal care. They can place disposable pads on the bed under the patient and remove them when soiled. Also, due to a slowing of kidney function and/or decreased fluid intake, there may be a decrease in the amount of urine. It may be dark and smell strong.

- Breathing patterns may become slower or faster, in cycles. The patient may not notice, but caregivers should let the doctor know if they are worried about the changes. There may be rattling or gurgling sounds that are caused by saliva and fluids collecting in the throat and upper airways. Although this can be very disturbing for caregivers, at this stage the patient is generally not experiencing any distress. Breathing may be easier if a person's body is turned to the side and pillows are placed behind the back and beneath the head. Caregivers can also ask the healthcare team about using a humidifier or external source of oxygen to make it easier for the patient to breathe, if the patient is short of breath.

- Skin may become bluish in color and feel cool as blood flow slows down. This is not painful or uncomfortable for the patient. Caregivers should avoid warming the patient with electric blankets or heating pads, which can cause burns. However, they may keep the patient covered with a light blanket.

What Are the Signs That the Person Has Died?

- The person is no longer breathing and doesn't have a pulse.

- Their eyes don't move or blink, and the pupils are dilated (enlarged). The eyelids may be slightly open.

- The jaw is relaxed and the mouth is slightly open.

- The body releases the bowel and bladder contents.

- The person doesn't respond to being touched or spoken to.

- The person's skin is very pale and cool to the touch.

What Needs to Be Done after the Person Has Died?

After the person has died, there is no need to hurry with arrangements. Family members and caregivers may wish to sit with the body, to talk, or to pray. When the family is ready, the following steps can be taken.

- Place the body on its back with one pillow under the head. If necessary, caregivers or family members may wish to put the person's dentures or other artificial parts in place.

- If the person is in a hospice program, follow the guidelines provided by the program. A caregiver or family member can request a hospice nurse to verify the death.

- Contact the appropriate authorities in accordance with local regulations. Contact the person's doctor and funeral home.

- When the patient's family members are ready, call other family members, friends, and clergy.

- Provide or obtain emotional support for family members and friends to cope with their loss.

Chapter 32

Information for Caregivers

Chapter Contents

Section 32.1

Self-Care Tips for Caregivers

This section includes text excerpted from "Module 1: Caregiver Self Care," U.S. Department of Veterans Affairs (VA), March 2013.

Your Role as Family Caregiver

In this section, we will focus on the importance of your role as a Family Caregiver and what you can do for yourself to keep life fulfilling and happy for you and your family. We know that caregiving does not occur in a vacuum. In addition to being the Family Caregiver of a Veteran, you may also look out for other family members, parents, siblings, in-laws and children. And, you may have a job, too.

We will share with you information about steps you can take to keep yourself physically and emotionally healthy. We also will offer you some tips related to your roles in meeting your family's needs and in the workplace. A theme to remember: resources exist all around you that can be of help to you and the Veteran you care for.

Over the past decade there has been more attention to the important role that Family Caregivers play in the lives of both Veterans and non-Veterans. We have learned a lot about what helps a Caregiver carry on this valuable role and how Caregivers themselves need support.

Staying Healthy

Why Is Your Health So Important?

Being a Caregiver requires stamina and good health. The journey is more of a marathon than a sprint and you need to be in the best condition you can be. Taking care of you is essential to your own well-being, and is crucial for the Veteran's health and comfort. Because caregiving can be very demanding, Caregivers often don't exercise enough, don't eat a healthy diet, or delay seeking healthcare for themselves. Yet the demands of caregiving are precisely why a healthy lifestyle is so important. If you are in good physical and mental health, you will be able to handle the challenges that present each day and provide the best care possible to the Veteran. If you ignore your own health, you risk becoming ill. Maintaining your own health is an investment that will pay off for your whole family.

Key Points to Staying Healthy

In this section we will take a closer look at the following actions you can take now to "take care of you:"

- Eat well

- Be physically active

- Prevent back injury

- Sleep enough

- Get preventive health services

Eating Well

Nutrition affects physical and emotional health. Proper diet helps protect the Caregiver from stress, while poor nutrition can lead to lower immunity and disease. Poor nutrition leads to fatigue, illness and disease. Small changes in diet can have benefits for health and wellbeing. You may be asking yourself, "With a very busy schedule, how can I eat well?" Or, "Where do I find the time to cook a proper meal?" Planning menus and making shopping lists ahead of time helps a lot. It makes grocery shopping quicker and preparation time shorter. Look for tasty, easy to prepare meals. When you cook, make extra and freeze portions to use later.

Nutrition Basics

Understanding the basics of good nutrition will help you navigate through the overwhelming amount of information about what you should and shouldn't eat. The information below will help you in making good choices.

Salt

Nearly all Americans consume more salt than is recommended. Since sodium added during the processing of foods provides more than three-fourths of total intake, it's important to read the sodium content on the food label on the back of the product when you are grocery shopping. Decreasing salt (sodium chloride) intake is advisable to reduce the risk of high blood pressure. The general goal is for adults to aim to consume less than 2,300 milligrams of sodium per day (about one teaspoon of salt). Intake should be reduced to 1500 milligrams for persons age 51 and older, and those of any age who are African American or have hypertension, diabetes or chronic kidney disease. This applies to about half of the U.S. population, including children and the majority of adults.

Saturated Fat

Saturated fats come from animal products such as meat, dairy products, and from coconut oil, palm/palm kernel oil and hydrogenated and partially hydrogenated oils. Some products that may be made with these oils are: fried chicken and fish, cakes, pies and cookies. In general, saturated fats are solid at room temperature. Saturated fats can raise blood cholesterol levels which are linked to higher risks of heart disease and stroke. Replace saturated fats in your diet with monounsaturated and polyunsaturated fats. Also try to consume less than 300mg of dietary cholesterol each day.

Carbohydrates

Reducing intake of added sugars (especially sugar sweetened beverages) may be helpful in weight control and balancing overall nutrition. A combined approach of reducing the intake of sugar and baked goods made with white flour will actually reduce your appetite, allowing for better weight control.

Whole Grains

The goal is to eat at least three servings per day of whole grains, preferably by replacing foods with refined grains (e.g., white flour) with foods made with whole grains.

Fruits, Vegetables, Dairy, and Protein

Table 32.1. Fruits, Vegetables, Dairy, and Protein

Fruits/Vegetables	To meet your need for vitamins and minerals a range of 5–13 servings of fruits and vegetables each day is recommended.

Table 32.1. Continued

Dairy	Most people need 2 to 3 cups of non-fat or low-fat milk, cheese, or yogurt each day.
Protein	Choose lean meat, poultry without skin, fish and dry beans and peas. Often, they are the choices lowest in fat. The suggested serving is 2–3 proteins per day.

Maintain a Balanced Diet

Here are some nutritional tips from ChooseMyPlate.gov to help you maintain a balanced diet.

Balance Calories:

- enjoy food but eat less,
- avoid oversized portions

Foods to Increase:

- make half your plate fruits and vegetables,
- make at least half your grains whole grains,
- switch to fat-free or low-fat (1%) milk

Foods to Reduce:

- compare sodium in foods like soup, bread and frozen meals
- choose foods with lowest amount of sodium
- drink water instead of sugary drinks.

Nutrition Tips

Try to stock up on healthy snacks and try not to purchase unhealthy ones. If you usually eat on the run, have fresh fruits, vegetables and proteins (like cheese wedges, roasted unsalted nuts or meat slices) ready in your kitchen to grab and go.

If you have five minutes, it really helps to wash and chop some healthy vegetables ahead of time, and then they'll be ready for you for a snack or when it's time to cook.

With everything you have to do, you may find yourself rushing through meals. This can cause overeating, because your brain doesn't get the chance to register the fact that your stomach is full. By slowing down and taking time to savor your food, you can reduce the risk of overeating and enhance your physical and emotional health.

Water

Water is a wonderful drink whenever you are thirsty. Bodies, particularly when stressed (as Caregivers' bodies often are), require water. Water cleanses, refreshes and also cuts down on the urge to indulge in mindless snacking or overeating for comfort. If you find yourself eating too much at a meal, drinking a full glass of water before the meal may work for you. This helps your brain register that your stomach is getting full. It will help you feel full with normal portions.

A Few More Tips

- Eat multiple small meals throughout the day, rather than three large meals.

- Don't skip meals.

- If you aren't sure you are eating properly, keep a journal and review this with your healthcare professional.

Physical Activity—Move Around!

You don't have to go to a gym to get the benefits of physical activity. The benefits of physical activity include: reduced stress, increased alertness, better sleep and more energy. Any way you move counts! You can choose activities that are appealing and meaningful to you such as:

- Stepping outside to do a little gardening.

- Taking a brisk walk around the block.

- Exercising to a DVD or video at home when you have time.

- Doing everyday chores has a health benefit.

- Listening to music while doing chores can help.

Walking

Walking is particularly good. It provides both exercise and relaxation; can be done almost anywhere; for any length of time. One way to increase the amount of walking in your day is to walk rather than drive short distances, or to park at the far end of the parking lot. Taking the stairs rather than the elevator is another good idea.

Exercise

- Five minutes of activity several times a day adds up to a good plan for obtaining moderate exercise.

- Moderate exercise improves blood flow, enhances energy and diminishes risk for disease and injury.

- Try to walk a total of 20 minutes a day, three days a week to start, and build up to 30 minutes, five days a week.

Protecting Your Back

Giving physical care increases the risk of getting a back injury. Lifting or helping a person shift from one place to another or moving a heavy or awkward object can seriously strain the back. The good news is that using back-protecting skills works.

The key is planning the lift. It's good to take these steps before starting:

1. Think through the whole move—plot it out.

2. Size up whether moving the object or person is truly manageable—if you can't comfortably handle the lift, you shouldn't do it.

3. Identify any obstacles in your way and remove them.

4. Bend your knees and lift with your legs, not your back.

5. Keep the object balanced as you lift.

Getting a Good Night's Sleep

As a Family Caregiver, you may be sacrificing your own sleep needs for the needs of your family, including caring for the Veteran. Lack of sleep can make you less alert, impair your productivity and ability to pay attention, reduce your ability to remember new information and slow your reaction times.

Experts say we need to make sleep a priority and put it on our "to do" lists like any other important task. Sleep is not what you do when everything else is done, rather it is essential and means leaving some things undone. Too little sleep is linked to:

- Car accidents.

- Obesity due to an increased appetite caused by sleep deprivation.

- Diabetes and heart problems.

- Depression.

Tips for Better Sleep

To open the door to better sleep, sleep specialists recommend having consistent sleep and-wake schedules, even on weekends, and offer the following tips:

- An hour or so before you expect to fall asleep, enjoy a regular, relaxing bedtime routine such as soaking in a hot bath or listening to soothing music.

- Submersing in warm water, or allowing it to flow over your body, is a known relaxant.

- Taking a bath or shower before bed prepares the mind and body for deep sleep.

- Create a sleep-friendly environment?a place that's dark, quiet and cool with a comfortable mattress and pillows.

- Using meditation or relaxation recordings helps some people sleep.

- White noise machines, or recordings of nature sounds, like the ocean, also can help.

Exercise and Sleep

Exercise regularly during the day. While exercising regularly will help you to sleep, it's usually best not to exercise close to bedtime, as this may keep you awake.

Bedtime Snacks and Sleep

It's generally best to finish eating a few hours before going to bed.

- Some people find that eating a small bedtime snack of sleep-promoting foods helps such as carbohydrates (like bananas or toast) or food containing tryptophan (like turkey or milk) is helpful.

- Foods containing caffeine, such as coffee or chocolate, can keep you awake if you have them within a few hours of bedtime.

Your Emotional Health

Why Emotional Health Is Important

When challenging things happen, emotional health lets you bounce back and move on. Most of us take emotional and mental health for granted and only focus on it when problems occur. But like physical health, it requires attention to build and maintain.

A Caregiver's emotional health is very important. Chronic stress that doesn't go away can lead to health problems. There are many different tools that can help you achieve balance in your life, with time to relax, enjoy relationships, work and have fun.

Let's talk about things Caregivers can do to maintain their emotional health. First, ask for help. Reach out to social contacts. Get some respite from the day-to-day stress and seek out support groups.

Ask For Help

Sometimes Caregivers have a difficult time saying they need help. They're expected to be, or expect themselves to be, the strong ones, taking care of others' needs. But one of the best things a Caregiver can do to maintain emotional health is to ask for help.

There's no shame in letting others know that you need assistance. A great place to start is in your faith community, your neighborhood or social groups where you already have a connection to others. Support might come in the form of direct help with care, or assistance with meals or chores around the house. Having supportive people in one's life can make all the difference in an emergency.

Reach Out to Social Contacts

A five-minute break to touch base with a compassionate friend, relative or neighbor, even by phone, or e-mail can lift your spirits.

Caregiving can feel lonely and isolating. Keeping up social contacts helps a lot in staying well. Hearing the sound of others' voices, reading their supportive words, or sharing thoughts with a kindred spirit requires only a short time in a busy caregiving day. Yet, this regular contact maintains your social support network.

Get Some Respite

Respite means having someone stand in for you so that you can take a break. Stepping away from caregiving for an hour or two, a full day or a week can help to relieve stress and restore your sense of well-being, when you know that the Veteran is in good hands during your absence.

The U.S. Department of Veterans Affairs (VA) provides enhanced respite support for Veterans and their primary Caregivers enrolled in the new Caregiver program as part of the Program of Comprehensive Assistance for Family Caregivers. VA respite options include:

- In-home respite, when someone comes into your home to provide caregiving for the Veteran while you are away.

- Adult day programs, where the Veteran can participate in a full day of programs and socialize.

- Out-of-home respite at the VA Medical Center (VAMC), VA Community Living Centers, or assisted living communities and community nursing homes.

Seek Out Support Groups

Your local VA Medical Center, churches, non-profit groups, community hospitals and other healthcare providers offer support groups specifically for Caregivers. Support groups are safe havens for exploring and expressing grief, fear, guilt, anger and loss, joys and sharing coping skills. They are also great places to exchange caregiving resources. A social worker or other professional often leads the group. Individual psychological counseling provides crucial support for some Caregivers. Many Caregivers find the combination of attending a support group and getting private counseling helps a lot in managing stress. In the Program of Comprehensive Assistance, primary and secondary Family Caregivers will be eligible to participate in individual and group therapy, counseling and peer support groups offered at the VA Medical Center. The counseling provided for the Family Caregiver is independent and not connected to the Veteran's care.

Section 32.2

Coping with Caregiving

This section includes text excerpted from "Coping
with Caregiving," *NIH News in Health*, National
Institutes of Health (NIH), December 2015.

It can be a labor of love, and sometimes a job of necessity. A total of
about 43 million U.S. adults provide unpaid care for someone with a
serious health condition each year. These often-unsung heroes provide
hours of assistance to others. Yet the stress and strain of caregiving
can take a toll on their own health. NIH-funded (National Institutes of
Health) researchers are working to understand the risks these caregivers face. And scientists are seeking better ways to protect caregivers'
health.

Many of us will end up becoming a caregiver at some point in our
lives. Chances are we'll be helping out older family members who can't
fully care for themselves. Such caregiving can include everyday tasks,
such as helping with meals, schedules, and bathing and dressing. It
can also include managing medicines, doctor visits, health insurance,
and money. Caregivers often give emotional support as well.

People who provide unpaid care for an elderly, ill, or disabled family
member or friend in the home are called informal caregivers. Most are
middle-aged. Roughly two-thirds are women. Nearly half of informal
caregivers assist someone who's age 75 or older. As the elderly population continues to grow nationwide, so will the need for informal
caregivers.

Studies have shown that some people can thrive when caring for
others. Caregiving may help to strengthen connections to a loved one.
Some find joy or fulfillment in looking after others. But for many,
the strain of caregiving can become overwhelming. Friends and family often take on the caregiving role without any training. They're
expected to meet many complex demands without much help. Most
care-givers hold down a full-time job in addition to the hours of unpaid
help they give to someone else.

"With all of its rewards, there is a substantial cost to caregiving—
financially, physically, and emotionally," says Dr. Richard J. Hodes,

director of National Institutes of Health's (NIH) National Institute on Aging. "One important insight from our research is that because of the stress and time demands placed on caregivers, they are less likely to find time to address their own health problems."

Informal caregivers, for example, may be less likely to fill a needed prescription for themselves or get a screening test for breast cancer. "Caregivers also tend to report lower levels of physical activity, poorer nutrition, and poorer sleep or sleep disturbance," says Dr. Erin Kent, an NIH expert on cancer caregiving.

Studies have linked informal caregiving to a variety of long-term health problems. Caregivers are more likely to have heart disease, cancer, diabetes, arthritis, and excess weight. Caregivers are also at risk for depression or anxiety. And they're more likely to have problems with memory and paying attention.

"Caregivers may even suffer from physical health problems related to caregiving tasks, such as back or muscle injuries from lifting patients," Kent adds.

Caregivers may face different challenges and risks depending on the health of the person they're caring for. Taking care of loved ones with cancer or dementia can be especially demanding. Research suggests that these caregivers bear greater levels of physical and mental burdens than caregivers of the frail elderly or people with diabetes.

"Cancer caregivers often spend more hours per day providing more intensive care over a shorter period of time," Kent says. "The health of cancer patients can deteriorate quickly, which can cause heightened stress for caregivers. And aggressive cancer treatments can leave patients greatly weakened. They may need extra care, and their medications may need to be monitored more often."

Cancer survivorship, too, can bring intense levels of uncertainty and anxiety. "A hallmark of cancer is that it may return months or even years later," Kent says. "Both cancer survivors and their caregivers may struggle to live with ongoing fear and stress of a cancer recurrence."

Dementia can also create unique challenges to caregivers. The healthcare costs alone can take an enormous toll. One recent study found that out-of-pocket spending for families of dementia patients during the last 5 years of life averaged $61,522, which was 81% higher than for older people who died from other causes.

Research has found that caregivers for people with dementia have particularly high levels of potentially harmful stress hormones. Caregivers and care recipients often struggle with the problems related to dementia, such as agitation, aggression, trouble sleeping, wandering, and confusion. These caregivers spend more days sick with an infectious disease, have a weaker immune response to the flu vaccine, and have slower wound healing.

One major successful and expanding effort to help ease caregiver stress is known as REACH (Resources for Enhancing Alzheimer's Caregiver Health). Nearly a decade ago, NIH-funded (National Institutes of Health) researchers showed that a supportive, educational program for dementia caregivers could greatly improve their quality of life and reduce rates of clinical depression. As part of the program, trained staff connected with caregivers over 6 months by making several home visits, telephone calls, and structured telephone support sessions.

"REACH showed that what caregivers need is support. They need to know that there are people out there and resources available to help them," says Dr. John Haaga, who oversees NIH's behavioral and social research related to aging.

The REACH program is now being more widely employed. It's been adapted for use in free community-based programs, such as in local Area Agencies on Aging (AAA). It's also being used by the U.S. Department of Veterans Affairs (VA) and by the Indian Health Service (IHS), in collaboration with the Administration for Community Living.

"We know how to support families caring for an older adult. But that knowledge is not easily accessible to the families who need it," says Dr. Laura Gitlin, a coauthor of the REACH study and an expert on caregiving and aging at Johns Hopkins University. "Caregivers need to know it's not only acceptable, but recommended, that they find time to care for themselves. They should consider joining a caregiver's support group, taking breaks each day, and keeping up with their own hobbies and interests."

Chapter 33

The Dying Process

What Are the Signs That Death Is Approaching, and What Can the Caregiver Do to Make the Person Comfortable during This Time?

Certain signs and symptoms can help a caregiver anticipate when death is near. They are described below, along with suggestions for managing them. However, each person's experience at the end of life is different. What may happen to one person may not happen for another.

Also, the presence of one or more of these symptoms doesn't necessarily mean that the patient is close to death. A member of the healthcare team can give family members and caregivers more information about what to expect.

Withdrawal from friends and family:

- People often focus inward during the last weeks of life. This doesn't necessarily mean that patients are angry or depressed or that they don't love their caregivers. It could be caused by decreased oxygen to the brain, decreased blood flow, and/or mental preparation for dying.

- They may lose interest in things they used to enjoy, such as favorite TV shows, friends, or pets.

This chapter includes text excerpted from "End-of-Life Care for People Who Have Cancer," National Cancer Institute (NCI), May 10, 2012. Reviewed October 2016.

- Caregivers can let the patient know they are there for support. The person may be aware and able to hear, even if they are unable to respond. Experts advise that giving them permission to "let go" may be helpful. If they do feel like talking, they may want to reminisce about joys and sorrows, or tie up loose ends.

Sleep changes:

- People may have drowsiness, increased sleep, intermittent sleep, or confusion when they first wake up.

- Worries or concerns may keep patients up at night. Caregivers can ask them if they would like to sit in the room with them while they fall asleep.

- Patients may sleep more and more as time passes. Caregivers should continue to talk to them, even if they're unconscious, for the patient may still hear them.

Hard-to-control pain:

- It may become harder to control pain as the cancer gets worse. It's important to provide pain medication regularly. Caregivers should ask to see a palliative care doctor or a pain specialist for advice on the correct medicines and doses. It may be helpful to explore other pain control methods such as massage and relaxation techniques.

Increasing weakness:

- Weakness and fatigue will increase over time. The patient may have good days and bad days, so they may need more help with daily personal care and getting around.

- Caregivers can help patients save energy for the things that are most important to them.

Appetite changes:

- As the body naturally shuts down, the person with cancer will often need and want less food. The loss of appetite is caused by the body's need to conserve energy and its decreasing ability to use food and fluids properly.

- Patients should be allowed to choose whether and when to eat or drink. Caregivers can offer small amounts of the foods the patient enjoys. Since chewing takes energy, they may prefer milkshakes, ice cream, or pudding. If the patient doesn't have trouble with swallowing, offer sips of fluids and use a flexible straw if they can't sit up. If a person can no longer swallow, offer ice chips. Keep their lips moist with lip balm and their mouth clean with a soft, damp cloth.

Awareness:

- Near the end of life, people often have episodes of confusion or waking dreams. They may get confused about time, place, and the identity of loved ones. Caregivers can gently remind patients where they are and who is with them. They should be calm and reassuring. But if the patient is agitated, they should not attempt to restrain them. Let the healthcare providers know if significant agitation occurs, as there are treatments available to help control or reverse it.

- Sometimes patients report seeing or speaking with loved ones who have died. They may talk about going on a trip, seeing lights, butterflies, or other symbols of reality we can't see. As long as these things aren't disturbing to the patient, caregivers can ask them to say more. They can let them share their visions and dreams, not trying to talk them out of what they believe they see.

The dying process:

- There may be a loss of bladder or bowel control due to the muscles relaxing in the pelvis. Caregivers should continue to provide clean, dry bedding and gentle personal care. They can place disposable pads on the bed under the patient and remove them when soiled. Also, due to a slowing of kidney function and/or decreased fluid intake, there may be a decrease in the amount of urine. It may be dark and smell strong.

- Breathing patterns may become slower or faster, in cycles. The patient may not notice, but caregivers should let the doctor know if they are worried about the changes. There may be rattling or gurgling sounds that are caused by saliva and fluids collecting in the throat and upper airways. Although this can be very disturbing for caregivers, at this stage the patient is generally not experiencing any distress. Breathing may be easier if a person's body is turned to the side and pillows are placed behind the back and beneath the head. Caregivers can also ask the healthcare team about using a humidifier or external source of oxygen to make it easier for the patient to breathe, if the patient is short of breath.

- Skin may become bluish in color and feel cool as blood flow slows down. This is not painful or uncomfortable for the patient. Caregivers should avoid warming the patient with electric blankets or heating pads, which can cause burns. However, they may keep the patient covered with a light blanket.

What Are the Signs That the Person Has Died?

- The person is no longer breathing and doesn't have a pulse.
- Their eyes don't move or blink, and the pupils are dilated (enlarged).
- The eyelids may be slightly open.
- The jaw is relaxed and the mouth is slightly open.
- The body releases the bowel and bladder contents
- The person doesn't respond to being touched or spoken to.
- The person's skin is very pale and cool to the touch.

What Needs to Be Done after the Person Has Died?

After the person has died, there is no need to hurry with arrangements. Family members and caregivers may wish to sit with the body, to talk, or to pray. When the family is ready, the following steps can be taken.

- Place the body on its back with one pillow under the head. If necessary, caregivers or family members may wish to put the person's dentures or other artificial parts in place.

- If the person is in a hospice program, follow the guidelines provided by the program. A caregiver or family member can request a hospice nurse to verify the death.

- Contact the appropriate authorities in accordance with local regulations. Contact the person's doctor and funeral home.

- When the patient's family members are ready, call other family members, friends, and clergy.

- Provide or obtain emotional support for family members and friends to cope with their loss.

Chapter 34

What to Do When Death Occurs

Death Is Unique

Just as every life is unique, so is each death—it can happen suddenly, or a person may become increasingly frail and slowly slip away. Listen closely to what a dying person's healthcare provider says. He or she may not come right out and say your loved one is close to death. You may have to ask if the end is near, and the provider can only give you a best estimate of how much time is left.

Common Signs of Death

The following are some common experiences that may mean the end is very near.

- shortness of breath (known as dyspnea)
- depression
- anxiety
- tiredness and sleepiness
- mental confusion
- constipation or incontinence

This chapter includes text excerpted from "End of Life," NIHSeniorHealth, National Institute on Aging (NIA), March 2014.

- nausea

- refusal to eat or drink

- parts of the body (hands, arms, feet, legs) becoming cool to the touch and/or darker or blue-colored

Each of these signs, taken alone, does not mean someone is dying. But when many are experienced by someone with a serious illness or declining health, it suggests a person is nearing the end of life.

As Death Approaches

It is common for breathing and heart rate to slow near the end. In fact, there may be times when the person doesn't breathe for many seconds, known as Cheyne-Strokes breathing. Some people hear a "death rattle" or noisy breathing that makes a gurgling or rattling sound. Finally, the chest stops moving, no air comes out of the nose, and there is no pulse. Eyes that are open can seem glassy.

After Death Occurs

After death, there may still be a few shudders or movements of the arms or legs. There could even be an uncontrolled cry because of muscle movements in the voice box. Sometimes there will be a release of urine or stool, but usually only a small amount since so little has probably been eaten in the last days of life.

If the person has an implantable cardioverter defibrillator (ICD) and it has not been deactivated, it may continue to deliver shocks that cause the body to jump slightly. If this occurs, you don't need to do anything, the ICD will stop on its own.

Note: If you are caring for a dying person at home, you may wish to check with your state concerning the need for a "non-hospital DNR." In many states, emergency medical technicians (EMTs) are legally required to perform Cardiopulmonary resuscitation (CPR) and similar techniques when called to a home where someone's heart has stopped beating. A "non-hospital DNR," signed by the dying person's healthcare provider, may be needed to allow the EMTs to not do CPR.

What to Do after Someone Dies

Immediately following death, nothing has to be done. Take the time you need to grieve. Some people want to stay in the room with the body, while others prefer to leave. How long you stay with the body depends on where death happens and if you wish to observe any special customs based on your religious, cultural, or ethnic background. If the death will take place in a facility (a hospital or nursing home), let the staff know about any customs or rituals early on, if possible. This will help ensure you have appropriate time with the body.

If you choose to leave the room, you may want to have someone make sure the body is lying flat before the joints become stiff and cannot be moved. Known as rigor mortis, this stiffness sets in during the first hours after death. You may have several people you wish to notify, who might want to come see the body before it is moved. Some people ask a member of the community or a spiritual counselor to come as well.

The Death Certificate

As soon as possible, the death must be "pronounced" by someone in authority, like the healthcare provider in a hospital or nursing home or a hospice nurse. This person fills out the forms certifying the cause, time, and place of death. If death happens at home without hospice, talk to the healthcare provider, local medical examiner (coroner), local health department, or funeral home representative to find out how to proceed.

The process of having an authority figure pronounce the death makes it possible for an official death certificate to be prepared. A death certificate is a legal form necessary for many reasons, such as filing a life insurance claim and settling financial and property issues. It is useful to obtain multiple copies of the death certificate so it can be provided to banks, insurance companies, credit card companies, and other institutions.

Arrangements for the Body

Arrangements will need to be made for the body to be picked up, usually by a funeral home, from wherever death takes place. Hospital or nursing home staff may call a funeral home for you. If at home, you will need to contact the funeral home directly, or ask a friend or family member to do that for you.

Autopsies

The healthcare provider may ask you if you want an autopsy. This is a medical procedure conducted by a specially trained doctor to learn more about what caused the death. For example, if the person who died was believed to have Alzheimer disease, a brain autopsy would help confirm the diagnosis.

If your religion or culture objects to autopsies, talk to the healthcare provider. Some people worry that asking for an autopsy means they will not be able to plan a funeral with a viewing, but in almost all cases, the physical signs of an autopsy will not show.

Organ Donation

At some point before death or right after it, a healthcare provider may ask if the dying person is an organ donor. This means he or she agreed, at death, to donate healthy organs, such as the heart, lungs, pancreas, kidneys, cornea, liver, and skin, to living people who need them.

Experts say that organs from one donor can save up to eight people. This is why it is often called "the gift of life." More than 114,000 people of all ages are on the waiting list for an organ.

People of any age can be an organ donor. In some states, this choice is included on a person's driver's license. If not, the decision has to be made quickly. There is no cost to the donor's family.

If the dying person has a Do Not Resuscitate (DNR) order but wants to donate organs, he or she might have to indicate that the desire to donate supersedes the DNR.

Part Six

Death and Children: Information for Parents

Chapter 35

Caring for a Terminally Ill Child

Taking care of a chronically ill child is one of the most draining and difficult tasks a parent can face. Beyond handling physical challenges and medical needs, you'll have to deal with your child's emotional needs and the impact that a prolonged illness can have on the entire family.

Luckily, this tough balancing act doesn't have to be done alone: support groups, social workers, and family friends often can lend a helping hand.

Explaining Long-Term Illness to a Child

Honest communication is vital to helping a child adjust to a serious medical condition. It's important for a child to know that he or she is sick and will be getting lots of care. The hospital, tests, and medicine may feel frightening, but they're part of helping your child feel better.

As you explain the illness and its treatment, give clear and honest answers to all questions in a way your child can understand. It's also important to accurately explain and prepare your child for treatments—and any possible discomfort that might go with along with those treatments.

Text in this chapter is excerpted from "Caring for a Seriously Ill Child," © 1995–2016. The Nemours Foundation/KidsHealth®. Reprinted with permission.

Avoid saying "This won't hurt" if the procedure is likely to be painful. Instead, be honest if a procedure may cause some discomfort, pain, pressure, or stinging. But then reassure your child that it will be temporary and that you'll be there to offer support.

Many hospitals give parents the option to speak to their child about a long-term diagnosis alone, or with the doctor or the entire medical team (doctors, social workers, nurses, etc.) present. Your doctor or other medical professional probably can offer advice on how to talk to your child about the illness.

Tackling Tough Emotions

Your child will have many feelings about the changes affecting his or her body, and should be encouraged and given opportunities to express those feelings and any concerns and fears. Ask what your child is experiencing and listen to the answers before bringing up your own feelings or explanations.

This kind of communication doesn't always have to be verbal. Music, drawing, or writing can often help kids express their emotions and escape through a fantasy world of their own design.

Kids also may need reminders that they're not responsible for the illness. It's common for them to fear that they brought their sickness on by something they thought, said, or did. Reassure your child that this is not the case, and explain in simple terms what is going on. (You also may want to reassure your other kids that nothing they said or did caused their sibling's illness.)

For many questions, there won't be easy answers. And you can't always promise that everything is going to be fine. But you can help your child feel better by listening, saying it's OK and completely understandable to have those feelings, and explaining that you and your family will make him or her as comfortable as possible.

If a child asks "why me?" it's OK to offer an honest "I don't know." Explain that even though no one knows why the illness occurred, the doctors do have treatments for it (if that's the case). If your child says "it's not fair that I'm sick," acknowledge that your child is right. It's important for kids to know it's OK to feel angry about the illness.

Your child may ask "am I going to die?" How you answer will depend not only on your child's medical situation, but also your child's age and maturity level. It's important to know, if possible, what specific fears or concerns your child has and to address them specifically.

If it is reassuring to your child, you may refer to your religious, spiritual, and cultural beliefs about death. You might want to stay away from euphemisms for death such as "going to sleep." Saying that may cause children to fear going to bed at night.

Regardless of their age, it's important for kids to know that there are people who love them and will be there for them, and that they'll be kept comfortable.

Just like any adult, a child will need time to adjust to the diagnosis and the physical changes and is likely to feel sad, depressed, angry, afraid, or even to deny that they are sick. Think about getting professional counseling if you see signs that these feelings are interfering with daily function, or your child seems withdrawn, depressed, and shows radical changes in eating and sleeping habits unrelated to the physical illness.

Behavioral Issues

Kids with chronic illnesses certainly require extra "tender loving care," but also need the routines of childhood. The foremost—and perhaps trickiest—task for worried parents is to treat a sick child as normally as possible.

Despite the circumstances, this means setting limits on unacceptable behavior, sticking to normal routines, and avoiding overindulgence. This may seem impossible, but spoiling or coddling can only make it harder for a child to return to daily activities. When your child leaves the hospital for home, normalcy is the goal.

Dealing with Siblings

Family dynamics can be severely tested when a child is sick. Clinic visits, surgical procedures, and frequent checkups can throw big kinks into everyone's schedules and take an emotional toll on the entire family.

To ease the pressure, seek help to keep the family routines as close to normal as possible. Friends and family members may be able to help handle errands, carpools, and meals. Siblings should continue to attend school and their usual recreational activities; the family should strive for normalcy and time for everyone to be together.

Flexibility is key. The "old normal" may have been the entire family around the table for a home-cooked meal at 6:00, while the "new normal" may be takeout pizza on clinic nights.

Also, consider talking with your other children's teachers or school counselors and let them know that a sibling in the family is ill. They can keep an eye out for behavioral changes or signs of stress among your kids.

It's common for siblings of a chronically ill child to become angry, sullen, resentful, fearful, or withdrawn. They may pick fights or fall behind in schoolwork. In all cases, parents should pay close attention, so that their other kids don't feel pushed aside by the demands of their sick brother or sister. It can help if parents reserve some special time for each sibling.

It can also help them to be included in the treatment process when possible. Depending on their ages and maturity level, visiting the hospital, meeting the nursing and physician staffs, or accompanying their sick sibling to the clinic for treatments can help make the situation less frightening and more understandable.

What they imagine about the illness and hospital visits are often worse than the reality. When they come to the hospital, they can develop a more realistic picture and see that, while unpleasant things may be part of the treatment, there are people who care about their brother or sister and do their best to help.

Lightening Your Load

The stress involved in caring for a child with a long-term illness is considerable, but these tips might ease the strain:

- Break problems into manageable parts. If your child's treatment is expected to be given over an extended time, view it in more manageable time blocks. Planning a week or a month at a time may be less overwhelming.

- Attend to your own needs. Get plenty of rest and, to the extent possible, pay attention to your relationship with your spouse, hobbies, and friendships.

- Depend on friends. Let them carpool siblings to soccer or theater practice. Let others—relatives, friends—share responsibilities of caring for your child. Remember that you can't do it all.

- Ask for help in managing the financial aspects of your child's illness.

- Recognize that everyone handles stress differently. If you and your spouse have distinct coping styles, talk about them and try to accommodate them. Don't pretend that they don't exist.

- Develop working partnerships with healthcare professionals. Realize that you are all part of the team. Ask questions and learn all you can about your child's illness.

- Consult other parents in support groups at your care center or hospital or online. They can offer information and understanding.

- Keep a journal.

- Utilize support staff offered at the treating hospital.

Chapter 36

Taking Care of You: Support for Caregivers

If your child has a serious illness, the caretaking that falls to you is undoubtedly intense. But of course you do it willingly. After all, you'd do anything for your child, including switching places in a minute if only that were possible.

Instead you give all that you can, in every other imaginable way. It's harder than anything you've ever done, and honestly, there are moments when the sheer magnitude of what you're up against is so overwhelming that you just want to run and hide.

Ask any parent who's done this before and you'll find out something very important: You're not alone.

The Caregiver's Dilemma

When you're the caregiver of a child who is seriously ill, it can feel as if the whole world is on your shoulders. Your sick child needs you. You may have other children who need you. Your spouse needs you. Your job—however pointless work might seem right now—needs you.

Yet there's only so much you can give before you will feel mentally, emotionally, and physically drained. That's why it's a necessity—not a luxury—to spend some time taking care of yourself so that you can recharge and feel empowered to continue to support and care for your child.

Tips for Caregivers

Many of these tips might seem easier said than done at first, and a few may seem downright frivolous. But to make it through the long haul, consider the wisdom of that air-safety rule about putting your own oxygen mask on first before helping others. Here are some ways to do that:

Take breaks. It's essential to regularly schedule a few times each week—even for just an hour or two—when you can get away while a family member, friend, or a health aide stays with your child. Once away, that time is yours, so don't feel guilty about how you spend it. Nap, read, have coffee with a friend, go shopping, whatever allows you to relax. While you're out, your child will probably enjoy having someone else to talk to and you'll feel refreshed when you get back.

Eat right. It's no surprise that living on coffee and picking at hospital leftovers can leave you feeling tired and run down. If you know you're going to be out, carry nutritious snacks with you, like fruit, granola bars, sandwiches, or nuts. And if friends offer to bring homemade meals to your home to help out, take them up on it.

Exercise. Whether through a brisk walk, a bike ride, or yoga, most people find that exercise helps clear the mind, boost energy levels, and improve sleep. Even 20 minutes can do the trick, so save a bit of time every day to get moving.

More Tips

Stay organized. Keep all the information you've accumulated about your child's illness in one place, including medication schedules, important phone numbers, and insurance information. When you think of questions for your doctor, write them down immediately so you won't forget. And since dealing with insurance companies can often seem like a full-time job in itself, enlist the help of your spouse or another trusted family member or friend to help keep it all straight. Use a notebook to keep all of the information in one place.

Ask for help. Your friends and family likely want to help you, but might not be sure about what you need. If someone says, "If there's anything I can do..."—and there is—say so. You'd be surprised at how running an errand, doing some laundry, or just sitting and listening to you talk about the day can not only benefit you, but also can make a loved one feel useful.

Find a support group. Ask your child's doctor, nurse, or social worker for information on local support groups related to your child's condition or caregiving in general. If you feel more comfortable sharing anonymously online, then look there. The important thing is to get beyond the feeling of isolation by reaching out to others who've been in your shoes.

Acknowledge your feelings. Your child is sick—of course you have feelings of anger and frustration, and days when you wish you didn't have to deal with it all. Does this make you a bad parent? No, it makes you human. Accept these negative feelings and the often painful fact that no matter how much time or energy you invest in your child's care, you can never be completely in control of your child's health and happiness.

Be aware of the signs of "caregiver burnout." Caregiver burnout is a true state of exhaustion, both physical and emotional. It tends to happen when caregivers try to "do it all" without getting the help or rest they need.

Because caregivers tend to be on autopilot, they're not usually quick to recognize burnout in themselves. Other people might notice the symptoms first, which can include changes in appetite and sleep patterns, withdrawal from social activities, increased anxiety, or emotions that are either heightened (such as excessive crying or irritability) or decreased (feeling empty or unconcerned). Take it seriously if someone you trust notices any of these things in you.

Getting Help

If you feel like you may be experiencing caregiver burnout, depression, or anxiety, explain your feelings and symptoms to your doctor, who may recommend that you see a counselor or therapist (especially one who specializes in caregiver needs).

Your doctor also may encourage you to take a temporary break from your duties by looking into respite care (the kind needed would depend on how ill your child is). Medications for anxiety or depression could be an option, too.

Finally, remember that you are not superhuman. You're a parent doing your best. So give your child your time, your encouragement, your attention, and your unconditional love. Just be sure to save a little bit for yourself.

Chapter 37

Pediatric Palliative Care

Palliative care provides comfort and support to your child and family. When a child is seriously ill, each person in the family is affected differently. That is why it is important that you, your child, and your family get the support and care you need during this difficult time. A special type of care called palliative care can help. Palliative care is a key part of care for children living with a serious illness. It is also an important source of support for their families. The information in this chapter will help you understand how your child and family can benefit from this type of care.

What Is Palliative Care?

Palliative care can ease the symptoms, discomfort, and stress of serious illness for your child and family. Palliative care can help with your child's illness and give support to your family. It can:

- Ease your child's pain and other symptoms of illness.

- Provide emotional and social support that respects your family's cultural values.

- Help your child's healthcare providers work together and communicate with one another to support your goals.

This chapter includes text excerpted from "Palliative Care: Conversations Matter®," National Institute of Nursing Research (NINR), February 4, 2016.

- Start open discussions with you, your child, and your healthcare team about options for care.

Palliative care provides comfort for your child. Palliative care can help children and teenagers living with many serious illnesses, including genetic disorders, cancer, neurologic disorders, heart and lung conditions, and others. Palliative care is important for children at any age or stage of serious illness. It can begin as soon as you learn about your child's illness. Palliative care can help prevent symptoms and give relief from much more than physical pain. It can also enhance your child's quality of life.

Palliative care gives you and your family an added layer of support. Serious illness in a child affects everyone in the family, including parents and siblings of all ages. Palliative care gives extra support for your whole family. It can ease the stress on all of your children, your spouse, and you during a hard time.

Palliative care surrounds your family with a team of experts who work together to support all of you. It is a partnership between your child, your family, and the healthcare team. This team listens to your preferences and helps you think through the care options for your family. They will work with you and your child to make a care plan for your family. They can also help when your child moves from one care setting (e.g., the hospital) to another (e.g., outpatient care or care at home).

Does Accepting Palliative Care Mean Our Family Is Giving up on Other Treatments?

No. The purpose of palliative care is to ease your child's pain and other symptoms and provide emotional and other support to your entire family. Palliative care can help children, from newborns to young adults, and their families—at any stage of a serious illness. Palliative care works alongside other treatments your child may be receiving. In fact, your child can start getting palliative care as soon as you learn about your child's illness.

Palliative Care Is Different from Hospice Care

Your child does not need to be in hospice to get palliative care. Your child can get palliative care wherever they receive care: in the hospital, during clinic visits, or at home. Hospice care focuses on a person's final months of life, but palliative care is available to your child at any time during a serious illness. Some children receive palliative care for many years. Some hospice programs require that patients are no longer getting treatments to cure their illness, but palliative care is different—it can be given at the same time as other treatments for your child's illness. Your child does not need to be in hospice to get palliative care. Your child can get palliative care wherever they receive care: in the hospital, during clinic visits, or at home. Hospice care focuses on a person's final months of life, but palliative care is available to your child at any time during a serious illness. Some children receive palliative care for many years. Some hospice programs require that patients are no longer getting treatments to cure their illness, but palliative care is different—it can be given at the same time as other treatments for your child's illness.

Palliative Care Helps Your Child Live a More Comfortable Life

Palliative care can provide direct support for your child by providing relief from distressing symptoms, such as:

- Pain
- Anxiety
- Shortness of breath
- Nausea
- Fatigue
- Loss of appetite
- Depression
- Problems with sleep

Palliative care can help your child deal with side effects from medicines and treatments. Perhaps most important, palliative care can help enhance your child's quality of life. For example, helping to cope with concerns about school and friends might be very valuable to your child.

Palliative care may also include direct support for families such as assistance with:

- Including siblings in conversations.

- Providing respite care for parents to be able to spend time with their other children.

- Locating community resources for services such as counseling and support groups.

Palliative care is effective. Scientists have studied how palliative care can help children living with serious illnesses. Studies show that patients who get palliative care say that it helps with:

- Pain and other distressing symptoms, such as nausea or short-ness of breath.

- Communication between healthcare providers and family members.

- Emotional support.

Other studies show that palliative care:

- Helps patients get the kinds of care they want.

- Meets the emotional, developmental, and spiritual needs of patients.

Palliative care focuses on the needs of your child and family.

How Do You Know If Your Child or Family Needs Palliative Care?

Children living with a serious illness often experience physical and emotional distress related to their disease. Emotional distress is also common among their parents, siblings, and other family members. If your child has a genetic disorder, cancer, neurologic disorder, heart or lung condition, or another serious illness, palliative care may help reduce pain and enhance quality of life.

Ask your child's healthcare provider about palliative care if your child or any member of your family (including you):

- Suffers from pain or other symptoms due to serious illness.

- Experiences physical pain or emotional distress that is not under control.

- Needs help understanding your child's health condition.

- Needs support coordinating your child's care.

Palliative care can start as soon as your child needs it. It's never too early to start palliative care. In fact, palliative care can take place at the same time as other treatments for your child's illness. It does not depend upon the course or stage of your child's illness.

If you feel your child, your family, or you could benefit from pallia-tive care, ask your child's healthcare provider about getting a referral for palliative care services. There is no reason to wait. The sooner you and your child seek palliative care services, the sooner a palliative care team can help your family manage the pain and other symptoms, and emotions that may come with a serious illness.

The palliative care team works with you, your child, and your care team. Together with your child's healthcare providers, palliative care professionals will work with you and your child to make a care plan that is right for your child, your family, and you. The team will help you and your child include pain and other symptom management into every part of your child's care.

Palliative care experts spend as much time with you and your family as it takes to help you fully understand your child's condition, care options, and other needs. They also make sure your child experiences a smooth transition between the hospital and other services, such as getting care at home.

Your team will listen to your preferences and work with you and your child to plan care for all of your child's symptoms throughout the illness. This will include care for your child's current needs and flexibility for future changes.

Your child's palliative care team is unique. Every palliative care team is different. Your child's palliative care team may include:

- Doctors
- Nurses
- Social workers
- Pharmacists
- Chaplains
- Counselors
- Child life specialists
- Nutritionists
- Art and music therapists

How Can Our Family Get Palliative Care?

The palliative care process can begin when your child's healthcare provider refers you to palliative care services. Or, you or your child can ask your provider for a referral if you feel that palliative care would be helpful for your child, your family, or yourself.

If We Start Palliative Care, Can My Child Still See the Same Primary Healthcare Provider?

Yes. Your child does not have to change to a new primary healthcare provider when starting palliative care. The palliative care team and your child's healthcare provider work together to help you and your child decide the best care plan for your child.

What If My Child's Healthcare Provider Is Unsure about Referring Us?

Some parents are afraid they might offend their child's current healthcare providers by asking about palliative care, but this is unlikely. Most healthcare providers appreciate the extra time and information the palliative care team provides to their patients. Occasionally, a clinician may not refer a patient for palliative care services. If this happens, ask for an explanation. Let your child's healthcare provider know why you think palliative care could help your family.

Who Pays for Palliative Care?

Many insurance plans cover palliative care. If you have questions or concerns about costs, you can ask your healthcare team to put you in touch with a social worker, care manager, or financial advisor at your hospital or clinic to look at payment options. Palliative care can begin at any time and be provided alongside other treatments your child may be receiving.

Where Can My Child Get Palliative Care?

Your palliative care team will help you to know what services are available in your community. Your child and family may receive palliative care in a hospital, during clinic visits, or at home. You and your child will likely first meet with your palliative care team in the hospital or at a clinic. After the first visit, some visits may still occur in the clinic or hospital. But many palliative care programs offer services at home and in the community. Home services can occur through telephone calls or home visits. If palliative care starts in the hospital, your care team can help your child make a successful move to your home or other healthcare setting. Home may feel most comfortable and safe to you and your child. Depending on your child's condition and treatment, the palliative care team may be able to help you find a nursing agency or community care agency to support palliative care for your child at home.

How Can My Child's Pain Be Managed?

The palliative care team can bring your child comfort in many ways. Treating pain often involves medication, but there are also other methods to address a child's discomfort. Your child may feel better with changes like low lighting, comfortable room temperatures, pleasant smells, guided relaxation, and deep breathing techniques. Your child may welcome additional activities like video chats, social media, soothing music, and massage and art therapy that may help decrease pain and anxiety. If your child has an illness that causes pain that is not relieved by drugs like acetaminophen (Tylenol®) or ibuprofen (Motrin® or Advil®), your child's palliative care team may recommend trying stronger medicines. There is no reason to wait before beginning these medications. Should your child's pain increase, the dose may be safely increased over time to provide relief. Pain relief can be offered in a hospital, at home, or in other healthcare settings. Your palliative care team will partner with you and your child to learn what is causing discomfort and how best to handle it. Don't wait to get your child and family the extra support they deserve. Talk to your loved ones and healthcare team about palliative care. If your child wants palliative care, or if you think palliative care could be helpful to any member of your family, ask for it now. Talk with your child's healthcare provider about palliative care.

Chapter 38

Children's Hospice and End-of-Life Care

Not every child is able to recover from a serious illness or injury. Sometimes a disease or condition continues to worsen, despite every attempt by the medical community to help the child get better. Other times, a successful cure might not be available when an illness is too widespread or severe.

When this happens, the primary aim of a child's care shifts from seeking a cure to making the child more physically and emotionally comfortable and as free from pain as possible. This is known as palliative care. Hospice care is a specific type of palliative care that helps children and families cope with terminal illness.

What Is Hospice Care?

Hospice care, sometimes called end-of-life palliative care, is designed for patients who are in the final stages of a terminal illness. A relatively new phenomenon in the United States, hospice care has grown from a volunteer-led movement to a significant part of the healthcare system that helps ensure that all dying patients receive comprehensive and compassionate care. Hospice care focuses not only on dying

Text in this chapter is excerpted from "End-of-Life Care for Children with Terminal Illness," © 1995–2016. The Nemours Foundation/KidsHealth®. Reprinted with permission.

as peacefully, comfortably, and with as much dignity as possible, but also on living as fully as possible until death occurs.

Usually, hospice care is offered to those who are expected to live no longer than 6 months and have stopped receiving curative treatments. The goal of hospice care is not to speed up the process of dying or to slow it down—but rather, to provide the best possible quality of life for dying patients and their families. It focuses on preventing and relieving pain and suffering and easing the fear and anxiety associated with the end of a person's life.

What Services Are Available?

Hospice care services are designed to meet the unique needs of a dying child and his or her family. Children receive pain management and counseling to learn to cope with the inevitable outcome of their condition. Families and loved ones receive support and counseling to help care for their child as well as to cope with the emotional strain of illness, loss, and grief.

At the center of the hospice care team are the child's parents and other family members. Keeping families involved in the decision-making allows them to feel more in control of their child's care. Care is provided by a team of professionals who have knowledge and experience in various disciplines, such as doctors, nurses, social workers, therapists, psychologists, teachers, home health aides, and spiritual advisors. The team also may include community volunteers who have been trained in the unique issues surrounding death and dying and are willing to help in any way they can.

A primary focus of hospice care is palliative care, which includes minimizing pain and other symptoms. Other hospice services for the child and family might include:

- emotional support
- information and advice
- nursing services
- nutritional counseling
- respite care, which offers temporary relief from the intense strain of hospice care to parents who are caring for children at home
- art, music, and play therapy, which helps children and families explore and express their feelings

- activities for siblings
- spiritual care, such as exploring the meaning of death and helping with religious ceremonies or rituals
- practical assistance with everyday tasks
- grief counseling and support, which helps parents and other family members through the bereavement process

Depending on the service, it may be offered on an emergent basis, either day or night, but most services can be scheduled in advance based on what is most convenient for families and patients.

Where Is Hospice Care Offered?

Many people think of hospice as a place; however, hospice care services can be provided in different places. Most hospice care is delivered in people's homes by community home health agencies or independently owned hospice programs. However, it also can be provided in hospice care facilities as well as in some hospitals, clinics, and long-term care facilities.

Who Pays for Hospice Care?

Most insurance plans, including Medicare and Medicaid, cover all or part of hospice care. In general, medical coverage is provided for patients who are expected to live for 6 months or less. If a child needs hospice services beyond that point, an insurance company usually will revaluate the child's condition and may continue to provide coverage for hospice care.

Is Hospice Care Right for Your Child?

Many parents are reluctant to accept hospice care for their children because they feel that doing so means that they're giving up hope. Similarly, some healthcare providers are reluctant to recommend hospice care because they're not willing to give up on finding a cure and want to do all they can to help a child live as long as possible. But hospice care is not about giving up hope; rather, it offers patients and caregivers hope for the best possible quality of life throughout a patient's remaining days.

Choosing hospice care for one's child is, no doubt, the hardest decision a parent will ever make. After you've considered your child's and your family's individual needs, it might help to talk to healthcare providers, spiritual advisors, social workers, counselors, or family members who can help you sort through your feelings and help you reach a decision. Depending on the age and maturity of your child, he or she also may want to be a part of this decision-making process.

Because this is such a difficult decision, sometimes families do not consider hospice care until shortly before their child dies. But seeking these services earlier in the process lets children and their families receive more of the available help and support.

If you're interested in learning about what hospice services are offered in your area, talk to your healthcare provider, social worker, or a representative from your local hospital. You also can research local hospice care services through the National Hospice and Palliative Care Organization by calling 1-800-658-8898.

Chapter 39

Sudden Infant Death Syndrome (SIDS)

What Is Sudden Infant Death Syndrome (SIDS)?

Sudden infant death syndrome (SIDS) is the sudden death of an infant younger than 1 year of age that stays unexplained after a complete investigation. This investigation can include an autopsy, a review of the death scene, and complete family and medical histories.

A diagnosis of SIDS is made by collecting information, conducting scientific or forensic tests, and talking with parents, other caregivers, and healthcare providers. If, after this process is complete, there is still no identifiable cause of death, the infant's death might be labeled as SIDS.

How Many Infants Die from SIDS or Are at Risk for SIDS?

Data from the Centers for Disease Control and Prevention (CDC) show that 2,063 infants died from SIDS in 2010 (the most recent year for which data are available). SIDS is the leading cause of death in children between 1 month and 1 year of age. The majority (90%) of

This chapter includes text excerpted from "Sudden Infant Death Syndrome (SIDS): Condition Information," *Eunice Kennedy Shriver* National Institute of Child Health and Human Development (NICHD), April 12, 2013.

SIDS deaths occur before a child is 6 months old, with most happening between 1 and 4 months.

What Factors Increase the Risk of SIDS?

Currently, there is no known way to completely prevent SIDS, but there are ways to reduce the risk. Several factors present before the infant is born, at birth, and throughout the first year can impact SIDS risk. Many of these factors can be controlled or changed to reduce the risk, but some cannot be controlled or changed.

The single most effective action that parents and caregivers can take to lower SIDS risk is to place their baby to sleep on his or her back for all sleep times. Research shows that:

- Stomach sleeping carries the highest risk for SIDS—between 1.7 and 12.9 times the risk of back sleeping.

- The side-lying position also increases the risk. It is unstable and babies can easily roll to their stomach.

- Back sleeping carries the lowest risk for SIDS and is safest. Other known risk factors for include the following:

- **Preterm birth.** Infants born before 39 weeks in the womb are at higher risk for SIDS than are infants born at full term.

- **Sex.** More boys die from SIDS than do girls.

- **Race/ethnic origin.** African American and American Indian/ Alaska Native infants are at higher risk for SIDS than are white, Hispanic American, or Asian/Pacific Islander American infants.

What Causes SIDS?

Healthcare providers and researchers don't know the exact cause, but there are many theories. More and more research evidence suggests that infants who die from SIDS are born with brain abnormalities or defects. These defects are typically found within a network of nerve cells that rely on a chemical called serotonin that allows one nerve cell to send a signal to another nerve cell. The cells are located in the part of the brain that probably controls breathing, heart rate, blood pressure, temperature, and waking from sleep.

But scientists believe that brain defects alone may not be enough to cause a SIDS death. Evidence suggests that other events must also occur for an infant to die from SIDS. Researchers use the Triple-Risk Model to explain this concept. In this model, all three factors have to occur for an infant to die from SIDS. Having only one of these factors may not be enough to cause death from SIDS, but when all three combine, the chances of SIDS are high.

These factors are:

- **At-risk infant.** An infant has an unknown problem—such as a genetic change or a brain defect—that puts him or her at risk for SIDS. Healthcare providers, parents, and caregivers don't know about these problems, so they don't know the infant is at risk.

- **Important time in infant's development.** During the first 6 months after birth, infants go through many quick phases of growth that can change how well the body controls or regulates itself. Also, infant's bodies are learning how to respond to their environment.

- **Stressors in the environment.** All infants have stressors in their environments—sometimes called external stressors because they are outside the body. Being placed to sleep on the stomach, overheating during sleep, and exposure to cigarette smoke are all examples of external stressors. Infants who have no problems like those explained above can usually correct or overcome external stressors to survive and thrive. But an infant who has an unknown problem and whose body systems are immature and unstable might not be able to overcome these stressors.

According to the Triple-Risk Theory, all three things have to be present for SIDS to occur. Removing one of these factors—such as external stressors—may tip the balance in favor of the infant's survival. Because the first two situations can't be seen or pinpointed, the most effective way to reduce the risk of SIDS is to remove or reduce environmental stressors.

How Can I Reduce the Risk of SIDS?

The following actions can reduce the risk for SIDS and other sleep-related causes of infant death (such as suffocation):

- Always place infants on their backs to sleep, for naps and at night, to reduce the risk of SIDS. The back sleep position is always the safest position for all infants, including preterm babies. Keep in mind that every sleep time counts.

- Use a firm sleep surface, covered by a fitted sheet, to reduce the risk of SIDS and other sleep-related causes of infant death. Firm sleep surfaces can include mattresses in safety-approved* cribs, bassinets, and portable play areas. Do not use a car seat, carrier, swing, or similar product as the baby's everyday sleep area. Never place babies to sleep on soft surfaces, such as on a couch or sofa, pillows, quilts, sheepskins, or blankets.

- Room sharing—keeping the baby's sleep area in the same room where you or others sleep—reduces the risk of SIDS and other sleep-related causes of infant death. Your baby should not sleep in an adult bed, on a couch, or on a chair alone, with you, or with anyone else. If you bring your baby into your bed to feed, make sure to put him or her back in the separate sleep area, such as a safety-approved crib, bassinet, or portable play area, in your room next to where you sleep when you are finished.

- Keep soft objects, toys, and loose bedding out of your baby's sleep area to reduce the risk of SIDS and other sleep-related causes of infant death. Don't use pillows, blankets, quilts, sheepskins, or crib bumpers anywhere in your baby's sleep area. Evidence does not support using crib bumpers to prevent injury. In fact, crib bumpers can cause serious injuries and even death. Keeping them out of baby's sleep area is the best way to avoid these dangers.

- To reduce the risk of SIDS, women should:

  - Get regular healthcare during pregnancy (prenatal care), and

  - Not smoke, drink alcohol, or use illegal drugs during pregnancy or after the baby is born.

- To reduce the risk of SIDS, do not smoke during pregnancy, and do not smoke or allow smoking around your baby.

- Breastfeed your baby to reduce the risk of SIDS. Breastfeeding has many health benefits for mother and infant. If you bring your baby into your bed to breastfeed, make sure to put him or her back in a separate sleep area, such as a safety-approved* crib, bassinet, or portable play area, in your room next to where you sleep when you are finished.

- Give your baby a dry pacifier that is not attached to a string for naps and at night to reduce the risk of SIDS. But don't force the baby to use it. If the pacifier falls out of the baby's mouth during sleep, there is no need to put the pacifier back in. Wait until the baby is used to breastfeeding before trying a pacifier.

- Do not let your baby get too hot during sleep. Dress your child in no more than one layer of clothing more than an adult would wear to be comfortable. Keep the room at a temperature that is comfortable for an adult.

- Follow healthcare provider guidance on your baby's vaccines and regular health checkups.

- Avoid products that claim to reduce the risk of SIDS and other sleep-related causes of infant death. These wedges, position- ers, and other products have not been tested for safety or effectiveness.

- Do not use home heart or breathing monitors to reduce the risk of SIDS. If you have questions about using monitors for other health conditions, talk with your child's healthcare provider. Keep in mind that monitors for health conditions are different from baby monitors that allow caregivers to hear and/or see an infant from another room. These baby monitors do not reduce or detect SIDS.

- Give your infant plenty of tummy time when he or she is awake and when someone is watching. Supervised tummy time helps the baby's neck, shoulder, and arm muscles get stronger. It also helps to prevent flat spots on the back of your baby's head. Hold- ing the baby upright and limiting time in carriers and bouncers can also help prevent flat spots on the back of the baby's head.

What Does a Safe Sleep Environment Look Like?

A safe sleep environment—one that is free of items and features that could be dangerous to infants—reduces the risk of SIDS and other sleep-related causes of infant death. Parents and caregivers can create a safe sleep environment in the following ways:

- Always place your baby on his or her back to sleep, for naps and at night.

- Use a firm sleep surface, such as a mattress in a safety-ap- proved* crib, covered only by a fitted sheet.

- Do not use pillows, blankets, sheepskins, or crib bumpers any- where in your baby's sleep area.

- Keep soft objects, toys, and loose bedding out of your baby's sleep area.

- Make sure nothing covers the baby's head or face.

- Dress your baby in light sleep clothing, such as a one-piece sleeper, and don't use a blanket.

- Do not smoke or let anyone smoke around your baby.

- Room-sharing—keeping baby's sleep area in the same room where you sleep—reduces the risk of SIDS and other sleep-related causes of infant death.

Will My Baby Choke If Placed on the Back to Sleep?

No. Healthy infants naturally swallow or cough up fluids—it's a reflex all people have. Where the opening to the windpipe is located in the body makes it unlikely for fluids to cause choking. Babies may actually clear such fluids better when on their backs.

When the baby is in the back sleep position, the windpipe lies on top of the esophagus, which leads to the stomach. Anything regurgitated or refluxed from the stomach through the esophagus has to work against gravity to enter the trachea and cause choking. When the baby is sleeping on its stomach, such fluids will exit the esophagus and pool at the opening for the trachea, making choking much more likely.

Cases of fatal choking are very rare except when related to a medical condition. The number of fatal choking deaths has not increased since back sleeping recommendations began. In most of the few reported cases of fatal choking, an infant was sleeping on his or her stomach.

Why Shouldn't I Use Bumpers in My Baby's Crib?

Current research shows that crib bumper pads or padded bassinets can cause injury or death to infants. Before crib safety was regulated, the spacing between the slats of the crib sides could be any width, which posed a danger to infants if they were too wide. Parents and caregivers used padded crib bumpers to protect infants. Now that cribs must meet safety standards, the slats don't pose the same dangers. As a result, the bumpers are no longer needed.

Evidence does not support using crib bumpers to prevent injuries. In addition, evidence shows that crib bumpers can cause serious injuries and death. Keeping them out of an infant's sleep area is the best way to avoid these dangers.

Does Back Sleeping Cause Flat Spots on the Back of the Head?

Infants' skulls are soft and are made up of several skull plates. These movable plates have spaces between them, called sutures, which allow the head to be flexible so that the brain can grow. If the head is left in the same position for long periods of time (such as lying on the back, or sitting in a car seat or carrier), the plates move in a way that may leave a flat spot. Positional plagiocephaly is the term used to describe a flattened or misshapen head. Healthcare providers also use the term brachycephaly to describe the flattening of the back of the skull. Positional plagiocephaly and brachycephaly often occur together.

Many cases of positional plagiocephaly can be prevented (and sometimes corrected) by repositioning the infant to remove the pressure from the back of his or her head. Repositioning includes the following:

- Providing "Tummy Time" when the infant is awake and when someone is watching. Tummy time not only helps prevent flat spots, but it also helps the head, neck, and shoulder muscles get stronger as part of normal development.

Parents and caregivers should try supervised tummy time several times a day, for short periods of time, until the infant gets used to being on the tummy. Once infants begin to enjoy the position, parents can try longer periods of time or increase frequency of tummy time.

- Changing the direction that the infant lies in the crib from one week to the next. For example, have the infant's feet point toward one end of the crib for a few days, and then change the position so his or her feet point toward the other end of the crib. This change will encourage the infant to turn his or her head in different directions to avoid resting in the same position all the time.

- Avoiding too much time in car seats, carriers, and bouncers while the infant is awake. Spend "cuddle time" with the child by holding him or her upright over one shoulder often during the day.

- Changing the location of the infant's crib in the room so that he or she has to look in different directions to see the door or the window.

It is important to note that although back sleeping may increase the risk of flat spots on the head, flat spots are much less serious than SIDS and can often be prevented and treated. Parents should not stop placing infants on their backs to sleep, but rather should be sure to offer tummy time while they are awake and use repositioning techniques. If you have concerns about the shape of your infant's head, talk with your child's healthcare provider.

Can Certain Breathing or Heart Monitors Detect SIDS before It Happens?

Some breathing and heart monitors claim to be able to detect SIDS before it happens. These products might be prescribed by healthcare providers to manage certain medical conditions, but research shows that these monitors are not effective at detecting SIDS or reducing SIDS risk. The *Eunice Kennedy Shriver* National Institute of Child Health and Human Development (NICHD)-led Collaborative Home Infant Monitoring Evaluation (CHIME) study evaluated infants at high risk for SIDS to determine whether these monitors could identify situations that are dangerous to infants and perhaps reduce the risk for SIDS. The research findings led the American Academy of Pediatrics (AAP) to recommend that these monitors not be used to prevent SIDS or identify infants at risk for SIDS.

Keep in mind that breathing, heart, and other home monitors are different from baby monitors that allow caregivers to hear and/or see the infant from another room. These baby monitors often are useful for alerting caregivers that a child is awake, but they do not reduce or detect SIDS.

Can Wedges and Other Products Reduce the Risk of SIDS?

Some products claim to prevent SIDS or safely position the infant for sleep. These products may include:

- Wedges

- Positioners

- Special mattresses

- Special sleep surfaces

The U.S. Consumer Product Safety Commission (CPSC), the U.S. Food and Drug Administration (FDA), and the American Academy of Pediatrics (AAP) warn against using these products because of the dangers they pose to infants and because there is no evidence that they reduce SIDS.

What Kind of Support Is Available for Parents Who Have Lost an Infant to SIDS?

One of the most important things to remember when an infant dies from SIDS is that the families themselves are not to blame. The causes of SIDS remain unknown. Even though there are ways to reduce the risk, there is no definitive way to prevent SIDS from occurring. There are a variety of resources available to help families who have lost an infant to SIDS. Talking to other parents or caregivers who have lost an infant to SIDS may be helpful. A healthcare provider may also be able to recommend local resources and groups.

Parents can also find support at the community and state level through the National SUID/SIDS Resource Center. The center offers resources for parents and caregivers grieving for their loss, including The Death of a Child: The Grief of the Parents, A Lifetime Journey.

Chapter 40

Stillbirth, Miscarriage, and Infant Death

Chapter Contents

Section 40.1

Stillbirth

This section includes text excerpted from "Facts about Stillbirth," Centers for Disease Control and Prevention (CDC), June 6, 2016.

What Is Stillbirth?

A stillbirth is the death of a baby before or during delivery. Both miscarriage and stillbirth are terms describing pregnancy loss, but they differ according to when the loss occurs. There is no universally accepted definition of when a fetal death is called a stillbirth, and the meaning of this term varies internationally. This lack of a consistent definition of stillbirth often makes it difficult to compare data on how frequently it occurs.

In the United States, a miscarriage usually refers to a fetal loss less than 20 weeks after a woman becomes pregnant, and a stillbirth refers to a loss 20 or more weeks after a woman becomes pregnant.

Stillbirth is further classified as either early, late, or term.

- An early stillbirth is a fetal death occurring between 20 and 27 completed weeks of pregnancy.

- A late stillbirth occurs between 28 and 36 completed pregnancy weeks.

- A term stillbirth occurs between 37 or more completed pregnancy weeks.

Occurrence

Stillbirth affects about 1% of all pregnancies, and each year about 24,000 babies are stillborn in the United States. That is about the same number of babies that die during the first year of life and it is more than 10 times as many deaths as the number that occur from Sudden Infant Death Syndrome (SIDS).

Because of advances in medical technology over the last 30 years, prenatal care (medical care during pregnancy) has improved, which has dramatically reduced the number of late and term stillbirth.

However, the rate of early stillbirth has remained about the same over time.

Causes

The causes of many stillbirths are unknown. Therefore, families are often left grieving without answers to their questions. Stillbirth is not a cause of death, but rather a term that means a baby's death during the pregnancy. Some women blame themselves, but rarely are these deaths caused by something a woman did or did not do. Known causes of stillbirth generally fall into one of three broad categories:

- Problems with the baby (birth defects or genetic problems)

- Problems with the placenta or umbilical cord (this is where the mother and baby exchange oxygen and nutrients)

- Certain conditions in the mother (for example, uncontrolled diabetes, high blood pressure, or obesity)

Stillbirth with an unknown cause is called "unexplained stillbirth." Having an unexplained stillbirth is more likely to occur the further along a woman is in her pregnancy.

Although stillbirth occurs in families of all races, ethnicities, and income levels, and to women of all ages, some women are at higher risk for having a stillbirth. Some of the factors that increase the risk for a stillbirth include the mother:

- being of black race

- being a teenager

- being 35 years of age or older

- being unmarried

- being obese

- smoking cigarettes during pregnancy

- having certain medical conditions, such as high blood pressure or diabetes

- having multiple pregnancies

- having had a previous pregnancy loss

These factors are also associated with other poor pregnancy outcomes, such as preterm birth.

What Can Be Done?

Although many causes of stillbirth remain unknown, more causes might be found if thorough investigations were performed, including an autopsy (a physical exam of a body after death), placental exam, genetic testing, and a detailed medical history. This information can be important in finding out whether there is a chance that a stillbirth could occur again and to provide appropriate medical care and counseling for future pregnancies. Even when a cause is not found, many families report that having an evaluation and looking for a cause was helpful in coping with their loss. After a stillbirth occurs, physicians can help by looking for a specific cause and arranging for grief counseling for the mother and family. If you or someone you know has experienced the loss of a baby due to stillbirth, please visit the organizations listed on our Other Resources page, many of which may be able to offer support.

Section 40.2

Miscarriage

This section includes text excerpted from "Pregnancy Loss: Condition Information," *Eunice Kennedy Shriver* National Institute of Child Health and Human Development (NICHD), July 15, 2013.

What Is Pregnancy Loss/Miscarriage?

A miscarriage, also called pregnancy loss or spontaneous abortion, is the unexpected loss of a fetus before the 20th week of pregnancy, or gestation. (Gestation is the period of pregnancy from conception to birth.) The loss of a pregnancy after the 20th week of gestation is called a stillbirth and can occur before or during delivery.

What Are the Symptoms of Pregnancy Loss/ Miscarriage?

Symptoms of miscarriage may include vaginal spotting or bleeding; abdominal pain or abdominal cramps; low back pain; or fluid, tissue, or clot-like material passing from the vagina. Although vaginal bleeding is a common symptom when a woman has a miscarriage, many pregnant women have spotting early during their pregnancy because of other factors but do not miscarry. Regardless, pregnant women who have any of the symptoms of miscarriage should contact their healthcare providers immediately.

How Many People Are Affected by or at Risk for Pregnancy Loss or Miscarriage?

The estimated rate of miscarriage is 15% to 20% in women who know they are pregnant, but as many as half of all fertilized eggs may spontaneously abort, often before the women realize they are pregnant. Women who have had previous miscarriages are at a higher risk for miscarriage. The risk of miscarriage also increases with maternal age beginning at age 30 and becoming greater after age 35.

What Causes Pregnancy Loss/Miscarriage?

Miscarriage occurs due to many different causes, some of them known and others unknown. Frequently, miscarriages occur when a pregnancy is not developing normally. More than half of all miscarriages are caused by a chromosomal abnormality in the fetus (typically due to the wrong number of chromosomes, the structures in a cell that contain the genetic information), which is more common with increasing age of the parents, particularly among women who are older than age 35.

Other possible causes of pregnancy loss or miscarriage are maternal health issues or exposure to chemicals. Maternal health issues include chronic disease, such as diabetes, thyroid disease, or polycystic ovary syndrome (PCOS), or problems associated with the immune system, such as an autoimmune disorder. Other maternal health issues that can increase the risk of miscarriage include infection, hormone problems, obesity, or problems of the placenta, cervix, or uterus. Exposure to environmental toxins, drug use or alcohol use, smoking, or the consumption of 200 milligrams or more of caffeine per day (equal to about one 12-ounce cup of coffee) also can increase the risk of miscarriage.

How Do Healthcare Providers Diagnose Pregnancy Loss or Miscarriage?

If a pregnant woman experiences any of the symptoms of miscarriage, such as crampy abdominal or back pain, light spotting, or bleeding, she should contact her healthcare provider immediately. For diagnosis, the woman may need to undergo a blood test to check for the level of hCG, the pregnancy hormone, or an internal pelvic examination to determine if her cervix is dilated or thinned, which can be a sign of a miscarriage; or depending on the length of time since her last menstrual period, and the level of pregnancy hormone in the blood, she may need to have an ultrasound test so that her healthcare provider can observe the pregnancy and the maternal reproductive organs, such as the uterus and placenta. If a woman has had more than one miscarriage, she may choose to have blood tests performed to check for chromosome abnormalities or hormone problems, or to detect immune system disorders that may interfere with a healthy pregnancy.

What Are the Treatments for Pregnancy Loss/ Miscarriage?

In most cases, no treatment is necessary for women who miscarry early in their pregnancy, because the bleeding associated with miscarriage usually empties the uterus of pregnancy-associated tissue. In some cases, however, a woman may need to undergo a surgical procedure called a dilation and curettage (D&C) to remove any pregnancy-associated tissue remaining in the uterus. A D&C is performed if the woman is bleeding heavily or if an ultrasound test detects any remaining tissue in the uterus.

An alternative to a D&C is the use of a medication called misoprostol that helps the tissue pass out of the uterus. The use of misoprostol has proven to be effective in 84% of the cases studied. Other treatments after a woman miscarries may include control of mild to moderate bleeding, prevention of infection, pain relief, and emotional support. If heavy bleeding occurs, the woman should contact her healthcare provider immediately.

Is There a Cure for Pregnancy Loss/Miscarriage?

In many cases, a woman can do little to prevent a miscarriage. However, having preconception and prenatal care (before becoming pregnant and during pregnancy) is the best prevention available for all complications associated with pregnancy. Miscarriages caused by systemic disease often can be prevented by detection and treatment of the disease before pregnancy occurs. A woman also can decrease her risk of miscarriage by avoiding environmental hazards, such as infectious diseases, X-rays, drugs and alcohol, and high levels of caffeine.

Is There Anything a Woman Can Do to Prevent a Pregnancy Loss?

Most of the time, a woman cannot do anything to prevent a miscarriage. Getting preconception care and prenatal care before becoming pregnant and during pregnancy can help prevent some complications before they occur.

What Health Conditions Contribute to Pregnancy Loss?

There are many different causes for miscarriage. In more than half of miscarriages, the developing fetus had a chromosomal abnormality that occurred randomly and was not inherited from the parents. These kinds of genetic errors are more likely as the mother gets older, especially after age 35.

However, there are some health conditions that may contribute to pregnancy loss, too. These are high blood pressure, diabetes, thyroid disease, inherited blood clotting disorders, certain disorders of the immune system, uterine or cervical abnormalities, abnormal levels of hormones, obesity, and maternal or fetal infection. Fetal death that occurs after the 20th week of gestation is called a stillbirth. In approximately one-half of all stillbirth cases reported, healthcare providers can find no cause for the loss. However, health conditions that may contribute to stillbirth are chromosomal abnormalities of the fetus; placental problems, such as placental abruption; poor fetal growth due to smoking or maternal high blood pressure; chronic health issues of the mother; umbilical cord accidents; and infection of the mother, fetus, or placenta.

What Lifestyle Factors Can Increase Risk for Pregnancy Loss?

Pregnant women who use illicit drugs, smoke, drink alcohol, or have more than 200 milligrams of caffeine every day (about the amount in a 12-ounce cup of coffee) may increase their risk of miscarriage. The consumption of less than 200 milligrams of caffeine per day does not seem to be related to risk of miscarriage or preterm birth.

How Soon after Pregnancy Loss Can a Woman Try Again for Another Infant?

It is typically safe for a woman to conceive after one normal menstrual cycle has occurred following a pregnancy loss. However, it is best to wait until she is physically and emotionally ready to become pregnant again and until any tests recommended by a healthcare provider to determine the cause of the miscarriage have been completed.

If a Woman Loses a Pregnancy, Does Her Risk for Another Pregnancy Loss Increase?

Miscarriage is typically a one-time occurrence. However, roughly 1% of women experience more than one miscarriage in a row, or repeated miscarriages. In some cases, an underlying problem causes repeated miscarriages. A healthcare provider may suggest a series of tests to determine, and treat if possible, the cause of repeated miscarriages.

What Is Repeated Miscarriage?

For every 100 women who have a miscarriage, one of them will have more than one miscarriage in a row. This is called repeated, or recurrent, miscarriage. Although most miscarriages are caused by a random genetic mistake in the egg or sperm that isn't likely to happen again, repeated miscarriages can sometimes have an underlying cause.

After about three repeated miscarriages, a woman's healthcare provider might suggest tests to try to find a cause. The provider will also ask detailed questions about the parents' medical histories. Potential causes of repeated miscarriage might include rearrangements in the parents' genetic material; structural problems, scarring, or fibroids in the uterus; or certain medical conditions in the mother. Some of these problems can be treated, which might improve the couple's chance of getting pregnant.

However, in about half to three-quarters of women with repeated miscarriages, doctors won't be able to find out a reason. Even if there's no apparent cause, the woman is still likely to be able to get pregnant and deliver a baby in the future: Almost two of every three women with recurrent miscarriage go on to give birth without any special treatment.

If a Woman Was Diagnosed with Preeclampsia In a Previous Pregnancy, Does She Have an Increased Risk for Miscarriage In a Subsequent Pregnancy?

Preeclampsia is a potentially serious condition that occurs only in pregnancy when a pregnant woman develops high blood pressure (also called hypertension) and protein in the urine. Research shows that a history of preeclampsia is not associated with an increase in the risk of miscarriage. Women diagnosed with preeclampsia during a previous pregnancy should work with their healthcare provider to get their blood pressure under control before becoming pregnant again.

Although preeclampsia is not associated with an increased risk of miscarriage, pregnancy complications as a result of high blood pressure include low birth weight, premature birth (before 37 weeks), and problems with the placenta.

Section 40.3

Infant Death

This section includes text excerpted from "Infant Mortality," Centers for Disease Control and Prevention (CDC), September 27, 2016.

Infant Mortality: A Cause of Concern

Over 23,000 infants died in the United States in 2014. The loss of a baby takes a serious toll on the health and well-being of families, as well as the nation. The death of a baby before his or her first birthday is called infant mortality. The infant mortality rate is the number of infant deaths that occur for every 1,000 live births. This rate is often used as an indicator to measure the health and well-being of a nation, because factors affecting the health of entire populations can also impact the mortality rate of infants. There are significant differences in infant mortality by race and ethnicity; for instance, the mortality rate for black infants is more than twice that of white infants.

What Are the Causes?

Most newborns grow and thrive. However, for every 1,000 babies that are born, almost six die during their first year. Most of these babies die as a result of:

- Birth defects
- Preterm birth (birth before 37 weeks gestation) and low birth weight

- Maternal complications of pregnancy

- Sudden Infant Death Syndrome (SIDS)

- Injuries (e.g., suffocation).

The top five leading causes of infant mortality together account for over half (57%) of all infant deaths that happened in the United States in 2014.

What Can Be Done?

Pregnancy outcomes are influenced by a woman's health and differ by factors such as race, ethnicity, age, location, healthcare access, education, and income.

Preconception health focuses on actions women can take before and between pregnancies to increase their chances of having a healthy baby, including thinking about their goals for having or not having children and how to achieve those goals, addressing health issues with their healthcare provider before getting pregnant, and adopting a healthy lifestyle.

Important steps women can take to improve their preconception health include:

- Take 400 micrograms of folic acid.

- Achieving and maintaining a healthy diet and weight.

- Being physically active regularly.

- Quitting tobacco use.

- Not drinking excessive amounts of alcohol and using "street" drugs.

- Talking to your healthcare provider about screening and proper management of chronic diseases, including depression.

- Talking with their healthcare provider about taking any medications.

- Visiting their healthcare provider at the recommended scheduled time periods for important exams, screenings, and vaccinations and discussing if or when they are considering becoming pregnant.

- Using effective contraception correctly and consistently if they are sexually active, but are not planning to become pregnant.

- Getting help for intimate partner violence.

- Learning about their family history and how this may affect their risks.

Healthcare providers and women can work together before and during pregnancy to address problems if they arise and improve women's chances for healthy outcomes.

Some women may be advised to give birth at special hospitals, especially if they are at risk of delivering a very small or very sick baby. These hospitals have staff and equipment needed to provide advanced newborn life support and medical services. Many states and localities have organized to provide this care under a system of "regionalization"—where this special hospital can serve a geographic region. These are known as "Level III" hospitals. Prospective parents should ask their providers about why Level III services may be important to the health of the woman and her baby and how they can prepare, if they have to deliver there.

Chapter 41

Grieving the Death of a Child

The Death of a Child the Grief of the Parents: A Lifetime Journey

There is no more devastating loss than the death of a child. Sudden death is a contradiction to everything that is known to be true in life. Losing a child to sudden death is a disruption in the natural law and order of life. It is a heartbreak like no other. Parental grief is different from other losses—it is intensified, exaggerated and lengthened.

"Children are not supposed to die...Parents expect to see their children grow and mature. Ultimately, parents expect to die and leave their children behind...This is the natural course of life events, the life cycle continuing as it should. The loss of a child is the loss of innocence, the death of the most vulnerable and dependent. The death of a child signifies the loss of the future, of hopes and dreams, of new strength, and of perfection" (Arnold and Gemma 1994, iv,9,39).

Grieving parents say that their grief is a lifelong process, a long and painful process... "a process in which [they] try to take and keep some meaning from the loss and life without the [child]" (Arnold and Gemma 1983, 57). After a child's death, parents embark on a long, sad journey that can be very frightening and extremely lonely—a journey

This chapter includes text excerpted from "The Death of a Child the Grief of the Parents: A Lifetime Journey," Health Resources and Services Administration (HRSA), U.S. Department of Health and Human Services (HHS), September 15, 2005. Reviewed October 2016.

that never really ends. The hope and desire that healing will come eventually is an intense and persistent one for grieving parents.

The child who died is considered a gift to the parents and family, and they are forced to give up that gift. Yet, as parents, they also strive to let their child's life, no matter how short, be seen as a gift to others. These parents seek to find ways to continue to love, honor, and value the lives of their children, and to make the child's presence known and felt in the lives of family and friends. Bereaved parents often try to live their lives more fully and generously because of this painful experience.

The Process of Grief

Grief is a process. Although parents would wish otherwise, grief cannot be bypassed or hurried; it must be allowed to happen. Parents do not go through grief and come out the other side as before the loss. Grief changes parents.

One approach to understanding bereavement, developed by Dr. J.W. Worden (2002), identifies grief not as a succession of phases through which a person passes with little or no control, but as four tasks for the bereaved person:

Accepting the reality of the loss: When someone dies, there is always a sense that it hasn't happened. The first task of grieving is to come full face with the reality that the child is dead, that the child is gone and will not return. The opposite of accepting the loss is not believing through some type of denial. Denial usually involves either the facts of the loss, the significance of the loss to the survivor, or the irreversibility of the loss. To accomplish this task, the parent must talk about the dead child and funeral, as well as the circumstances around the death.

Working through the pain of grief: It is necessary to acknowledge and work through the pain of grief or it will manifest itself through some symptoms or atypical behavior. Not everyone experiences the same intensity of pain or feels it in the same way, but it is impossible to lose someone with whom you have been deeply attached without experiencing some level of pain. The negation of this second task is not to feel.

People may avoid feeling pain by using thought stopping procedures or by avoiding reminders of the child. Many emotions such as shock, anger, guilt and depression may be expressed. The bereaved need to allow themselves to indulge in the pain: to feel it and know that one day it will pass. Some say it is easier to express emotions with someone who knew the child or who can relate to the experience directly.

Adjusting to an environment in which the deceased is missing: Caring for a child takes an amazing amount of time and energy. Parents and other caregivers once consumed with the constant task of meeting the needs of a child are suddenly forced into inactivity. Where responsibility was, is now emptiness. During this adaptation to loss, people can work to avoid promoting their own helplessness by gradually reforming schedules and responsibilities. Creating meaningful rituals like a special memorial or keeping a journal or writing poetry are helpful components of completing this task.

Emotionally relocating the deceased and moving on with life: Survivors sometimes think that if they withdraw their emotional attachment, they are somehow dishonoring the memory of the child. In some cases, parents are frightened by the prospect of having another baby because he or she might also die. For many people, this task is the most difficult one to accomplish. They may get stuck at this point and later realize that their life in some way stopped at the point the loss occurred.

Some bereavement experts note the grieving process includes not only the parent adapting to the loss and returning to functioning in their life, but also includes changing and maintaining their relationship with the infant or child. It is normal for parents to report that they having an ongoing relationship with their child through their memories and mental life.

Factors that may interfere with the grief process:

- Avoiding emotions

- Over activity leading to exhaustion

- Use of alcohol or other drugs

- Unrealistic promises made to the deceased

- Unresolved grief from a previous loss

- Judgmental relationships

- Resentment of those who try to help

Complicated grief is delayed or incomplete adaptation to loss. In complicated grief, there is a failure to return, over time, to pre-loss levels of functioning, or to the previous state of emotional well-being. Grief may be more difficult in younger parents, women, and persons with limited social support, thus increasing their risk for complicated grief. The grief surrounding a child's death is unique in its challenges and may necessitate professional counseling from the clergy, grief counselor, family physician, or mental health professional.

Fathers and Grief

"When is it my turn to cry? I'm not sure society or my upbringing will allow me a time to really cry, unafraid of the reaction and repercussion that might follow. I must be strong, I must support my wife, because I am a man. I must be the cornerstone of our family because society says so, my family says so, and, until I can reverse my learned nature, I say so" (A father in DeFrain, J., L. Ernst, D. Jakub, and J. Taylor, J. 1991, 112).

Although both mothers and fathers grieve deeply when such a tragedy occurs, they grieve differently. Fathers are expected to be strong for their partners, to be the "rock" in the family. All too often fathers are considered to be the ones who should attend to the practical but not the emotional aspects surrounding the death; they are expected to be the ones who should not let emotions show or tears fall outwardly, the ones who will not and should not fall apart. Men are often asked how their wives are doing, but not asked how they are doing.

Such expectations place an unmanageable burden on men and deprive them of their rightful and urgent need to grieve. This need will surface eventually if it is not expressed. It is not unusual for grieving fathers to feel overwhelmed, ignored, isolated, and abandoned, but many say that such strong emotions are very difficult to contain after their child's death.

A father's grief needs to be verbalized and understood by his partner, other family members, professionals, coworkers and friends, and by anyone who will listen. Fathers repeatedly say that for their own peace of mind, they (and those who care about them) need to move away from this mind set and allow themselves to grieve as they need to.

Families Needing Additional Support

The tragedy of a child's death brings profound pain to all affected, and it presents incredibly difficult and unusual problems for all grieving parents. For some parents, the effects of such a complicated and devastating tragedy can be further compounded when the death occurs in a family already experiencing added stress in their lives, such as substance abuse or domestic violence. There are some parents for whom there is no "circle of concern" or extended family. There are also families who choose not to seek out a support network for their own reasons.

It is important to assess each family's special needs and preferences. Additional resources for families include hospice organizations, local health departments, bereavement support programs, and community or religious leaders or healers. Each family's cultural beliefs and practices must be honored during the bereavement process.

Non-Traditional Families

When a non-traditional family experiences the death of an infant, the community's response may be less supportive to that family. It may be necessary to assist the family to seek out support networks that will best address their needs. Examples of a non-traditional family include:

- Single parent

- Unmarried parents

- Teenage parents

- Step-parents

- Parents in blended families

- Adoptive and foster parents

- Gay and lesbian parents

All of these parents and those in traditional families may find their grief unusually complicated. Regardless of the family's composition, parental experience, coping strategies, and cultural practices are unique for each family.

Ways to Comfort a Grieving Parent

- Acknowledge the child's death by telling the parent(s) of your sadness for them and by expressing love and support and trying to provide comfort.

- Allow the parent(s) to express feelings without imposing your views or feelings about what is appropriate behavior. Avoid telling the parent(s) you know just how they feel.

- Allow the parent(s) to cry—it is appropriate to cry with them.

- Visit and talk with the family about the child who died; ask to see pictures or memories the family may have. Refer to the child by name.

- Extend gestures of concern such as bringing flowers or writing a personal note expressing your feelings, letting the parent(s) know of your sadness for them.

- Attend the child's funeral or memorial service.

- Offer to go with the parent(s) to the cemetery in the days and weeks after the funeral, or find other special ways to extend personal or sensitive gestures of concern.

- Remember anniversaries and special days.

- Donate to a specific memorial in honor of the child.

- Make practical and specific suggestions, such as offering to stop by at a convenient time, bringing a meal, purchasing a comforting book, offering to take the other children for a special outing, or treating the parent(s) to something special.

- Respect the dynamics of each person's grief. The often visible expressions of pain and confusion shown by the grieving parent(s) are normal. Grief is an ongoing and demanding process.

- Keep in mind that the parent(s) may not be able to ask for help or tell you what they need.

From One Bereaved Parent to Another

When are you ready to live again? There is no list of events or anniversaries to check off. In fact, you are likely to begin living again before you realize you are doing it. You may catch yourself laughing. You may pick up a book for recreational reading again. You may start playing lighter, happier music. When you do make these steps toward living again, you are likely to feel guilty at first. "What right have I, you may ask yourself, to be happy when my child is dead?" And yet something inside feels as though you are being nudged in this positive direction. You may even have the sense that this nudge is from your child, or at least a feeling that your child approves of it (Horchler and Morris, 2003, 178).

All newly bereaved parents must find ways to get through, not over, their grief—to go on with their lives. Each is forced to continue life's journey in an individual manner.

Many bereaved parents find solace in their religion. Seeking spiritual comfort in a time of grief does not mean repressing the grief.

Many grieving parents also find comfort in rituals. Funerals or memorial services have served many parents as beautiful and meaningful ways of saying goodbye, providing a sense of closure after the child's death. For others, sending announcement cards about the baby's death, writing poems, keeping journals or writing down personal reflections or prayers, or volunteering with a parental bereavement group become ways to remember and honor the child who died.

Grief is the natural response to any loss. Healing for bereaved parents can begin to occur by acknowledging and sharing their grief.

Friends and caregivers who care should grieve and mourn with the parents; and be willing to listen. Bereaved parents need to know that their child will be remembered, not just by them but also by family and friends. They need to have the child acknowledged and referred to by name. They want that child's life to matter. They do not want to forget and they don't want others to forget.

Ways That Help Parents Cope and Heal from the Sudden Loss of a Child

- Admitting to themselves and others that their grief is overwhelming, unpredictable, painful, draining, and exhausting—that th eir grief should not be diminished or ignored.

- Allowing themselves to be angry and acknowledging that they are vulnerable, helpless, and feeling disoriented.

- Trying to understand that to grieve is to heal and that integrating grief into their lives is a necessity.

- Acknowledging the need and desire to talk about the child who died as well as the moments and events that will be missed and never experienced with the child.

- Maintaining a belief in the significance of their child's life, no mattcr how short.

- Creating memorial services and other rituals as ways to commemorate the child's life.

- Deriving support from religious beliefs, a sense of spirituality, or a personal faith.

- Expressing feelings in journals, poetry, prayers, or other reflective writings or in art, music, or other creative activities.

- Trying to be patient and forgiving with themselves and others and refraining from making hasty decisions.

- Counting on, confiding in, and trusting those who care, listen, and hear, those who will walk with them, and not be critical of them, those who will try to understand their emotional and physical limitations, while also trying to understand and respect the limitations of their caretakers.

- Increasing their physical activity and maintaining a healthful diet.

- Volunteering their services to organizations concerned with support for bereaved parents.

- Obtaining help from traditional support systems, such as family, friends, professionals or religious groups, undergoing professional counseling, joining a parent support group, or acquiring information on the type of death that occurred as well as about their own grief.

- Reassuring themselves and others that they were and still are loving parents.

- Letting go of fear and guilt when the time seems right and the grief seems less.

- Accepting that they are allowed to feel pleasure and continue their lives, knowing their love for the child transcends death.

Chapter 42

Helping Children Cope with Death

When a loved one dies, children feel and show their grief in different ways. How kids cope with the loss depends on things like their age, how close they felt to the person who died, and the support they receive.

Here are some things parents can do to help a child who has lost a loved one:

When talking about death, use simple, clear words. To break the news that someone has died, approach your child in a caring way. Use words that are simple and direct. For example, "I have some sad news to tell you. Grandma died today." Pause to give your child a moment to take in your words.

Listen and comfort. Every child reacts differently to learning that a loved one has died. Some kids cry. Some ask questions. Others seem not to react at all. That's OK. Stay with your child to offer hugs or reassurance. Answer your child's questions or just be together for a few minutes.

Put emotions into words. Encourage kids to say what they're thinking and feeling in the days, weeks, and months following the loss. Talk about your own feelings: It helps kids be aware of and feel

---

comfortable with theirs. Say things like, "I know you're feeling very sad. I'm sad, too. We both loved Grandma so much, and she loved us, too."

Tell your child what to expect. If the death of a loved one means changes in your child's life, head off any worries or fears by explaining what will happen. For example, "Aunt Sara will pick you up from school like Grandma used to." Or, "I need to stay with Grandpa for a few days. That means you and Dad will be home taking care of each other. But I'll talk to you every day, and I'll be back on Sunday."

Talk about funerals and rituals. Allow children to join in rituals like viewings, funerals, or memorial services. Tell your child ahead of time what will happen. For example, "Lots of people who loved Grandma will be there. We will sing, pray, and talk about Grandma's life. People might cry and hug. People will say things like, 'I'm sorry for your loss,' or, 'My condolences.' Those are polite and kind things to say to the family at a funeral. We can say, 'Thank you,' or, 'Thanks for coming.' You can stay near me and hold my hand if you want."

You might need to explain burial or cremation. For example, "After the funeral, there is a burial at a cemetery. The person's body is in a casket (or coffin) that gets buried in the ground with a special ceremony. This can feel like a sad goodbye, and people might cry." Share your family's beliefs about what happens to a person's soul or spirit after death.

Explain what happens after the service as a way to show that people will feel better. For example, "We all will go eat food together. People will laugh, talk, and hug some more. Focusing on the happy memories about Grandma and on the good feeling of being together helps people start to feel better."

Give your child a role. Having a small, active role can help kids master an unfamiliar and emotional situation such as a funeral or memorial service. For example, you might invite your child to read a poem, pick a song to be played, gather some photos to display, or make something. Let kids decide if they want to take part, and how.

Help your child remember the person. In the days and weeks ahead, encourage your child to draw pictures or write down favorite stories of their loved one. Don't avoid mentioning the person who died. Recalling and sharing happy memories helps heal grief and activate positive feelings.

Respond to emotions with comfort and reassurance. Notice if your child seems sad, worried, or upset in other ways. Ask about feelings and listen. Let your child know that it takes time to feel better after a loved one dies. Some kids may temporarily have trouble concentrating or sleeping, or have fears or worries. Support groups and counseling can help kids who need more support.

Help your child feel better. Provide the comfort your child needs, but don't dwell on sad feelings. After a few minutes of talking and listening, shift to an activity or topic that helps your child feel a little better. Play, make art, cook, or go somewhere together.

Give your child time to heal from the loss. Grief is a process that happens over time. Be sure to have ongoing conversations to see how your child is feeling and doing. Healing doesn't mean forgetting about the loved one. It means remembering the person with love, and letting loving memories stir good feelings that support us as we go on to enjoy life.

Chapter 43

Guiding Children through Grief

Children and Grief

A Child's Grief Process Is Different from an Adult's.

Children do not react to loss in the same ways as adults. These are some of the ways children's grief is different:

- Children may seem to show grief only once in a while and for short times. This may be because a child is not able to feel strong emotions for long periods of time. A grieving child may be sad one minute and playful the next. Often families think the child doesn't really understand the loss or has gotten over it quickly. Usually, neither is true. Children's minds protect them from what is too much for them to handle emotionally.

- Mourning is a process that continues over years in children. Feelings of loss may occur again and again as the child gets older. This is common at important times, such as going to camp, graduating from school, getting married, or having children.

This chapter includes text excerpted from "Grief, Bereavement, and Coping with Loss (PDQ®)–Patient Version," National Cancer Institute (NCI), March 6, 2013.

- Grieving children may not show their feelings as openly as adults. Grieving children may throw themselves into activities instead of withdrawing or showing grief.

- Children cannot think through their thoughts and feelings like adults. Children have trouble putting their feelings about grief into words. Strong feelings of anger and fears of death or being left alone may show up in the behavior of grieving children. Children often play death games as a way of working out their feelings and worries. These games give children a safe way to express their feelings.

- Grieving adults may withdraw and not talk to other people about the loss. Children, however, often talk to the people around them (even strangers) to see how they react and to get clues for how they should respond to the loss.

- Children may ask confusing questions. For example, a child may ask, "I know grandpa died, but when will he come home?" This is a way of testing reality and making sure the story of the death has not changed.

Several Factors Can Affect How a Child Will Cope with Grief.

Although grief is different for each child, several factors can affect the grief process of a child:

- The child's age and stage of development.

- The child's personality.

- The child's previous experiences with death.

- The child's relationship with the deceased.

- The cause of death.

- The way the child acts and communicates within the family.

- How stable the family life is after the loss.

- How the child continues to be cared for.

- Whether the child is given the chance to share and express feelings and memories.

- How the parents cope with stress.

- Whether the child has ongoing relationships with other adults.

Children at Different Stages of Development Have Different Understandings of Death and the Events near Death.

Infants

Infants do not recognize death, but feelings of loss and separation are part of developing an awareness of death. Children who have been separated from their mother may be sluggish and quiet, may not respond to a smile or a coo, may have physical symptoms (such as weight loss), and may sleep less.

Age 2-3 years

Children at this age often confuse death with sleep and may feel anxiety as early as age 3. They may stop talking and appear to feel overall distress.

Age 3-6 years

At this age children see death as a kind of sleep; the person is alive, but only in a limited way. The child cannot fully separate death from life. Children may think that the person is still living, even though he or she might have been buried. The child may ask questions about the deceased (for example, how does the deceased eat, go to the toilet, breathe, or play?). Young children know that death is physical, but think it is not final.

The child's understanding of death may involve "magical thinking." For example, the child may think that his or her thoughts can cause another person to become sick or die.

Grieving children under 5 may have trouble eating, sleeping, and controlling the bladder and bowel.

Age 6-9 years

Children at this age are often very curious about death, and may ask questions about what happens to the body when it dies. Death is thought of as a person or spirit separate from the person who was alive, such as a skeleton, ghost, angel, or bogeyman. They may see death as final and scary but as something that happens mostly to old people (and not to themselves).

Grieving children can become afraid of school, have learning problems, show antisocial or aggressive behavior, or become overly worried about their own health and complain of imaginary symptoms. Children this age may either withdraw from others or become too attached and clingy.

Boys often become more aggressive and destructive (for example, acting out in school), instead of showing their sadness openly.

311

When one parent dies, children may feel abandoned by both the deceased parent and the living parent, whose grief may make him or her unable to emotionally support the child.

Age 9 and older

Children aged 9 and older know that death cannot be avoided and do not see it as a punishment. By the time a child is 12 years old, death is seen as final and something that happens to everyone.

Grief and Developmental Stages

Table 43.1.

Age	Understanding of Death	Expressions of Grief
Infancy to 2 years	Is not yet able to understand death.	Quietness, crankiness, decreased activity, poor sleep, and weight loss.
	Separation from mother causes changes.	
2-6 years	Death is like sleeping.	Asks many questions (How does she go to the bathroom? How does she eat?).
		Problems in eating, sleeping, and bladder and bowel control.
		Fear of being abandoned.
		Tantrums.
	Dead person continues to live and function in some ways.	"Magical thinking" (Did I think or do something that caused the death? Like when I said I hate you and I wish you would die?).
	Death is not final.	
	Dead person can come back to life.	
6-9 years	Death is thought of as a person or spirit (skeleton, ghost, bogeyman).	Curious about death.
		Asks specific questions.
		May have fears about school.
	Death is final and scary.	May have aggressive behavior (especially boys).
		Worries about imaginary illnesses.
	Death happens to others, it won't happen to me.	May feel abandoned.

Table 43.1. Continued

Age	Understanding of Death	Expressions of Grief
9 and older	Everyone will die.	Strong emotions, guilt, anger, shame.
		Increased anxiety over own death.
		Mood swings.
	Death is final.	Fear of rejection; not wanting to be different from peers.
	Even I will die.	Changes in eating habits.
		Sleeping problems.
		Regressive behavior (loss of interest in outside activities).
		Impulsive behavior.
		Feels guilty about being alive (especially related to death of a brother, sister, or peer).

Most Children Who Have Had a Loss Have Three Common Worries about Death.

Children coping with a loss often have these three questions:

Did I make the death happen?

Children often think that they have "magical powers." If a mother is irritated and says, "You'll be the death of me" and later dies, her child may wonder if he or she actually caused the mother's death. Also, when children argue, one may say (or think), "I wish you were dead." If that child dies, the surviving child may think that those thoughts caused the death.

Is it going to happen to me?

The death of another child may be very hard for a child. If the child thinks that the death may have been prevented (by either a parent or a doctor) the child may fear that he or she could also die.

Who is going to take care of me?

Since children depend on parents and other adults to take care of them, a grieving child may wonder who will care for him or her after the death of an important person.

Talking honestly about the death and including the child in rituals may help the grieving child.

Explain the death and answer questions.

Talking about death helps children learn to cope with loss. When talking about death with children, describe it simply. Each child should be told the truth using as much detail as he or she is able to understand. Answer questions in language the child can understand.

Children often worry that they will also die, or that their surviving parent will go away. They need to be told that they will be safe and taken care of.

Use the correct language.

When talking with the child about death, include the correct words, such as "cancer," "died," and "death." Using other words or phrases (for example, "he passed away," "he is sleeping," or "we lost him") can confuse children and cause them to misunderstand.

Include the child in planning and attending memorial ceremonies.

When a death occurs, children may feel better if they are included in planning and attending memorial ceremonies. These events help children remember the loved one. Children should not be forced to be involved in these ceremonies, but encourage them to take part when they feel comfortable doing so. Before a child attends a funeral, wake, or memorial service, give the child a full explanation of what to expect. A familiar adult or family member may help with this if the surviving parent's grief makes him or her unable to.

Part Seven

Legal and Economic Issues
at the End of Life

Chapter 44

Getting Your Affairs in Order

Plan for the Future

No one ever plans to be sick or disabled. Yet, it's this kind of planning that can make all the difference in an emergency. Long before she fell, Louise put all her important papers in one place and told her son where to find them. She gave him the name of her lawyer, as well as a list of people he could contact at her bank, doctor's office, insurance company, and investment firm. She made sure he had copies of her Medicare and other health insurance cards. She added her son's name to her checking account and safe deposit box at the bank. Louise made sure Medicare and her doctor had written permission to talk with her son about her health and insurance claims.

On the other hand, Ben always took care of family money matters, and he never talked about the details with Shirley. No one but Ben knew that his life insurance policy was in a box in the closet or that the car title and deed to the house were filed in his desk drawer. Ben never expected that his wife would have to take over. His lack of planning has made a tough job even tougher for Shirley.

What Exactly Is an "Important Paper"?

The answer to this question may be different for every family. Remember, this is a starting place. You may have other information to

This chapter includes text excerpted from "Getting Your Affairs in Order," National Institute on Aging (NIA), National Institutes of Health (NIH), July 2016.

add. For example, if you have a pet, you will want to include the name and address of your veterinarian. Include complete information about:

Personal Records

- Full legal name
- Social Security number
- Legal residence
- Date and place of birth
- Names and addresses of spouse and children
- Location of birth and death certificates and certificates of marriage, divorce, citizenship, and adoption
- Employers and dates of employment
- Education and military records
- Names and phone numbers of religious contacts
- Memberships in groups and awards received
- Names and phone numbers of close friends, relatives, doctors, lawyers, and financial advisors
- Medications taken regularly (be sure to update this regularly)
- Location of living will and other legal documents

Financial Records

- Sources of income and assets (pension from your employer, IRAs, 401(k)s, interest, etc.)
- Social Security and Medicare/Medicaid information
- Insurance information (life, health, long-term care, home, car) with policy numbers and agents' names and phone numbers
- Names of your banks and account numbers (checking, savings, credit union)
- Investment income (stocks, bonds, property) and stockbrokers' names and phone numbers
- Copy of most recent income tax return
- Location of most up-to-date will with an original signature

- Liabilities, including property tax—what is owed, to whom, and when payments are due

- Mortgages and debts—how and when they are paid

- Location of original deed of trust for home

- Car title and registration

- Credit and debit card names and numbers

- Location of safe deposit box and key

Steps for Getting Your Affairs in Order

- **Put your important papers and copies of legal documents in one place.** You can set up a file, put everything in a desk or dresser drawer, or list the information and location of papers in a notebook. If your papers are in a bank safe deposit box, keep copies in a file at home. Check each year to see if there's anything new to add.

- **Tell a trusted family member or friend where you put all your important papers.** You don't need to tell this friend or family member about your personal affairs, but someone should know where you keep your papers in case of an emergency. If you don't have a relative or friend you trust, ask a lawyer to help.

- **Give permission in advance for your doctor or lawyer to talk with your caregiver as needed.** There may be questions about your care, a bill, or a health insurance claim. Without your consent, your caregiver may not be able to get needed information. You can give your okay in advance to Medicare, a credit card company, your bank, or your doctor. You may need to sign and return a form.

Legal Documents

There are many different types of legal documents that can help you plan how your affairs will be handled in the future. Many of these documents have names that sound alike, so make sure you are getting the documents you want. Also, State laws vary, so find out about the rules, requirements, and forms used in your State.

Wills and trusts let you name the person you want your money and property to go to after you die.

Advance directives let you make arrangements for your care if you become sick. There are two ways to do this:

- A living will gives you a say in your healthcare if you become too sick to make your wishes known. In a living will, you can state what kind of care you do or don't want. This can make it easier for family members to make tough healthcare decisions for you.

- A durable power of attorney for healthcare lets you name the person you want to make medical decisions for you if you can't make them yourself. Make sure the person you name is willing to make those decisions for you.

For legal matters, there are two ways to give someone you trust the power to act in your place:

- A general power of attorney lets you give someone else the authority to act on your behalf, but this power will end if you are unable to make your own decisions.

- A durable power of attorney allows you to name someone to act on your behalf for any legal task, but it stays in place if you become unable to make your own decisions.

Resources

You may want to talk with a lawyer about setting up a general power of attorney, durable power of attorney, joint account, trust, or advance directive. Be sure to ask about the lawyer's fees before you make an appointment.

You should be able to find a directory of local lawyers at your library, or you can contact your local bar association for lawyers in your area. Your local bar association can also help you find what free legal aid options your State has to offer. An informed family member may be able to help you manage some of these issues.

Chapter 45

Patients' Rights

Chapter Contents

Section 45.1

Informed Consent

This section contains text excerpted from the following sources:
Text in this section begins with excerpts from "Patient Rights,"
U.S. Department of Health and Human Services (HHS), August
31, 2016; Text beginning with the heading "Basic Premise of
Informed Consent" is excerpted from "Informed Consent," Indian
Health Service (IHS), U.S. Department of Health and Human
Services (HHS), April 27, 2007. Reviewed October 2016.

As a patient, you have certain rights. Some are guaranteed by
federal law, such as the right to get a copy of your medical records,
and the right to keep them private. Many states have additional laws
protecting patients, and healthcare facilities often have a patient bill
of rights.

An important patient right is informed consent. This means that
if you need a treatment, your healthcare provider must give you the
information you need to make a decision. Many hospitals have patient
advocates who can help you if you have problems. Many states have
an ombudsman office for problems with long term care. Your state's
department of health may also be able to help.

Basic Premise of Informed Consent

The basic premise of informed consent dates back to the early part
of this century, and centers on the principle of battery. Courts have
clearly ruled that "every human being of adult years and sound mind
has a right to determine what shall be done with his own body." Most
states now have specific informed consent statutes, yet even in the
absence of such laws physicians have a common law duty to ensure
that diagnostic, medical, and surgical procedures are authorized by the
knowledgeable consent of the patient or his/her legal representative.
A physician who fails to obtain his/her patient's consent to treatment
commits a battery.

It is very important to realize that courts have increasingly held that
informed consent is a process, not just a piece of paper. A written and
signed consent form will not necessarily withstand a legal challenge

if it can be shown that the patient was not adequately informed about the treatment, risks, and alternative procedures available.

Informed Consent Standards

Courts generally use one of two informed consent standards. The older "professional disclosure" standard is followed in about half the states. This standard requires the physician to disclose to the patient everything that is customary in the profession to disclose under the same or similar circumstances. In court, plaintiffs in these states must produce an expert witness to testify that the defendant's actions fell below the standard of customary disclosure.

The newer "reasonable patient standard" has been adopted in the remaining states. Under this standard, physicians are required to tell their patients everything that would reasonably bear on a decision to submit to treatment. Because expert testimony is not needed, it is generally easier to sue on informed consent grounds in states using this standard. In the case of federal court malpractice suits, the standard of the state in which the facility is located is used.

Most courts also require proximate cause. This means that plaintiffs must also prove that a reasonable person would not have gone through with the procedure if they had been fully informed of the risks and alternatives. In the case of elective surgery, it is easier for a patient to prove that he/she would not want the procedure if additional information had been provided; for more urgent or life saving procedures, the plaintiff's argument must be much more convincing. As a general rule, the more elective the procedure (and hence the greater the number of therapeutic alternatives), the more detailed the disclosure should be.

Required Elements: No matter what standard is applicable, there are five basic elements that must be disclosed to patients in language that a lay individual reasonably can be expected to understand:

1. The diagnosis, including the disclosure of any reservations the provider has concerning the diagnosis;

2. The nature and purpose of the proposed procedure or treatment;

3. The risks and consequences of the proposed procedure or treatment. This includes only those risks and consequences of which the physician has, or reasonably should have, knowledge. It is not necessary to disclose every potential minor risk or side effect.

4. Reasonable treatment alternatives. This includes other treatment modalities that are considered to be appropriate for the situation, even though they may not be the personal preference of the disclosing physician.

5. Prognosis without treatment. The patient must be informed of the potential consequences, if he/she elects not to have the recommended procedure.

Therapeutic Privilege: Under limited circumstances, courts have recognized that a physician may be justified in withholding information if it can be shown to be in the patient's best interest. This privilege applies only when a patient is unusually sensitive, anxious, or emotional.

Patient hypersensitivity should never be presumed. There must be ample justification for withholding information and the physician should carefully document his/her reasoning in the medical record. If the physician's use of the therapeutic privilege is challenged, it must be determined whether the physician acted appropriately. The use of this therapeutic privilege should be relied upon only in rare circumstances.

Implied Consent: Consent is either expressed (verbally or written) or implied. Consent may be implied under a variety of circumstances. For example, when a patient comes to see a physician for a particular ailment, it is implied that they consent to be examined. If a patient has a fractured arm, it is implied that he consents to casting. In general, physicians can assume that most patients would readily consent to care or treatments that are customary, noninvasive, and non-experimental.

Implied consent also relates to the performance of additional procedures when medically justified. When a physician is performing a hysterectomy, for example, an incidental appendectomy cannot be performed without the patient's expressed consent to do so. However, if the appendix is diseased, it is reasonable to assume that the patient would allow the procedure, unless the patient had expressly prohibited the appendix from being removed.

The use of general or blanket consent forms is not sound practice. These types of consent forms do not represent true informed consent as they are often solicited by an admission clerk, adequate information is not given, and they are not specific to any particular treatment or procedure. Blanket consent forms only serve as evidence of the patient's voluntary submission to treatment in general, which is usually self evident (implied), but these types of forms do not demonstrate that the patient understood specific indications and risks of any proposed invasive procedures. Again, it is recommended that blanket consent forms not be used.

Who May Give Consent: If the patient is a competent adult, the authority to give consent to treatment rests exclusively with the patient, unless the patient formally delegates that authority to someone else. Through the use of a document called a "power of attorney," executed in writing, a competent adult can delegate the responsibility for healthcare decisions to another competent adult.

A power of attorney in most states becomes ineffective when the person granting it becomes incompetent. For this reason, many states now recognize a "durable power of attorney," which generally remains effective even after the person granting the power becomes incompetent. In the healthcare setting, a durable power of attorney is the preferred document. Healthcare providers should always be careful to ensure that the proposed treatment lies within the scope of the expressed authorization.

Individuals who have not attained the legal age of majority (in most states, age 18) cannot legally give consent except in the following situations:

1. The patient is an emancipated minor (e.g., the minor is married, lives away from their parent's home, or is financially independent);

2. The state has fixed a lower limit of age for certain healthcare decisions (such as in the case of abortion, pregnancy, and treatment of venereal disease);

3. The state recognizes a "mature minor" exception, which allows minors to give consent to healthcare when there is a pressing need and the parent or guardian is unavailable. It is recommended that the reader be familiar with the laws in the state in which you practice.

The law holds that the closest available relative or legal guardian can authorize necessary and reasonable care when the patient is incapable of giving consent because of age, incompetency, or incapacity. A healthcare provider acting on the reasonable belief that a person is the patient's next of kin is legally protected if the authorizing person turns out not to be a close relative.

Emergency Situations: When the need for care is urgent, the patient is unable to give consent, and it is not feasible to contact the patient's next of kin, then the law does allow the physician to proceed with life saving diagnostic and therapeutic procedures without informed consent. The emergency consent exception is based on the following concepts:

1. The healthcare provider is entitled to presume that the patient would have chosen the care others would have chosen under similar circumstances, unless the provider has information to the contrary;

2. The exception only applies to situations where immediate action is necessary to preserve life (or in some states "to prevent serious physical harm");

3. The circumstances justifying the emergency consent exception are well documented, including all attempts to notify the next of kin before treatment is begun.

Informed Refusal: The issue of documenting informed refusal is a relatively recent development. It is clear, as noted above, that patients have both the right to determine what is done to their body, and what is not. However, a patient should be very well informed if he/she is going to refuse a well established, common procedure such as a cancer screening test. On more than one occasion when patients have sued over a delayed diagnosis of cancer, courts have held that the physician was liable because he/she failed to adequately inform a patient about the consequences of the patient's prior refusal to accept standard cancer screening procedures.

For this reason, it is becoming more common for physicians to send registered letters to patients who decline certain types of care, informing them of the consequences in detail. Alternatively there may be circumstances where it would be wise to have the patient sign a written "informed refusal" document. Is this necessary every time a patient declines a test? No, but it would seem prudent to assess each situation carefully.

Document, Document, Document: All physicians should accept the doctrine of informed consent. It has b ethical and moral backing, it emanates from the right of self-determination and the right to privacy, and healthcare providers should not expect the courts to lose interest in patient rights.

In most states, verbal consent to treatment is legally sound, but it is very difficult for the provider to prove what the patient was told in the event that an adverse outcome leads to a malpractice claim.

There is no question that written documentation enhances a physician's credibility. It therefore makes for good defensive medicine to carefully document the informed consent process, which includes, but is not limited to, a form that details the information disclosed to the patient, signed by both the patient and provider, and witnessed by a third party. It is helpful to have a third person (preferably a healthcare provider) present at the counseling session to witness the exchange of information, help solicit and answer questions, verify that the patient understands the information, and attest that the session took place. By signing the consent form, the third party is serving as a witness, and he/ she is not liable for the quality and sufficiency of the information given.

The patient-counseling session must be documented. There should be ample written evidence that informed consent was given to the patient, and the process by which it was given. In addition to a signed consent form, a progress note should include the fact that a counseling session took place, the mode of information delivery, and any additional clinically important details not specified on the consent form.

The American College of Surgeons recommends that the following principles be adhered to when documenting informed consent:

1. There should be a clear explanation of each medical term in lay language;

2. There should be a listing of commonly occurring risks of the procedure;

3. Never describe a procedure as "simple," "uncomplicated," or "minor." The consent form should include a statement that no result has been guaranteed;

4. Avoid the use of national statistics, as the operating surgeon's own experience may vary from the national norm;

5. Indicate on the consent form if the patient has been given an informational brochure or shown a video;

6. The patient should acknowledge on the consent form that the information disclosed has been understood, that an opportunity to ask questions has been provided, and that all questions have been answered to the patient's satisfaction;

7. The signature of both the patient and operating surgeon should be on the consent form, timed and dated;

8. The form should include a statement indicating that "unexpected risks or complications not discussed may occur," and that "unforeseen conditions may be revealed requiring the performance of additional procedures, and I authorize such procedures to be performed."

Section 45.2

Health Information Privacy Rights

This section contains text excerpted from the following sources:
Text beginning with the heading "Health Insurance Portability
and Accountability Act (HIPAA)" is excerpted from "What Does the
HIPAA Privacy Rule Do?" U.S. Department of Health and Human
Services (HHS), July 26, 2013; Text under the heading "Rights and
Protections for Everyone with Medicare" is excerpted from "Medicare
Rights and Protections," Medicare.gov, Centers for Medicare and
Medicaid Services (CMS), July 15, 2014.

Health Insurance Portability and Accountability Act (HIPAA)

Most of us feel that our health information is private and should be protected. That is why there is a federal law that sets rules for healthcare providers and health insurance companies about who can look at and receive our health information. This law, called the Health Insurance Portability and Accountability Act of 1996 (HIPAA), gives you rights over your health information, including the right to get a copy of your information, make sure it is correct, and know who has seen it.

Get It. You can ask to see or get a copy of your medical record and other health information. If you want a copy, you may have to put your request in writing and pay for the cost of copying and mailing. In most cases, your copies must be given to you within 30 days.

Check It. You can ask to change any wrong information in your file or add information to your file if you think something is missing or incomplete. For example, if you and your hospital agree that your file has the wrong result for a test, the hospital must change it. Even if the hospital believes the test result is correct, you still have the right to have your disagreement noted in your file. In most cases, the file should be updated within 60 days.

Know Who Has Seen It. By law, your health information can be used and shared for specific reasons not directly related to your care, like making sure doctors give good care, making sure nursing homes are clean and safe, reporting when the flu is in your area, or reporting as required by state or federal law. In many of these cases, you can find out who has seen your health information. You can:

Learn how your health information is used and shared by your doctor or health insurer. Generally, your health information cannot be used for purposes not directly related to your care without your permission. For example, your doctor cannot give it to your employer, or share it for things like marketing and advertising, without your written authorization. You probably received a notice telling you how your health information may be used on your first visit to a new healthcare provider or when you got new health insurance, but you can ask for another copy anytime.

Let your providers or health insurance companies know if there is information you do not want to share. You can ask that your health information not be shared with certain people, groups, or companies. If you go to a clinic, for example, you can ask the doctor not to share your medical records with other doctors or nurses at the clinic. You can ask for other kinds of restrictions, but they do not always have to agree to do what you ask, particularly if it could affect your care. Finally, you can also ask your healthcare provider or pharmacy not to tell your health insurance company about care you receive or drugs you take, if you pay for the care or drugs in full and the provider or pharmacy does not need to get paid by your insurance company.

Ask to be reached somewhere other than home. You can make reasonable requests to be contacted at different places or in a different way. For example, you can ask to have a nurse call you at your office instead of your home or to send mail to you in an envelope instead of on a postcard.

If you think your rights are being denied or your health information is not being protected, you have the right to file a complaint with your provider, health insurer, or the U.S. Department of Health and Human Services.

Employers and Health Information in the Workplace

The Privacy Rule controls how a health plan or a covered health-care provider shares your protected health information with an employer.

Employment Records

The Privacy Rule does not protect your employment records, even if the information in those records is health-related. In most cases, the Privacy Rule does not apply to the actions of an employer.

If you work for a health plan or a covered healthcare provider:

- The Privacy Rule does not apply to your employment records.

- The Rule does protect your medical or health plan records if you are a patient of the provider or a member of the health plan.

Requests from Your Employer

Your employer can ask you for a doctor's note or other health information if they need the information for sick leave, workers' compensation, wellness programs, or health insurance.

However, if your employer asks your healthcare provider directly for information about you, your provider cannot give your employer the information without your authorization unless other laws require them to do so.

Generally, the Privacy Rule applies to the disclosures made by your healthcare provider, not the questions your employer may ask.

For employer issues, contact:

- Department of Labor: (866) 4-USA-DOL

- Equal Employment Opportunity Commission: (800) 669-4000

Personal Representatives

Generally, an HIPAA-covered healthcare provider or health plan must allow your personal representative to inspect and receive a copy of protected health information about you that they maintain.

Naming a Personal Representative

Your personal representative can be named several ways; state law may affect this process.

If a person can make healthcare decisions for you using a healthcare power of attorney, the person is your personal representative.

Children

The personal representative of a minor child is usually the child's parent or legal guardian.? State laws may affect guardianship.?

In cases where a custody decree exists, the personal representative is the parent(s) who can make healthcare decisions for the child under the custody decree.

Deceased Persons

When an individual dies, the personal representative for the deceased is the executor or administrator of the deceased individual's estate, or the person who is legally authorized by a court or by state law to act on the behalf of the deceased individual or his or her estate.

Exceptions

A provider or plan may choose not to treat a person as your personal representative if the provider or plan reasonably believes that the person might endanger you in situations of domestic violence, abuse, or neglect.

Family Members and Friends

The Privacy Rule does not require a healthcare provider or health plan to share information with your family or friends, unless they are your?personal representatives.

However, the provider or plan can share your information with family or friends if:

- They are involved in your healthcare or payment for your healthcare,

- You tell the provider or plan that it can do so,

- You do not object to sharing of the information, or

- If, using its professional judgment, a provider or plan believes that you do not object.

Examples

- If you do not object, your doctor could talk with the friend who goes with you to the hospital or with a family member who pays your medical bill.?

- If you send your friend to pick up your prescription for you, the pharmacist can assume that you do not object to their being given the medication. ?

- When you are not there or when you are injured and cannot give your permission, a provider may share information with these people if it seems like this would be in your best interest.

Court Orders and Subpoenas

Court Order

A HIPAA-covered healthcare provider or health plan may share your protected health information if it has a court order. This includes the order of an administrative tribunal. However, the provider or plan may only disclose the information specifically described in the order.

Subpoena

A subpoena issued by someone other than a judge, such as a court clerk or an attorney in a case, is different from a court order.

A HIPAA-covered provider or plan may disclose information to a party issuing a subpoena only if the notification requirements of the Privacy Rule are met. Before responding to the subpoena, the provider or plan should receive evidence that there were reasonable efforts to:

Notify the person who is the subject of the information about the request, so the person has a chance to object to the disclosure, or

Seek a qualified protective order for the information from the court.

Notice of Privacy Practices

What Is the HIPAA Notice I Receive from My Doctor and Health Plan?

Your healthcare provider and health plan must give you a notice that tells you how they may use and share your health information. It must also include your health privacy rights. In most cases, you should receive the notice on your first visit to a provider or in the mail from your health plan. You can also ask for a copy at any time.

Why Do I Have to Sign a Form?

The law requires your doctor, hospital, or other healthcare provider to ask you to state in writing that you received the notice.

- The law does not require you to sign the "acknowledgement of receipt of the notice."
- Signing does not mean that you have agreed to any special uses or disclosures (sharing) of your health records.
- Refusing to sign the acknowledgement does not prevent a provider or plan from using or disclosing health information as HIPAA permits.
- If you refuse to sign the acknowledgement, the provider must keep a record of this fact.

What Is in the Notice?

The notice must describe:

- How the Privacy Rule allows provider to use and disclose protected health information. It must also explain that your permission (authorization) is necessary before your health records are shared for any other reason
- The organization's duties to protect health information privacy
- Your privacy rights, including the right to complain to HHS and to the organization if you believe your privacy rights have been violated
- How to contact the organization for more information and to make a complaint

When and How Can I Receive a Notice of Privacy Practices?

You'll usually receive notice at your first appointment. In an emergency, you should receive notice as soon as possible after the emergency.

The notice must also be posted in a clear and easy to find location where patients are able to see it, and a copy must be provided to anyone who asks for one.

If an organization has a website, it must post the notice there.

A health plan must give its notice to you at enrollment. It must also send a reminder at least once every three years that you can ask for the notice at any time.

A health plan can give the notice to the "named insured" (subscriber for coverage). It does not also have to give separate notices to spouses and dependents.

Rights and Protections for Everyone with Medicare

No matter how you get your Medicare, you have certain rights and protections designed to:

- Protect you when you get healthcare.

- Make sure you get the healthcare services that the law says you can get.

- Protect you against unethical practices.

- Protect your privacy.

You have these rights:

- Be treated with dignity and respect at all times.

- Be protected from discrimination.

- Discrimination is against the law. Every company or agency that works with Medicare must obey the law, and can't treat you differently because of your race, color, national origin, disability, age, or sex.

- Have your personal and health information kept private.

If you have Original Medicare, see the "Notice of Privacy Practices for Original Medicare." You can view this notice in the "Medicare & You" handbook.

If you have a Medicare Advantage Plan (like an HMO or PPO), other Medicare health plan, or a Medicare Prescription Drug Plan, read your plan materials.

Get information in a way you understand from Medicare, healthcare providers, and contractors.

Get clear and simple information about Medicare to help you make healthcare decisions, including:

- What's covered.

- What Medicare pays.

- How much you have to pay.

- What to do if you want to file a complaint or an appeal.

- Have your questions about Medicare answered.

- Call 1-800-MEDICARE (1-800-633-4227). TTY users should call 1-877-486-2048.

- Call your State Health Insurance Assistance Program (SHIP). To get the most up-to-date SHIP phone numbers, call 1-800-MEDICARE.

- Call your plan if you have a Medicare Advantage Plan, other Medicare health plan, or a Medicare Prescription Drug Plan.

- Have access to doctors, specialists, and hospitals.

- Learn about your treatment choices in clear language that you can understand, and participate in treatment decisions. You have the right to participate fully in all your healthcare decisions. If you can't fully participate, ask a family member, friend, or someone you trust to help you make a decision about what treatment is right for you.

- Get healthcare services in a language you understand an a culturally sensitive way.

- Get emergency care when and where you need it.

- If your health is in danger because you have a bad injury, sudden illness, or an illness that quickly gets much worse, call 911. You can get emergency care anywhere in the United States.

If you have a Medicare Advantage Plan or other Medicare health plan, your plan materials describe how to get emergency care. You don't need to get permission from your primary care doctor (the doctor you see first for health problems) before you get emergency care. If you're admitted to the hospital, you, a family member, or your primary care doctor should contact your plan as soon as possible.

If you get emergency care, you'll have to pay your regular share of the cost (copayment). Then, your plan will pay its share. If your plan doesn't pay its share for your emergency care, you have the right to appeal.

- Get a decision about healthcare payment, coverage of services, or prescription drug coverage. When you request coverage for items or services, or a claim is filed for items or services you got, you'll get a notice from Medicare or be notified by your Medicare Advantage Plan, other Medicare health plan, or Medicare Prescription Drug Plan letting you know what it will and won't cover. If you disagree with this decision, you have the right to file an appeal.

- Request a review (appeal) of certain decisions about healthcare payment, coverage of services, or prescription drug coverage. If you disagree with a decision about your claims or services, you have the right to appeal.

For more information on appeals:

- Call 1-800-MEDICARE (1-800-633-4227) to find out if a copy can be mailed to you. TTY users should call 1-877-486-2048.

- If you have a Medicare Advantage Plan, other Medicare health plan, or a Medicare Prescription Drug Plan, read your plan materials.

- Call the SHIP in your state. To get the most up-to-date SHIP phone numbers.

- File complaints (sometimes called "grievances"), including complaints about the quality of your care.

- You can file a complaint about services you got, other concerns or problems you have in getting healthcare, or the quality of the healthcare you got.

- If you're concerned about the quality of the care you received, you have the right to file a complaint.

- If you have Original Medicare, call your Beneficiary and Family Centered Care Quality Improvement Organization (BFCC-QIO). Call 1-800-MEDICARE to get your BFCC-QIO's phone number.

- If you have a Medicare Advantage Plan (like an HMO or PPO), Medicare drug plan, or other Medicare health plan, call the BFCC-QIO, your plan, or both.

If you have End-Stage Renal Disease (ESRD) and have a complaint about your care, call the ESRD Network for your state. ESRD is permanent kidney failure that requires a regular course of dialysis or a kidney transplant. Call 1-800-MEDICARE.

Section 45.3

Informed Consent for Clinical Trials

This section includes text excerpted from "Informed Consent for Clinical Trials," U.S. Food and Drug Administration (FDA), February 25, 2016.

To many, the term informed consent is mistakenly viewed as the same as getting a research participant's signature on the consent form. The U.S. Food and Drug Administration (FDA) believes that obtaining a research participant's verbal or written informed consent is only part of the process. Informed consent involves providing a potential participant with:

- adequate information to allow for an informed decision about participation in the clinical investigation.

- facilitating the potential participant's understanding of the information.

- an appropriate amount of time to ask questions and to discuss with family and friends the research protocol and whether you should participate.

- obtaining the potential participant's voluntary agreement to participate.

- continuing to provide information as the clinical investigation progresses or as the subject or situation requires.

To be effective, the process must provide sufficient opportunity for the participant to consider whether to participate. FDA considers this to include allowing sufficient time for participants to consider the information and providing time and opportunity for the participant to ask questions and have those questions answered. The investigator (or other study staff who are conducting the informed consent interview) and the participant should exchange information and discuss the contents of the informed consent document. This process must occur under circumstances that minimize the possibility of coercion or undue influence.

337

What Is Informed Consent?

As new medical products are being developed, no one knows for sure how well they will work, or what risks they will find. Clinical trials are used to answer questions such as:

- Are new medical products safe enough to outweigh the risks related to the underlying condition?

- How should the product be used? (for example, the best dose, frequency, or any special precautions necessary to avoid problems),

- How effective is the medical product at relieving symptoms, treating or curing a condition?

The main purpose of clinical trials is to "study" new medical products in people. It is important for people who are considering participation in a clinical trial to understand their role, as a "subject of research" and not as a patient.

While research subjects may get personal treatment benefit from participating in a clinical trial, they must understand that they:

- may not benefit from the clinical trial,

- may be exposed to unknown risks,

- are entering into a study that may be very different from the standard medical practices that they currently know

To make an informed decision about whether to participate or not in a clinical trial, people need to be informed about:

- what will be done to them,

- how the protocol (plan of research) works,

- what risks or discomforts they may experience,

- participation being a voluntary decision on their part.

This information is provided to potential participants through the informed consent process. Informed consent means that the purpose of the research is explained to them, including what their role would be and how the trial will work.

A central part of the informed consent process is the informed consent document. The U.S. Food and Drug Administration (FDA) does not dictate the specific language required for the informed consent document, but does require certain basic elements of consent be included.

Before enrolling in a clinical trial, the following information must be given to each potential research subject:

- A statement explaining that the study involves research.

- An explanation of the purposes of the research.

- The expected length of time for participation.

- A description of all the procedures that will be completed during enrollment on the clinical trial.

- Information about all experimental procedures the will be completed during the clinical trial.

- A description of any predictable risks.

- Any possible discomforts (e.g., injections, frequency of blood test, etc.) that could occur as a result of the research.

- Any possible benefits that may be expected from the research.

- Information about any alternative procedures or treatment (if any) that might benefit the research subject.

- A statement describing:
  - the confidentiality of information collected during the clinical trial,
  - how records that identify the subject will be kept
  - the possibility that the FDA may inspect the records.

- For research involving more than minimal risk information including:
  - an explanation as to whether any compensation or medical treatments are available if injury occurs,
  - what they consist of, or
  - where more information may be found.
  - questions about the research,
  - research subjects' rights,
  - injury related to the clinical trial.

- Research subject participation is voluntary,

- Research subjects have the right to refuse treatment and will not losing any benefits for which they are entitled,

- Research subjects may choose to stop participation in the clinical trial at any time without losing benefits for which they are entitled.

When Appropriate, one or more of the following elements of information must also be provided in the informed consent document:

- A statement that the research treatment or procedure may involve unexpected risks (to the subject, unborn baby, if the subject is or may become pregnant).

- Any reasons why the research subject participation may be ended by the clinical trial investigator (e.g., failing to follow the requirements of the trial or changes in lab values that fall outside of the clinical trial limits).

- Added costs to the research subject that may result from participating in the trial.

- The consequence of leaving a trial before it is completed (e.g., if the research and procedures require a slow and organized end of participation).

- A statement that important findings discovered during the clinical trial will be provided to the research subject.

- The approximate number of research subjects that will be enrolled in the study.

A potential research subject must have an opportunity to:

- read the consent document

- ask questions about anything they do not understand

Usually, if one is considering participating in a clinical trial, he or she may take the consent document home to discuss with family, friend or advocate.

An investigator should only get consent from a potential research subject if:

- enough time was given to the research subject to consider whether or not to participate

- the investigator has not persuaded or influenced the potential research subject.

The information must be in language that is understandable to the research subject.

Informed consent may not include language that:

- the research subject is made to ignore or appear to ignore any of the research subject's legal rights,

- releases or appears to release the investigator, the sponsor, the institution, or its agents from their liability for negligence.

Participating in clinical trials is voluntary. You have the right not to participate, or to end your participation in the clinical trial at any time. Read the informed consent document carefully. Ask questions about any information you don't understand or find confusing.

Chapter 46

Advance Directives

What Are Advance Directives?

Advance directives are legal papers that tell your loved ones and doctors what kind of medical care you want if you can't tell them yourself. The papers let you say ahead of time how you want to be treated and to select someone who will make sure your wishes are carried out. It's best to fill these out when you're healthy in case you become ill or unable to make these decisions in the future. Think about taking action now to give someone you trust the right to make medical decisions for you. This is one of the most important things you can do.

Types of Advance Directives

Living Will

This is a document used for people to state whether or not they would like to receive certain types of medical care if they become unable to speak for themselves. The most common types of care addressed by a living will are:

- The use of machines to keep you alive. Examples include dialysis machines and ventilators (also called respirators)

This chapter includes text excerpted from "Advance Directives," National Cancer Institute (NCI), March 10, 2015.

343

- "Do not resuscitate" (DNR) orders. These instruct the healthcare team not to use cardiopulmonary resuscitation (CPR) if your breathing or heartbeat stops

- Tube feeding

- Withholding food and fluids

- Organ and tissue donation

Medical Power of Attorney

This is a document that allows people to name another person to make decisions about their medical care if they are unable to make these decisions for themselves. (It is also called a healthcare proxy or durable power of attorney for healthcare.) People often appoint someone they know well and trust to carry out their wishes. This person may be called a healthcare agent, surrogate, or proxy.

Why Advance Directives Are Important

Filling out advance directives gives people control over their healthcare. Choices about end-of-life care can be hard to make even when people are healthy. But if they are already seriously ill, such decisions can seem overwhelming. Some cancer patients want to try every drug or treatment in the hope that something will be effective. Others will choose to stop treatment. Although patients may turn to family and friends for advice, ultimately it is the patient's decision.

It's important to keep in mind that if a day comes where you choose not to receive or to stop treatment to control your disease, medical care to promote your well-being (palliative care) continues. This type of care includes treatment to manage pain and other physical symptoms, as well as support for psychosocial and spiritual needs. You have the right to make your own decisions about treatment. Filling out advance directives gives you a way to be in control.

When to Fill out Advance Directives

Ideally, these documents should be completed when you're healthy. Yet many people connect filling out advance directives to making decisions near the end of life. But you don't need to wait until being diagnosed with a serious illness to think about your wishes for care. In fact, making these choices when you're healthy can reduce the burden on you and your loved ones later on. Talking about these issues ensures that when the time comes, you will face the end of your life with dignity and with treatment that reflects your values.

Talk to your doctor, nurse, or social worker for advice or help with filling out advance directives. Most healthcare facilities have someone who can help. As you prepare your advance directives, you should talk about your decisions with family members and loved ones and explain the reasons behind your choices.

It's hard to talk about these issues. But the benefits of talking to the people close to you about the kind of care you want are:

- Your wishes are known and can be followed.

- It often comforts family members to know what you want.

- It saves family members from having to bring up the subject themselves.

- You may also gain peace of mind. You are making the choices for yourself instead of leaving them to your loved ones.

- It can help you and your loved ones worry less about the future and live each day to the fullest.

If talking with your family and other loved ones is too hard, consider having a family meeting and invite a social worker or member of the faith community to guide the discussion.

Reviewing and Signing Your Advance Directives

Once your advance directives have been completed, the next steps are:

- Review them with a member of your healthcare team or other healthcare professional for accuracy before signing. Most states require a witness to be present at the signing of the documents.

- Provide copies to your doctor, hospital, and family members after you sign them.

- Store copies in a safe, accessible place.

- Consider keeping a card in your wallet with a written statement declaring you have a living will and medical power of attorney and describing where the documents can be found.

Some organizations will store advance directives and make them available on the patient's behalf.

Changing Your Advance Directives

Even after advance directives have been signed, you can change your mind at any time. As a matter of fact, the process of discussing advance directives should be ongoing, rather than taking place just once. This way you can review the documents from time to time and modify them if your situation or wishes change.

To update your document, you should talk to your healthcare providers and loved ones about the new decisions you would like to make. When new advance directives have been signed, the old ones should be destroyed.

Advance Directives and State Laws

Each state has its own laws regarding advance directives. Therefore, special care should be taken to follow the laws of the state where you live or are being treated. A living will or medical power of attorney that is accepted in one state may not be accepted in another state. State-specific advance directives can be downloaded from the National Hospice and Palliative Care Organization.

More Information about Advance Directives

There are a number of organizations that can answer questions and give you more information about advance directives. Two well-known ones are:

Aging with Dignity

Aging with Dignity is a national nonprofit organization that worked with the American Bar Association to develop an easy-to-read living will called Five Wishes. This document is legal in 42 states and the District of Columbia, and is available in 26 languages, including Spanish and Braille. The organization has also created an advance care planning guide for adolescents and young adults called Voicing My Choices. Both these, and other resources, can be accessed online or ordered in hard copy format.

1–888–594–7437 (1–888–5WISHES)
1–850–681–2010

National Hospice and Palliative Care Organization

The National Hospice and Palliative Care Organization (NHPCO) represents programs and professionals that provide hospice and palliative care in the United States. Caring Connections is a national consumer and community engagement program of NHPCO that works to improve care at the end of life. Caring Connections provides a toll-free number, website, and a wide range of free materials about end-of-life care (such as hospice and palliative care information, advance care planning, and caregiving). Caring Connections provides free advance directives with instructions for each state. Some Spanish-language publications are available, and staff can answer calls in Spanish.

1–800–658–8898 (helpline)
1–877–658–8896 (multilingual line)

Chapter 47

Financial Assistance at the End of Life

People nearing the end of life often need a great deal of care—and this kind of healthcare is typically expensive. How people pay for end-of-life care depends on their financial situation and the kinds of services they want to use. Care services at the end of life can include:

- palliative care
- at-home care
- hospice care
- facility-based care, such as a nursing home

Although some people are cared for at home, most people are in hospitals or long-term care facilities such as nursing homes at the end of their lives. Palliative care is being offered more widely and, increasingly, people are choosing hospice care at the end of life. It is important to plan for the cost of these services as far in advance as possible.

This chapter includes text excerpted from "End of Life: Paying for Care," NIHSeniorHealth, National Institute on Aging (NIA), March 2014.

Sources of Payment

To pay for end-of-life care, people rely on a variety of payment sources, including:

- personal funds

- government health insurance programs, such as Medicare and Medicaid

- private financing options, such as long-term care insurance.

Review Your Personal Funds

Think about your financial resources and how you feel about using them to pay for end-of-life care. These resources may include:

- Social Security

- a pension or other retirement fund

- personal savings

- income from stocks and bonds

Your home is another type of asset that could be used if needed. For instance, if the home is fully paid for, a reverse mortgage might raise enough money to pay for a considerable amount of in-home care. Unlike a conventional mortgage, none of the reverse mortgage loan amount has to be repaid until the homeowner dies or permanently leaves the home.

- It's a good idea to review your insurance coverage. Many health insurance plans provide little, if any, coverage for long-term or end-of-life care.

Government Health Insurance Programs

Another source of funds for end-of-life care is government insurance programs like Medicare and Medicaid.

- **Medicare** is Federal health insurance for people age 65 and older, younger people with certain disabilities, and all people with late-stage kidney failure.

- **Medicaid** is Federal health insurance for people of any age with limited income. To be eligible, you must meet certain financial and health requirements. People with financial resources above a certain limit are unlikely to qualify unless they first use their own resources to pay for care, which is called "spending down."

Eligibility for Medicaid and what services are covered varies from state to state. As the Affordable Care Act of 2010 is implemented, Medicaid coverage in many states will change. This includes reforms to hold insurance companies accountable for services provided, to enhance the quality and availability of services, and to expand coverage.

Medicare End-of-Life Benefits

Medicare covers medically necessary care and focuses on medical acute care, such as doctor visits, drugs, and hospital stays. Medicare also provides coverage for short-term services for conditions that are expected to improve, such as physical therapy to help you regain your function after a fall or a stroke.

Medicare and Palliative Care

- Medicare does not use the term "palliative," but standard Medicare Part B benefits cover certain palliative treatments and medications, as well as visits from palliative care specialists and social workers. The palliative care provider (the organization offering you the services) will bill Medicare for services provided, but be sure you understand what copays or fees, if any, you will be asked to pay. Ask about your responsibility for fees and request a fee schedule before agreeing to receive services.

Medicare and Hospice Care

You are eligible for Medicare's Hospice benefit when you meet all of the following conditions.

- You are eligible for Medicare Part A (Hospital Insurance).

- Your doctor and the hospice medical director certify that you have a life-limiting illness and, if the disease runs its normal course, death may be expected in six months or less.

- You sign a statement choosing hospice care instead of routine Medicare-covered benefits for your illness.

- You receive care from a Medicare-approved hospice program.

Medicare defines a set of hospice core services. This means that hospices are required to provide these services to every person they serve, regardless of the person's insurance policy.

Medicare-Covered Hospice Services

Medicare covers the following hospice services and pays nearly all of their costs.

- doctor services

- nursing care

- medical equipment (such as wheelchairs or walkers)

- medical supplies (such as bandages and catheters)

- drugs for symptom control and pain relief

- short-term care in the hospital, including respite and inpatient care for pain and symptom management

- home health aide and homemaker services

- physical and occupational therapy

- speech therapy

- social work services

- dietary counseling

- grief support to help you and your family

You will have to pay part of the cost of outpatient drugs and inpatient respite care.

Length of Medicare Hospice Coverage

- Medicare can continue to pay for hospice services for longer than six months if the healthcare provider continues to certify that the person is still close to dying. It is also possible to leave hospice for a while and later return if the healthcare provider still believes the patient has less than six months to live.

- If your health provider thinks it is too soon for Medicare to cover hospice services, you can explore other ways to pay for the care that is needed. Some private health insurance plans also cover hospice care, but you will need to check with your insurance provider.

Medigap Policies

- "Medigap" policies, which supplement Medicare, are not designed to meet end-of-life care needs. But some policies cover copayments for nursing home stays that qualify for Medicare coverage.

Medicaid End-of-Life Benefits

Medicaid provides coverage for several services that can help someone near the end of life. These include personal care, home healthcare, and nursing home care.

Medicaid and Palliative Care

- Like Medicare, Medicaid does not use the term "palliative." Depending on the state, Medicaid may cover certain palliative treatments and medications as well as visits from palliative care specialists.

- The palliative care provider (the organization offering you the services) will bill Medicaid for services provided, but be sure you understand what copays or fees, if any, you will be asked to pay. Ask about your responsibility for fees and request a fee schedule before agreeing to receive services.

Medicaid and Hospice Care

- The Medicaid Hospice Benefit is identical to the Medicare Hospice Benefit in states where it is offered. Some states impose limitations on the length of time coverage is offered or who is considered eligible, however, so it is important to check with your state's Department of Health or Agency on Aging.

Long-Term Care Insurance Can Fill in Gaps

Long-term care insurance helps fill in the gaps where Medicare and Medicaid coverage stops. Long-term care insurance policies provide a great deal of choice and flexibility. You can select from a range of care options and benefits, including palliative and hospice care, that allow you to get the services you need, when and where you need them. The cost of your long-term care policy is based on the type and amount of services you choose to cover, how old you are when you buy the policy, and any optional benefits you choose, such as benefits that increase with inflation. If you are in poor health or already receiving end-of-life care services, you may not qualify for long-term care insurance. In some cases, you may be able to buy a limited amount of coverage, or coverage at a higher "non-standard" rate. You can also purchase nursing home-only coverage or a comprehensive policy that includes both home care and facility care. Many companies sell long-term care insurance. It is a good idea to shop around and compare policies.

Paying for Nursing Home Care

Many people spend their final days in a nursing home. Because nursing homes cost so much—thousands of dollars a month—most people who live in them for more than six months cannot pay the entire bill on their own. Instead, they "spend down" their resources until they qualify for Medicaid. There are rules for spending down resources. Nursing home care generally costs more than home-based care unless you need extensive services at home.

For More Information

The National Clearinghouse for Long-Term Care Information has information about long-term care planning and services. To find out what long-term care services are in your community, call Eldercare Locator at 800-677-1116.

Chapter 48

Social Security Issues

You should let Social Security know when a person dies as soon as possible. Usually, the funeral director will report the person's death to Social Security. You'll need to give the deceased's Social Security number to the funeral director so he or she can make the report. Some of the deceased's family members may be able to receive Social Security benefits if the deceased person worked long enough under Social Security to qualify for benefits. Contact Social Security as soon as you can to make sure the family gets all the benefits they're entitled. Please read the following information carefully to learn what benefits may be available.

- One-time payment of $255 to the surviving spouse if he or she was living with the deceased. If living apart and getting certain Social Security benefits on the deceased's record, the surviving spouse may still be able to get this one-time payment. If there's no surviving spouse, a child who's eligible for benefits on the deceased's record in the month of death can get this payment.

This chapter contains text excerpted from the following sources: Text in this chapter begins with excerpts from "How Social Security Can Help You When a Family Member Dies," U.S. Social Security Administration (SSA), November 15, 2015; Text beginning with the heading "What Is a Burial Fund?" is excerpted from "Spotlight on Burial Funds—2016," U.S. Social Security Administration (SSA), July 14, 2015; Text under the heading "Survivors Planner: How Much Would Your Benefit Be?" is excerpted from "Survivors Planner: How Much Would Your Benefit Be?" U.S. Social Security Administration (SSA), October 28, 2014.

- Certain family members may be eligible to receive monthly benefits, including:
  - A widow or widower age 60 or older (age 50 or older if disabled);
  - A widow or widower any age caring for the deceased's child who is under age 16 or disabled;
- An unmarried child of the deceased who is:
  - Younger than age 18 (or up to age 19 if he or she is a full-time student in an elementary or secondary school); or
  - Age 18 or older with a disability that began before age 22;
- A stepchild, grandchild, step grandchild, or adopted child under certain circumstances;
- Parents, age 62 or older, who were dependent on the deceased for at least half of their support; and
- A surviving divorced spouse, under certain circumstances.

If the deceased was receiving Social Security benefits, you must return the benefit received for the month of death or any later months. For example, if the person dies in July, you must return the benefit paid in August. If received by direct deposit, contact the bank or other financial institution and ask them to return any funds received for the month of death or later. If paid by check, do not cash any checks received for the month the person dies or later. Return the checks to Social Security as soon as possible. However, eligible family members may be able to receive death benefits for the month the beneficiary died.

What Is a Burial Fund?

A burial fund is money set aside to pay for burial expenses. For example, this money can be in a bank account, other financial instrument, or a prepaid burial arrangement. Some states allow an individual to pre-pay their burial by contracting with a funeral home and paying in advance for their funeral. You should discuss this with your local Social Security office.

Does a Burial Fund Count as a Resource for Supplemental Security Income (SSI)?

Generally, you and your spouse can set aside up to $1,500 each to pay for burial expenses. In most cases, this money will not count as a resource for Supplemental Security Income (SSI). If you (and your spouse) own life insurance policies or have other burial arrangements in addition to your $1,500 burial funds, some of the money in the burial fund may count toward the resource limit of $2,000 for an individual or $3,000 for a couple.

Does Interest Earned on Your (and Your Spouse's) Burial Fund Count as a Resource or Income for SSI?

No. Interest earned on your (or your spouse's) burial fund that you leave in the fund does not count as a resource or income for SSI and does not affect your SSI benefit.

How Can You Set up a Burial Fund?

Any account you set up must clearly show that the money is set aside to pay burial expenses. You can do this either by:

- titling the account as a burial fund; or
- signing a statement saying:
    - how much has been set aside for burial expenses,
    - for whose burial the money is set aside,
    - how the money has been set aside, and
    - the date you first considered the money set aside for burial expenses.

What Happens When You Spend Money from a Burial Fund?

If you spend any money from a burial fund on items unrelated to burial expenses, there may be a penalty.

Survivors Planner: How Much Would Your Benefit Be?

Your survivor benefit amount would be based on the earnings of the person who died. The more they paid into Social Security, the higher your benefits would be. The monthly amount you would get is a percentage of the deceased's basic Social Security benefit. It depends on your age and the type of benefit you would be eligible to receive.

If the person who died was receiving reduced benefits, we base your survivor's benefit on that amount. The maximum survivors benefit amount is limited to what they would receive if they were still alive.

These are examples of the benefits that survivors may receive:

- Widow or widower, full retirement age or older—100 percent of the deceased worker's benefit amount;

- Widow or widower, age 60—full retirement age—71½ to 99 percent of the deceased worker's basic amount;

- Disabled widow or widower aged 50 through 59—71½ percent;

- Widow or widower, any age, caring for a child under age 16—75 percent.

- A child under age 18 (19 if still in elementary or secondary school) or disabled—75 percent.

- Dependent parent(s) of the deceased worker, age 62 or older:

  - One surviving parent—82½ percent.

  - Two surviving parents—75 percent to each parent.

Percentages for a surviving divorced widow or widower would be the same as above. There may also be a special lump-sum death benefit.

Maximum Family Amount

There's a limit to the amount that family members can receive each month. The limit varies, but it is generally equal to about 150 to 180 percent of the basic benefit rate.

If the sum of the benefits payable to family members is greater than this limit, the benefits will be reduced proportionately. (Any benefits paid to a surviving divorced spouse based on disability or age won't count toward this maximum amount.)

Note: Although you can use our benefit calculators to see how much your survivors could receive on your record, you cannot use them to calculate your potential benefits on someone else's record.

You need to contact your local Social Security office or call our toll-free number, 1-800-772-1213, (TTY 1-800-325-0778) to learn how much you could receive on the other record.

Other Things You Need To Know

There are limits on how much survivors may earn while they receive benefits.

Benefits for a widow, widower or surviving divorced spouse may be affected by several additional factors:

If You Remarry

- If you remarry before you reach age 60 (age 50 if disabled), you cannot receive benefits as a surviving spouse while you are married.

- If you remarry after you reach age 60 (age 50 if disabled), you will continue to qualify for benefits on your deceased spouse's Social Security record.

However, if your current spouse is a Social Security beneficiary, you may want to apply for spouse's benefits on their record. If that amount is more than your widow's or widower's benefit, you will receive a combination of benefits that equals the higher amount.

If You Are Eligible for Retirement Benefits on Your Own Record

If you receive benefits as a widow or widower or as a surviving divorced spouse, you can switch to your own retirement benefit as early as age 62. This assumes you are eligible for retirement benefits and your retirement rate is higher than your rate as a widow, widower or surviving divorced spouse.

In many cases, a widow or widower can begin receiving one benefit at a reduced rate and then, at full retirement age, switch to the other benefit at an unreduced rate.

If You Will Receive a Pension Based on Work Not Covered by Social Security

If you will also receive a pension based on work not covered by Social Security, such as government or foreign work, your Social Security benefits as a survivor may be affected.

Chapter 49

Duties of an Executor /
Personal Representative

Personal Representative's Authority to Make Healthcare Decisions

Naming a Personal Representative

Your personal representative can be named several ways; state law may affect this process. If a person can make healthcare decisions for you using a healthcare power of attorney, the person is your personal representative.

Children

The personal representative of a minor child is usually the child's parent or legal guardian? State laws may affect guardianship. In

---

This chapter contains text excerpted from the following sources: Text under the heading "Personal Representative's Authority to Make Healthcare Decisions" is excerpted from "Personal Representatives," U.S. Department of Health and Human Services (HHS), July 26, 2013; Text under the heading "Who Must Be Recognized as the Individual's Personal Representative" is excerpted from "Personal Representatives," U.S. Department of Health and Human Services (HHS), March 1, 2003. Reviewed October 2016; Text beginning with the heading "General Responsibilities of an Estate Administrator" is excerpted from "Deceased Taxpayers—Understanding the General Duties as an Estate Administrator," Internal Revenue Service (IRS), April 19, 2016.

cases where a custody decree exists, the personal representative is the parent(s) who can make healthcare decisions for the child under the custody decree.

Deceased Persons

When an individual dies, the personal representative for the deceased is the executor or administrator of the deceased individual's estate, or the person who is legally authorized by a court or by state law to act on the behalf of the deceased individual or his or her estate.

Who Must Be Recognized as the Individual's Personal Representative?

The following table displays who must be recognized as the personal representative for a category of individuals:

Table 49.1. Who Must Be Recognized as the Individual's Personal Representative

If the Individual Is:	The Personal Representative Is:
An Adult orAn Emancipated Minor	A person with legal authority to make healthcare decisions on behalf of the individual Examples: Healthcare power of attorneyCourt appointed legal guardianGeneral power of attorney or durable power of attorney that includes the power to make healthcare decisions Exceptions: See abuse, neglect, and endangerment situations discussion below.
An Unemancipated Minor	A parent, guardian, or other person acting in loco parentis with legal authority to make healthcare decisions on behalf of the minor child Exceptions: See parents and unemancipated minors, and abuse, neglect and endangerment situations discussion below.
Deceased	A person with legal authority to act on behalf of the decedent or the estate (not restricted to persons with authority to make healthcare decisions) Examples: Executor or administrator of the estateNext of kin or other family member (if relevant law provides authority)

General Responsibilities of an Estate Administrator

When a person dies a probate proceeding may be opened. Depending on state law, probate will generally open within 30 to 90-days from the date of death.

One of the probate court's first actions will be to appoint a legal representative for the decedent and his or her estate. The legal representative may be a surviving spouse, other family member, executor named in the decedent's will or an attorney. The term "estate administrator" refers to the appointed legal representative. The probate court will issue Letters Testamentary authorizing the estate administrator of the decedent to act on the decedent's behalf. You will need the Letters Testamentary to handle the decedent's tax and other matters.

In general, the responsibilities of an estate administrator are to collect all the decedent's assets, pay creditors and distribute the remaining assets to heirs or other beneficiaries. As an estate administrator your first responsibility is to provide the probate court with an accounting of the decedent's assets and debts. Some assets may need to be appraised to determine their value. All debts will need to be verified and creditor claims against the estate must be filed.

Tax Responsibilities of an Estate Administrator

A decedent and their estate are separate taxable entities. So if filing requirements are satisfied, an estate administrator may have to file different types of tax returns.

First, an estate administrator may need to file income tax returns for the decedent. The decedent's Form 1040 for the year of death, and for any preceding years for which a return was not filed, are required if the decedent's income for those years was above the filing requirement.

Second, an estate administrator may need to file income tax returns for the estate). To file this return you will need to get a tax identification number for the estate (called an employer identification number or EIN). An estate is required to file an income tax return if assets of the estate generate more than $600 in annual income. For example, if the decedent had interest, dividend or rental income when alive, then after death that income becomes income of the estate and may trigger the requirement to file an estate income tax return.

If the estate operates a business after the owner's death, the estate administrator is required to secure a new employer identification number for the business, report wages or income under the new EIN and pay any taxes that are due. Some or all of the information you need to file income tax returns for the decedent and their estate may be in the decedent's personal records. The IRS (Internal Revenue Service) can help by providing copies of income documents and copies of filed tax returns or transcripts of tax accounts.

Third, an estate administrator may need to file an estate tax return. Estate tax is a tax on the transfer of assets from the decedent to their heirs and beneficiaries. In general, estate tax only applies to large estates.

Chapter 50

Understanding the Family and Medical Leave Act (FMLA)

Whether you are unable to work because of your own serious health condition, or because you need to care for your parent, spouse, or child with a serious health condition, the The Family and Medical Leave Act (FMLA) provides unpaid, job-protected leave. Leave may be taken all at once, or may be taken intermittently as the medical condition requires. This section provides a simple overview of how the FMLA may benefit you. In your time of need, sometimes you just need time.

Who Can Use FMLA Leave?

In order to take FMLA leave, you must first work for a covered employer. Generally, private employers with at least 50 employees are covered by the law. Private employers with fewer than 50 employees are not covered by the FMLA, but may be covered by state family and medical leave laws. Government agencies (including local, state and federal employers) and elementary and secondary schools are covered by the FMLA, regardless of the number of employees. If you work for

This chapter includes text excerpted from "The Employee's Guide to the Family and Medical Leave Act," U.S. Department of Labor (DOL), June 2015.

a covered employer, you need to meet additional criteria to be eligible to take FMLA leave. Not everyone who works for a covered employer is eligible.

First, you must have worked for your employer for at least 12 months. You do not have to have worked for 12 months in a row (so seasonal work counts), but generally if you have a break in service that lasted more than seven years, you cannot count the period of employment prior to the seven-year break.

Second, you must have worked for the employer for at least 1250 hours in the 12 months before you take leave. That works out to an average of about 24 hours per week over the course of a year.

Lastly, you must work at a location where the employer has at least 50 employees within 75 miles of your worksite. So even if your employer has more than 50 employees, if they are spread out and there are not 50 employees within 75 miles of where you work, you will not be eligible to take FMLA leave.

When Can I Use FMLA Leave?

If you work for an employer that is covered by the FMLA, and you are an eligible employee, you can take up to 12 weeks of FMLA leave in any 12-month period for a variety of reasons, including:

Serious Health Condition

You may take FMLA leave to care for your spouse, child or parent who has a serious health condition, or when you are unable to work because of your own serious health condition.

The most common serious health conditions that qualify for FMLA leave are:

1. conditions requiring an overnight stay in a hospital or other medical care facility;

2. conditions that incapacitate you or your family member (for example, unable to work or attend school) for more than three consecutive days and require ongoing medical treatment (either multiple appointments with a healthcare provider, or a single appointment and follow-up care such as prescription medication);

3. chronic conditions that cause occasional periods when you or your family member are incapacitated and require treatment by a healthcare provider at least twice a year; and

4. pregnancy (including prenatal medical appointments, incapacity due to morning sickness, and medically required bed rest).

Military Family Leave

The FMLA also provides certain military family leave entitlements. You may take FMLA leave for specified reasons related to certain military deployments. Additionally, you may take up to 26 weeks of FMLA leave in a single 12-month period to care for a covered servicemember with a serious injury or illness.

Expanding Your Family

You may take FMLA leave for the birth of a child and to bond with the newborn child, or for the placement of a child for adoption or foster care and to bond with that child. Men and women have the same right to take FMLA leave to bond with their child but it must be taken within one year of the child's birth or placement and must be taken as a continuous block of leave unless the employer agrees to allow intermittent leave (for example, a part-time schedule).

What Can the FMLA Do for Me?

If you are faced with a health condition that causes you to miss work, whether it is because of your own serious health condition or to care for a family member with a serious health condition, you may be able to take up to 12 weeks of job-protected time off under the FMLA.

If you take FMLA leave, your employer must continue your health insurance as if you were not on leave (you may be required to continue to make any normal employee contributions).

As long as you are able to return to work before you exhaust your FMLA leave, you must be returned to the same job (or one nearly identical to it). This job protection is intended to reduce the stress that you may otherwise feel if forced to choose between work and family during a serious medical situation.

Time off under the FMLA may not be held against you in employment actions such as hiring, promotions or discipline.

You can take FMLA leave as either a single block of time (for example, three weeks of leave for surgery and recovery) or in multiple, smaller blocks of time if medically necessary (for example, occasional absences due to diabetes). You can also take leave on a part-time basis if medically necessary (for example, if after surgery you are able to return to work only four hours a day or three days a week for a period of time). If you need multiple periods of leave for planned medical treatment such as physical therapy appointments, you must try to schedule the treatment at a time that minimizes the disruption to your employer.

FMLA leave is unpaid leave. However, if you have sick time, vacation time, personal time, etc., saved up with your employer, you may use that leave time, along with your FMLA leave so that you continue to get paid. In order to use such leave, you must follow your employer's normal leave rules such as submitting a leave form or providing advance notice. Even if you don't want to use your paid leave, your employer can require you to use it during your FMLA leave. For example, if you are out for one week recovering from surgery, and you have two weeks of paid vacation saved up, your employer can require you to use one week of your vacation time for your FMLA leave. When you use paid leave for an FMLA-covered reason (whether at your request or your employer's), your leave time is still protected by the FMLA.

How Do I Request FMLA Leave?

To take FMLA leave, you must provide your employer with appropriate notice. If you know in advance that you will need FMLA leave (for example, if you are planning to have surgery or you are pregnant), you must give your employer at least 30 days advance notice. If you learn of your need for leave less than 30 days in advance, you must give your employer notice as soon as you can (generally either the day you learn of the need or the next work day). When you need FMLA leave unexpectedly (for example, if a family member is injured in an accident), you MUST inform your employer as soon as you can. You must follow your employer's usual notice or call-in procedures unless you are unable to do so (for example, if you are receiving emergency medical care).

While you do not have to specifically ask for FMLA leave for your first leave request, you do need to provide enough information so your employer is aware it may be covered by the FMLA. Once a condition has been approved for FMLA leave and you need additional leave for that condition (for example recurring migraines or physical therapy appointments), your request must mention that condition or your need for FMLA leave. If you don't give your employer enough information to know that your leave may be covered by the FMLA, your leave may not be protected.

You do not have to tell your employer your diagnosis, but you do need to provide information indicating that your leave is due to an

FMLA-protected condition (for example, stating that you have been to the doctor and have been given antibiotics and told to stay home for four days).

Communication with Your Employer

Ongoing communication between you and your employer will make the FMLA process run much more smoothly. Each of you has to follow guidelines about notifying the other when FMLA leave is being used.

You will need to inform your employer if your need for FMLA leave changes while you are out (for example, if your doctor determines that you can return to work earlier than expected).

Your employer may also require you to provide periodic updates on your status and your intent to return to work. Your employer must notify you if you are eligible for FMLA leave within five business days of your first leave request. If the employer says that you are not eligible, it has to state at least one reason why you are not eligible (for example, you have not worked for the employer for a total of 12 months).

At the same time that your employer gives you an eligibility notice, it must also give you a notice of your rights and responsibilities under the FMLA. This notice must include all of the following:

- A definition of the 12-month period the employer uses to keep track of FMLA usage. It can be a calendar year, 12 months from the first time you take leave, a fixed year such as your anniversary date, or a rolling 12-month period measured backward from the date you use FMLA leave. You need to know which way your employer measures the 12-month window so that you can be sure of how much FMLA leave you have available when you need it.

- Whether you will be required to provide medical certification from a healthcare provider.

- Your right to use paid leave.

- Whether your employer will require you to use your paid leave.

- Your right to maintain your health benefits and whether you will be required to make premium payments.

- Your right to return to your job at the end of your FMLA leave.

When your employer has the information necessary to determine if your leave is FMLA protected, it must notify you whether the leave will be designated as FMLA leave and, if possible, how much leave will be counted against your FMLA entitlement. If your employer determines that your leave is not covered by FMLA, it must notify you of that determination.

Medical Certification

If your employer requests medical certification, you only have 15 calendar days to provide it in most circumstances. You are responsible for the cost of getting the certification from a healthcare provider and for making sure that the certification is provided to your employer. If you fail to provide the requested medical certification, your FMLA leave may be denied.

The medical certification must include some specific information, including:

- contact information for the healthcare provider;

- when the serious health condition began;

- how long the condition is expected to last;

- appropriate medical facts about the condition (which may include information on symptoms, hospitalization, doctors visits, and referrals for treatment);

- whether you are unable to work or your family member is in need of care; and

- whether you need leave continuously or intermittently. (If you need to take leave a little bit at a time, the certification should include an estimate of how much time you will need for each absence, how often you will be absent, and information establishing the medical necessity for taking such intermittent leave.)

If your employer finds that necessary information is missing from your certification, it must notify you in writing of what additional information is needed to make the certification complete. You must provide the missing information within seven calendar days.

If your employer has concerns about the validity of your certification, it may request a second opinion, but it must cover the cost. Your employer may request a third opinion if the first and second opinion differ, but it must cover the cost.

If your need for leave continues for an extended period of time, or if it changes significantly, your employer may require you to provide an updated certification.

Returning to Work

When you return to work, the FMLA requires that your employer return you to the same job that you left, or one that is nearly identical. If you are not returned to the exact same job, the new position must:

- involve the same or substantially similar duties, responsibilities, and status;

- include the same general level of skill, effort, responsibility and authority;

- offer identical pay, including equivalent premium pay, overtime and bonus opportunities;

- offer identical benefits (such as life insurance, health insurance, disability insurance, sick leave, vacation, educational benefits, pensions, etc.); and

- offer the same general work schedule and be at the same (or a nearby) location.

Please keep in mind that if you exhaust your FMLA leave entitlement and are unable to return to work, your employer is not required to restore you to your position.

Part Eight

Final Arrangements

Chapter 51

Funeral Services: An Overview

When a loved one dies, grieving family members and friends often are confronted with dozens of decisions about the funeral—all of which must be made quickly and often under great emotional duress. What kind of funeral should it be? What funeral provider should you use? Should you bury or cremate the body, or donate it to science? What are you legally required to buy? What about the availability of environmentally friendly or "green" burials? What other arrangements should you plan? And, practically, how much is it all going to cost?

Funeral Planning Tips

Many funeral providers offer various "packages" of goods and services for different kinds of funerals. When you arrange for a funeral, you have the right to buy goods and services separately. That is, you do not have to accept a package that may include items you do not want. Here are some tips to help you shop for funeral services:

- Shop around in advance. Compare prices from at least two funeral homes. Remember that you can supply your own casket or urn.

This chapter includes text excerpted from "Shopping for Funeral Services," Federal Trade Commission (FTC), July 2012. Reviewed October 2016.

- Ask for a price list. The law requires funeral homes to give you written price lists for products and services.

- Resist pressure to buy goods and services you don't really want or need.

- Avoid emotional overspending. It's not necessary to have the fanciest casket or the most elaborate funeral to properly honor a loved one.

- Recognize your rights. Laws regarding funerals and burials vary from state to state. It's a smart move to know which goods or services the law requires you to purchase and which are optional.

- Apply the same smart shopping techniques you use for other major purchases. You can cut costs by limiting the viewing to one day or one hour before the funeral, and by dressing your loved one in a favorite outfit instead of costly burial clothing.

- Shop in advance. It allows you to comparison shop without time constraints, creates an opportunity for family discussion, and lifts some of the burden from your family.

The Federal Trade Commission (FTC) Funeral Rule

The Funeral Rule, enforced by the Federal Trade Commission (FTC), makes it possible for you to choose only those goods and services you want or need and to pay only for those you select, whether you are making arrangements when a death occurs or in advance. The Rule allows you to compare prices among funeral homes, and makes it possible for you to select the funeral arrangements you want at the home you use. (The Rule does not apply to third-party sellers, such as casket and monument dealers, or to cemeteries that lack an on-site funeral home.)

Your Rights under the Funeral Rule

The Funeral Rule gives you the right to:

- Buy only the funeral arrangements you want. You have the right to buy separate goods (such as caskets) and services (such as embalming or a memorial service). You do not have to accept a package that may include items you do not want.

- Get price information on the telephone. Funeral directors must give you price information on the telephone if you ask for it. You don't have to give them your name, address, or telephone number first. Although they are not required to do so, many funeral homes mail their price lists, and some post them online.

- Get a written, itemized price list when you visit a funeral home. The funeral home must give you a General Price List (GPL) that is yours to keep. It lists all the items and services the home offers, and the cost of each one.

- See a written casket price list before you see the actual caskets. Sometimes, detailed casket price information is included on the funeral home's GPL. More often, though, it's provided on a separate casket price list. Get the price information before you see the caskets, so that you can ask about lower-priced products that may not be on display.

- See a written outer burial container price list. Outer burial containers are not required by state law anywhere in the United States, but many cemeteries require them to prevent the grave from caving in. If the funeral home sells containers, but doesn't list their prices on the GPL, you have the right to look at a separate container price list before you see the containers. If you don't see the lower-priced containers listed, ask about them.

- Receive a written statement after you decide what you want, and before you pay. It should show exactly what you are buying and the cost of each item. The funeral home must give you a statement listing every good and service you have selected, the price of each, and the total cost immediately after you make the arrangements.

- Get an explanation in the written statement from the funeral home that describes any legal cemetery or crematory requirement that requires you to buy any funeral goods or services.

- Use an "alternative container" instead of a casket for cremation. No state or local law requires the use of a casket for cremation. A funeral home that offers cremations must tell you that alternative containers are available, and must make them available. They might be made of unfinished wood, pressed wood, fiberboard, or cardboard.

- Provide the funeral home with a casket or urn you buy elsewhere. The funeral provider cannot refuse to handle a casket or urn you bought online, at a local casket store, or somewhere else—or charge you a fee to do it. The funeral home cannot require you to be there when the casket or urn is delivered to them.

- Make funeral arrangements without embalming. No state law requires routine embalming for every death. Some states require embalming or refrigeration if the body is not buried or cremated within a certain time; some states don't require it at all. In most cases, refrigeration is an acceptable alternative. In addition, you may choose services like direct cremation and immediate burial, which don't require any form of preservation. Many funeral homes have a policy requiring embalming if the body is to be publicly viewed, but this is not required by law in most states. Ask if the funeral home offers private family viewing without embalming. If some form of preservation is a practical necessity, ask the funeral home if refrigeration is available.

Funeral Costs and Pricing Checklist

Funeral costs include basic services fee for the funeral director and staff, charges for other services and merchandise, and cash advances. Make copies of the checklist at the end of this article. Use it when you shop with several funeral homes to compare costs.

Funeral Fees

The Funeral Rule allows funeral providers to charge a basic services fee that customers have to pay. The basic services fee includes services that are common to all funerals, regardless of the specific arrangement. These include funeral planning, securing the necessary permits and copies of death certificates, preparing the notices, sheltering the remains, and coordinating the arrangements with the cemetery, crematory or other third parties. The fee does not include charges for optional services or merchandise.

Charges for other services and merchandise, include costs for optional goods and services such as transporting the remains; embalming and other preparation; use of the funeral home for the viewing, ceremony or memorial service; use of equipment and staff for a graveside service; use of a hearse or limousine; a casket, outer burial container or alternate container; and cremation or interment.

Cash advances are fees charged by the funeral home for goods and services it buys from outside vendors on your behalf, including flowers, obituary notices, pallbearers, officiating clergy, and organists and soloists. Some funeral providers charge you their cost for the items they buy on your behalf. Others add a service fee to the cost. The Funeral Rule requires those who charge an extra fee to disclose that fact in writing, although it doesn't require them to specify the amount of their markup. The Rule also requires funeral providers to tell you if there are refunds, discounts, or rebates from the supplier on any cash advance item.

Calculating the Actual Cost of a Funeral

The funeral provider must give you an itemized statement of the total cost of the funeral goods and services you have selected when you are making the arrangements. If the funeral provider doesn't know the cost of the cash advance items at the time, he or she is required to give you a written "good faith estimate." This statement also must disclose any legal cemetery or crematory requirements that you purchase specific funeral goods or services.

The Funeral Rule does not require any specific format for this information. Funeral providers may include it in any document they give you at the end of your discussion about funeral arrangements.

Embalming

Many funeral homes require embalming if you're planning a viewing or visitation. But embalming generally is not necessary or legally required if the body is buried or cremated shortly after death. Eliminating this service can save you hundreds of dollars. Under the Funeral Rule, a funeral provider:

- may not provide embalming services without permission.

- may not falsely state that embalming is required by law.

- must disclose in writing that embalming is not required by law, except in certain special cases.

- may not charge a fee for unauthorized embalming unless embalming is required by state law.

- must disclose in writing that you usually have the right to choose a disposition, like direct cremation or immediate burial, that does not require embalming if you do not want this service.

- must disclose in writing that some funeral arrangements, such as a funeral with viewing, may make embalming a practical necessity and, if so, a required purchase.

Caskets

For a "traditional" full-service funeral:

A casket often is the single most expensive item you'll buy if you plan a "traditional" full-service funeral. Caskets vary widely in style and price and are sold primarily for their visual appeal. Typically, they're constructed of metal, wood, fiberboard, fiberglass or plastic. Although an average casket costs slightly more than $2,000, some mahogany, bronze or copper caskets sell for as much as $10,000.

When you visit a funeral home or showroom to shop for a casket, the Funeral Rule requires the funeral director to show you a list of caskets the company sells, with descriptions and prices, before showing you the caskets. Industry studies show that the average casket shopper buys one of the first three models shown, generally the middle-priced of the three.

So it's in the seller's best interest to start out by showing you higher-end models. If you haven't seen some of the lower-priced models on the price list, ask to see them—but don't be surprised if they're not prominently displayed, or not on display at all.

Traditionally, caskets have been sold only by funeral homes. But more and more, showrooms and websites operated by "third-party" dealers are selling caskets. You can buy a casket from one of these dealers and have it shipped directly to the funeral home. The Funeral Rule requires funeral homes to agree to use a casket you bought elsewhere, and doesn't allow them to charge you a fee for using it.

No matter where or when you're buying a casket, it's important to remember that its purpose is to provide a dignified way to move the body before burial or cremation. No casket, regardless of its qualities or cost, will preserve a body forever. Metal caskets frequently are described as "gasketed," "protective" or "sealer" caskets. These terms mean that the casket has a rubber gasket or some other feature that is designed to delay the penetration of water into the casket and prevent rust. The Funeral Rule forbids claims that these features help preserve the remains indefinitely because they don't. They just add to the cost of the casket.

Most metal caskets are made from rolled steel of varying gauges—the lower the gauge, the thicker the steel. Some metal caskets come with a warranty for longevity. Wooden caskets generally are not gasketed and don't have a warranty for longevity. They can be hardwood like mahogany, walnut, cherry or oak, or softwood like pine. Pine caskets are a less expensive option, but funeral homes rarely display them. Manufacturers of both wooden and metal caskets usually offer warranties for workmanship and materials.

For cremation:

Many families that choose to have their loved ones cremated rent a casket from the funeral home for the visitation and funeral, eliminating the cost of buying a casket. If you opt for visitation and cremation, ask about the rental option. For those who choose a direct cremation without a viewing or other ceremony where the body is present, the funeral provider must offer an inexpensive unfinished wood box or alternative container, a non-metal enclosure—pressboard, cardboard or canvas—that is cremated with the body.

Under the Funeral Rule, funeral directors who offer direct cremations:

- may not tell you that state or local law requires a casket for direct cremations, because none do;

- must disclose in writing your right to buy an unfinished wood box or an alternative container for a direct cremation; and

- must make an unfinished wood box or other alternative container available for direct cremations.

Burial Vaults or Grave Liners

Burial vaults or grave liners, also known as burial containers, are commonly used in "traditional" full-service funerals. The vault or liner is placed in the ground before burial, and the casket is lowered into it at burial. The purpose is to prevent the ground from caving in as the casket deteriorates over time. A grave liner is made of reinforced concrete and will satisfy any cemetery requirement. Grave liners cover only the top and sides of the casket. A burial vault is more substantial and expensive than a grave liner. It surrounds the casket in concrete or another material and may be sold with a warranty of protective strength.

State laws do not require a vault or liner, and funeral providers may not tell you otherwise. However, keep in mind that many cemeteries require some type of outer burial container to prevent the grave from sinking in the future. Neither grave liners nor burial vaults are designed to prevent the eventual decomposition of human remains. It is illegal for funeral providers to claim that a vault will keep water, dirt, or other debris from penetrating into the casket if that's not true.

Before showing you any outer burial containers, a funeral provider is required to give you a list of prices and descriptions. It may be less expensive to buy an outer burial container from a third-party dealer than from a funeral home or cemetery. Compare prices from several sources before you select a model.

Preservation Processes and Products

As far back as the ancient Egyptians, people have used oils, herbs and special body preparations to help preserve the bodies of their dead. Yet, no process or products have been devised to preserve a body in the grave indefinitely. The Funeral Rule prohibits funeral providers from telling you that it can be done. For example, funeral providers may not claim that either embalming or a particular type of casket will preserve the body of the deceased for an unlimited time.

Types of Funerals

Every family is different, and not everyone wants the same type of funeral. Funeral practices are influenced by religious and cultural traditions, costs, and personal preferences. These factors help determine whether the funeral will be elaborate or simple, public or private, religious or secular, and where it will be held. They also influence whether the body will be present at the funeral, if there will be a viewing or visitation, and if so, whether the casket will be open or closed, and whether the remains will be buried or cremated.

"Traditional" Full-Service Funeral

This type of funeral, often referred to by funeral providers as a "traditional" funeral, usually includes a viewing or visitation and formal funeral service, use of a hearse to transport the body to the funeral site and cemetery, and burial, entombment, or cremation of the remains.

It is generally the most expensive type of funeral. In addition to the funeral home's basic services fee, costs often include embalming and dressing the body; rental of the funeral home for the viewing or service; and use of vehicles to transport the family if they don't use their own. The costs of a casket, cemetery plot or crypt and other funeral goods and services also must be factored in.

Direct Burial

The body is buried shortly after death, usually in a simple container. No viewing or visitation is involved, so no embalming is necessary. A memorial service may be held at the graveside or later. Direct burial usually costs less than the "traditional" full-service funeral.

Costs include the funeral home's basic services fee, as well as transportation and care of the body, the purchase of a casket or burial container and a cemetery plot or crypt. If the family chooses to be at the cemetery for the burial, the funeral home often charges an additional fee for a graveside service.

Direct Cremation

The body is cremated shortly after death, without embalming. The cremated remains are placed in an urn or other container. No viewing or visitation is involved. The remains can be kept in the home, buried, or placed in a crypt or niche in a cemetery, or buried or scattered in a favorite spot. Direct cremation usually costs less than the "traditional" full-service funeral. Costs include the funeral home's basic services fee, as well as transportation and care of the body. A crematory fee may be included or, if the funeral home does not own the crematory, the fee may be added on. There also will be a charge for an urn or other container. The cost of a cemetery plot or crypt is included only if the remains are buried or entombed.

Funeral providers who offer direct cremations also must offer to provide an alternative container that can be used in place of a casket.

Chapter 52

Planning a Funeral

Choosing a Funeral Provider

Many people don't realize that in most states they are not legally required to use a funeral home to plan and conduct a funeral. However, because they have little experience with the many details and legal requirements involved and may be emotionally distraught when it's time to make the plans, they find the services of a professional funeral home to be a comfort.

People often select a funeral home or cemetery because it's close to home, has served the family in the past, or has been recommended by someone they trust. But limiting the search to just one funeral home may risk paying more than necessary for the funeral or narrowing their choice of goods and services.

Comparison Shopping for a Funeral Home/Provider

Comparison shopping doesn't have to be difficult, especially if it's done before the need for a funeral arises. Thinking ahead can help you make informed and thoughtful decisions about funeral arrangements. It allows you to choose the specific items you want and need, and to compare the prices several funeral providers charge.

If you visit a funeral home in person, the funeral provider is required by law to give you a general price list (GPL) itemizing the

This chapter includes text excerpted from "Shopping for Funeral Services," Federal Trade Commission (FTC), July 2012. Reviewed October 2016.

cost of the items and services the home offers. If the GPL does not include specific prices of caskets or outer burial containers, the law requires the funeral director to show you the price lists for those items before showing you the items.

Sometimes it's more convenient and less stressful to "price shop" funeral homes by telephone. The Funeral Rule requires funeral directors to provide price information on the phone to any caller who asks for it. In addition, many funeral homes are happy to mail you their price lists, although that is not required by law.

When comparing prices, be sure to consider the total cost of all the items together, in addition to the costs of single items. Every funeral home should have price lists that include all the items essential for the different types of arrangements it offers. Many funeral homes offer package funerals that may cost less than buying individual items or services. Offering package funerals is permitted by law, as long as an itemized price list also is provided. But you can't accurately compare total costs unless you use the price lists.

In addition, there's a trend toward consolidation in the funeral home industry, and many neighborhood funeral homes may appear to be locally owned when in fact, they're owned by a national corporation. If this issue is important to you, you may want to ask if the funeral home is independent and locally owned.

Buying a Cemetery Site

When you buy a cemetery plot, the cost is not the only consideration. The location of the cemetery and whether it meets the requirements of your family's religion are important, as well.

Specific Considerations

Additional considerations include what, if any, restrictions the cemetery places on burial vaults purchased elsewhere, the type of monuments or memorials it allows, and whether flowers or other remembrances may be placed on graves.

And then there's cost. Cemetery plots can be expensive, especially in metropolitan areas. Most, but not all, cemeteries require you to purchase a grave liner, which will cost several hundred dollars. Note that there are charges—usually hundreds of dollars—to open a grave for interment and additional charges to fill it in. Perpetual care on a cemetery plot sometimes is included in the purchase price, but it's important to clarify that point before you buy the site or service. If it's not included, look for a separate endowment care fee for maintenance and groundskeeping.

If you plan to bury your loved one's cremated remains in a mausoleum or columbarium, you can expect to purchase a crypt and pay opening and closing fees, as well as charges for endowment care and other services. The Federal Trade Commission (FTC)'s Funeral Rule does not cover cemeteries and mausoleums unless they sell both funeral goods and funeral services.

Veterans Cemeteries

All veterans are entitled to a free burial in a national cemetery and a grave marker. This eligibility also extends to some civilians who have provided military-related service and some Public Health Service personnel. Spouses and dependent children also are entitled to a lot and marker when buried in a national cemetery. There are no charges for opening or closing the grave, for a vault or liner, or for setting the marker in a national cemetery. The family generally is responsible for other expenses, including transportation to the cemetery.

In addition, many states have established veterans cemeteries. Eligibility requirements and other details vary.

You may see ads for so-called "veterans' specials" by commercial cemeteries. These cemeteries sometimes offer a free plot for the veteran, but charge exorbitant rates for an adjoining plot for the spouse, as well as high fees for opening and closing each grave. Evaluate the bottom-line cost to be sure the special is as special as you may be led to believe.

Planning Your Own Funeral

To help relieve their families, an increasing number of people are planning their own funerals, designating their funeral preferences, and sometimes paying for them in advance. They see funeral planning as an extension of will and estate planning.

Funeral Planning Tips

Thinking ahead can help you make informed and thoughtful decisions about funeral arrangements. It allows you to choose the specific items you want and need, and compare the prices offered by several funeral providers. It also spares your survivors the stress of making these decisions under the pressure of time and strong emotions. You can make arrangements directly with a funeral establishment.

An important consideration when planning a funeral pre-need is where the remains will be buried, entombed, or scattered. In the short time between the death and burial of a loved one, many family members find themselves rushing to buy a cemetery plot or grave—often without careful thought or a personal visit to the site. That's why it's in the family's best interest to buy cemetery plots before you need them.

You may wish to make decisions about your arrangements in advance, but not pay for them in advance. Keep in mind that over time, prices may go up and businesses may close or change ownership. However, in some areas with increased competition, prices may go down over time. It's a good idea to review and revise your decisions every few years, and to make sure your family is aware of your wishes.

Put your preferences in writing, give copies to family members and your attorney, and keep a copy in a handy place. Don't designate your preferences in your will, because a will often is not found or read until after the funeral. And avoid putting the only copy of your preferences in a safe deposit box. That's because your family may have to make arrangements on a weekend or holiday, before the box can be opened.

Prepaying

Millions of Americans have entered into contracts to arrange their funerals and prepay some or all of the expenses involved. Laws of individual states govern the prepayment of funeral goods and services; various states have laws to help ensure that these advance payments are available to pay for the funeral products and services when they're needed. But protections vary widely from state to state, and some state laws offer little or no effective protection. Some state laws require the funeral home or cemetery to place a percentage of the prepayment in a state-regulated trust or to purchase a life insurance policy with the death benefits assigned to the funeral home or cemetery.

- If you're thinking about prepaying for funeral goods and services, it's important to consider these issues before putting down any money:

- What are you are paying for? Are you buying only merchandise, like a casket and vault, or are you purchasing funeral services as well?

- What happens to the money you've prepaid? States have different requirements for handling funds paid for prearranged funeral services.

- What happens to the interest income on money that is prepaid and put into a trust account?

- Are you protected if the firm you dealt with goes out of business?

- Can you cancel the contract and get a full refund if you change your mind?

- What happens if you move to a different area or die while away from home? Some prepaid funeral plans can be transferred, but often at an added cost.

Be sure to tell your family about the plans you've made; let them know where the documents are filed. If your family isn't aware that you've made plans, your wishes may not be carried out. And if family members don't know that you've prepaid the funeral costs, they could end up paying for the same arrangements. You may wish to consult an attorney on the best way to ensure that your wishes are followed.

Chapter 53

Military Funeral Planning

For Burial in a National Cemetery

Burial benefits available include a gravesite in any of the 135 national cemeteries with available space, opening and closing of the grave, perpetual care, a Government headstone or marker, a burial flag, and a Presidential Memorial Certificate, at no cost to the family. Some Veterans may also be eligible for Burial Allowances. Cremated remains are buried or inurned in national cemeteries in the same manner and with the same honors as casketed remains.

Burial benefits available for spouses and dependents buried in a national cemetery include burial with the Veteran, perpetual care, and the spouse or dependents name and date of birth and death will be inscribed on the Veteran's headstone, at no cost to the family. Eligible spouses and dependents may be buried, even if they predecease the Veteran.

The Veterans family should make funeral or cremation arrangements with a funeral provider or cremation office. Any item or service obtained from a funeral home or cremation office will be at the family's expense.

Preparing in Advance

Gravesites in the U.S. Department of Veterans Affairs (VA) national cemeteries cannot be reserved in advance.

This chapter includes text excerpted from "National Cemetery Administration," U.S. Environmental Protection Agency (EPA), August 10, 2016.

You should advise your family of your wishes and where your discharge papers are kept. These papers are very important in establishing your eligibility.

At the time of need your family would contact a funeral home who will assist them with making burial arrangements at the national cemetery. You may wish to make pre-need arrangements with a funeral home.

To schedule a burial, first fax all discharge documentation to the National Cemetery Scheduling Office at 1-866-900-6417 or scan and email the documentation to NCA.Scheduling@va.gov with the name of the decedent in the subject line. Follow-up with a phone call to 1-800-535-1117 and have the following information readily available when you call:

- Cemetery of choice

- First or subsequent burial (Veteran or dependent already buried)

  - If subsequent interment, who is already interred, section and site number (if known)

- Decedent's:

  - Full name;

  - Gender;

  - Social Security Number (SSN);

  - Date of death;

  - Date of birth; and

  - Relationship (Veteran or dependent)

- Funeral director's contact information:

  - Funeral director's name;

  - Funeral home's name;

  - Address; and

  - Email address of the funeral home

- Next of kin information:

  - Name;

  - Relationship to deceased;

- SSN;
- Telephone number; and
- Address
- Type of religious emblem for headstone (if known)
- Did the decedent reside within 75 miles of requested cemetery?
- ZIP code of decedent at time of death
- County of decedent at time of death
- Type of burial:
  - Casket;
  - Casket size/liner size
  - Cremation
  - Urn size/urn vault size
- Marital status of deceased (if Veteran is buried in a private cemetery, must provide documentation of marital status of spouse at time of death)
- Is surviving spouse a Veteran?
- Any disabled children for future interment (must provide name and date of birth). If requesting immediate interment (must provide marital status, doctor's statement stating type of illness, date of onset of illness and capability of self-support).
- Military Honors requested

Donating Burial Flags in National Cemeteries

Most of the U.S. Department of Veterans Affairs national cemeteries display an Avenue of Flags on patriotic holidays and during special events. The Avenues consist of burial flags donated by the families of deceased Veterans and provide a unique visible tribute to all of our Nation's Veterans.

A Certificate of Appreciation is presented to the donor for providing their loved ones' burial flag to a national cemetery.

Please contact the cemetery of your choice for information on how to donate a Veteran's burial flag.

For Burial in a Private Cemetery

Burial benefits available for Veterans buried in a private cemetery may include a Government headstone, marker or medallion, a burial flag, and a Presidential Memorial Certificate, at no cost to the family. Some Veterans may also be eligible for Burial Allowances. There are not any VA benefits available to spouses and dependents buried in a private cemetery.

Chapter 54

Cremation Explained

Cremation is the second most common method of disposition in the United States and gains in popularity every year. It is the most common option in Japan, India, England, and other countries. For most individuals, the selection of cremation is motivated by religious practice and cultural preference. Additional reasons for choosing cremation over traditional burial are lower cost, ease, more options for memorialization, and environmental considerations. Cremation is generally less expensive than traditional burial.

Some consumers perceive cremation to be simpler than traditional burial, and this simplicity appeals to a growing share of the market. There are fewer transactions in the cremation process; a consumer may only have to interact with a funeral director rather than with cemeteries and other agencies. Funeral directors provide most legal services as part of the cremation fee, reducing the burden on families.

Cremation also provides more options for memorialization. Remains can be stored in an urn at someone's home, a cemetery, or mausoleum. The remains can also be scattered at sea, in a park, or at other locations (where permitted by law) per the deceased's request. Finally, cremated remains do not require the relatively large burial plots needed for traditional burial, reducing the cemeteries' pressure on the environment. When cremains are buried, the individual plot is significantly smaller than the plot used in traditional burial.

This chapter includes text excerpted from "Economic Impact Analysis of Proposed Other Solid Waste Incinerator Regulation," U.S. Environmental Protection Agency (EPA), September 1999. Reviewed October 2016.

Cremation Process

There are many different classes of crematories; however, the technology employed by each unit-type is essentially the same. The technology has changed little in the latter half of the twentieth century. Crematories vary according to size and capacity. They are typically large, front-loaded units that weigh between 20,000 and 30,000 pounds. Combustion takes place in two chambers at an average rate of 100 to 150 pounds per hour. Crematories use natural gas, electricity, and propane to power the unit and facilitate the combustion process.

The primary chamber is preheated to about 700 °C. The body is enclosed in a combustible container, such as a wooden coffin, cardboard box, or plastic bag. The operator increases the temperature to between 900 and 1,100 °C. The body stays in the primary chamber between 1 and 2 hours, depending on body size. After the remains have cooled, the bones are crushed to the consistency of coarse sand. Finally, all the remains are placed in either an urn or a plastic bag for transport.

Cremated human remains, or "cremains," are of about the same consistency as sand. After the cremains are removed, the ash is set aside and the bones pulverized. Both powders are then mixed and placed in an appropriate receptacle. If the cremains are not immediately placed in an urn, they are carefully packaged in a plastic bag encased in a plain cardboard box. Depending on the size of the body, cremation results in 3 to 9 pounds of cremains.

Chapter 55

Medical Certification of Death

Importance of Death Registration and Fetal Death Reporting

The death certificate is a permanent record of the fact of death, and depending on the State of death, may be needed to get a burial permit. The information in the record is considered as prima facie evidence of the fact of death that can be introduced in court as evidence. State law specifies the required time for completing and filing the death certificate.

The death certificate provides important personal information about the decedent and about the circumstances and cause of death. This information has many uses related to the settlement of the estate and provides family members' closure, peace of mind, and documentation of the cause of death.

The death certificate is the source for State and national mortality statistics and is used to determine which medical conditions receive research and development funding, to set public health goals, and to measure health status at local, State, national, and international levels.

This chapter includes text excerpted from "Medical Examiners' and Coroners' Handbook on Death Registration and Fetal Death Reporting," Centers for Disease Control and Prevention (CDC), April 2003. Reviewed October 2016.

These mortality data are valuable to physicians indirectly by influencing funding that supports medical and health research (which may alter clinical practice) and directly as a research tool. Research topics include identifying disease etiology, evaluating diagnostic and therapeutic techniques, examining medical or mental health problems that may be found among specific groups of people, and indicating areas in which medical research can have the greatest impact on reducing mortality.

Analyses typically focus on a single condition reported on the death certificate, but some analyses do consider all conditions mentioned. Such analyses are important in studying certain diseases and conditions and in investigating relationships between conditions reported on the same death certificate (for example, types of fatal injuries and automobile crashes or types of infections and human immunodeficiency virus (HIV).

Because statistical data derived from death certificates can be no more accurate than the information provided on the certificate, it is very important that all persons concerned with the registration of deaths strive not only for complete registration, but also for accuracy and promptness in reporting these events. Furthermore, the potential usefulness of detailed specific information is greater than more general information.

The fetal death report is recommended as a legally required statistical report designed primarily to collect information for statistical and research purposes. In most States, these reports are not maintained in the official files of the State health department, and certified copies of these reports are rarely issued. However, in a number of States, it remains a legal certificate. The record, whether a certificate or a report, provides valuable health and research data. The information is used to study the causes of poor pregnancy outcome. These data are also essential in planning and evaluating prenatal care services and obstetrical programs. They are also used to examine the consequences of possible environmental and occupational exposures of parents on the fetus.

U.S. Standard Certificates and Reports

The registration of deaths and fetal deaths is a State function supported by individual State laws and regulations. The original certificates are filed in the States and stored in accordance with State practice. Each State has a contract with National Center for Health Statistics (NCHS) that allows the Federal Government to use information from the State records to produce national vital statistics. The national data program is called the National Vital Statistics System (NVSS).

To ensure consistency in the NVSS, NCHS provides leadership and coordination in the development of a standard certificate of death for the States to use as a model. The standard certificate is revised periodically to ensure that the data collected relate to current and anticipated needs. In the revision process, stakeholders review and evaluate each item on the standard certificate for its registration, legal, genealogical, statistical, medical, and research value. The associations on the stakeholder panel that recommended the current U.S. Standard Certificate of Death included the American Medical Association (AMA), the National Association of Medical Examiners (NAME), the College of American Pathologists (CAP), and the American Hospital Association (AHA). For the U.S. Standard Report of Fetal Death, the associations included the American Academy of Pediatrics (AAP), American College of Obstetricians and Gynecologists (ACOG), Association of State and Territorial Health Officers (Maternal and Child Health Affiliate), American Medical Association (AMA), and American College of Nurse Midwives (ACNM).

Most State certificates conform closely in content and arrangement to the standard. Minor modifications are sometimes necessary to comply with State laws or regulations or to meet specific information needs. Having similar forms promotes uniformity of data and comparable national statistics. They also allow the comparison of individual State data with national data and data from other States. Uniformity of death certificates among the States also increases their acceptability as legal records.

Confidentiality of Vital Records

To encourage appropriate access to vital records, NCHS promotes the development of model vital statistics laws concerning confidentiality. State laws and supporting regulations define which persons have authorized access to vital records. Some States have few restrictions on access to death certificates. However, there are restrictions on access to death certificates in the majority of States. Legal safeguards to the confidentiality of vital records have been strengthened over time in some States.

The fetal death report is designed primarily to collect information for statistical and research purposes. In many States these records are not maintained in the official files of the State health department. Most States never issue certified copies of these records; the other States issue certified copies very rarely.

Responsibility of the Medical Examiner or Coroner

Death Registration

The principal responsibility of the medical examiner or coroner in death registration is to complete the medical part of the death certificate. Before delivering the death certificate to the funeral director, he or she may add some personal items for proper identification such as name, residence, race, and sex. Under certain circumstances and in some jurisdictions, he or she may provide all the information, medical and personal, required on the certificate.

The funeral director, or other person in charge of interment, will otherwise complete those parts of the death certificate that call for personal information about the decedent. He or she is also responsible for filing the certificate with the registrar where the death occurred. Each State prescribes the time within which the death certificate must be filed with the registrar.

In general, the duties of the medical examiner or coroner are to:

- Complete relevant portions of the death certificate.

- Deliver the signed or electronically authenticated death certificate to the funeral director promptly so that the funeral director can file it with the State or local registrar within the State's prescribed time period.

- Assist the State or local registrar by answering inquiries promptly.

- Deliver a supplemental report of cause of death to the State vital statistics office when autopsy findings or further investigation reveals the cause of death to be different from what was originally reported.

When the cause of death cannot be determined within the statutory time limit, a death certificate should be filed with the notation that the report of cause of death is "deferred pending further investigation." A permit to authorize disposal or removal of the body may then be obtained.

If there are other reasons for a delay in completing the medical portion of the certificate, the registrar should be given written notice of the reason for the delay.

When the circumstances of death (accident, suicide, or homicide) cannot be determined within the statutory time limit, the cause-of-death section should be completed and the manner of death should be shown as "pending investigation."

As soon as the cause of death and circumstances or manner of death are determined, the medical examiner or coroner should file a supplemental report with the registrar or correct or amend the death certificate according to State and local regulations regarding this procedure.

When a body has been found after a long period of time, the medical examiner or coroner should estimate the date and time of death as accurately as possible. If an estimate is made, the information should be entered as "APPROX—date" and/or "APPROX—time."

If completed properly, the cause of death will communicate the same essential information that a case history would. For example, the following cause-of-death statement is complete:

I   a. Septic shock

    b. Infected decubitus ulcers

    c. Complications of cerebral infarction

    d. Cerebral artery atherosclerosis

II   Insulin-dependent diabetes mellitus

If not completed properly, information may be missing from the cause-of death section, so someone reading the cause of death would not know why the condition on the lowest used line developed. For example:

I   a. Pneumonia

    b. Malnutrition

II   This example does not explain what caused malnutrition. A variety of different circumstances could cause malnutrition, so the statement is incomplete and ambiguous.

In some cases, the medical-legal officer will be contacted to verify information reported on a death certificate or to provide additional information to clarify what was meant. The original cause-of-death statement may not be wrong from a clinical standpoint, but may not include sufficient information for assigning codes for statistical purposes. Following guidelines in this handbook should minimize the frequency with which the medical examiner or coroner will need to spend additional time answering follow-up questions about a patient's cause of death.

Fetal Death Reporting

In some jurisdictions the medical-legal officer is required to complete reports of fetal death when the fetal death occurred without medical attendance or occurred under strange or unusual circumstances or was a result of an accident, suicide, or homicide. When completing a report of fetal death, the medical examiner or coroner is to:

- Complete the cause-of-fetal-death section

- Return the fetal death report to the person or institution charged by State law with the responsibility for filing the report.

- If the medical-legal officer is required by State law to fill out a report of fetal death when the fetal death occurs outside a hospital or other institution, complete such a report and send it directly to the local or State registrar.

When an abandoned infant or apparent newborn is found dead, a problem may arise as to whether the event should be registered as a fetal death or an infant death. If the infant is considered to have lived, even for a very short time, following delivery, then the medical examiner or coroner will use the death certificate usually employed. He or she must also ensure that the birth of this infant is properly registered. If the infant is considered to be a fetal death or stillborn, then the appropriate fetal death report must be completed.

Medical Certification of Death

Certifying the Cause of Death

The medical examiner or coroner's primary responsibility in death registration is to complete the medical part of the death certificate. The medical certification includes:

- Date and time pronounced dead;

- Date and time of death;

- Question on whether the case was referred to the medical examiner or coroner;

- Cause-of-death section including cause of death, manner of death, tobacco use, and pregnancy status items;

- Injury items for cases involving injuries;

- Certifier section with signatures.

The proper completion of this section of the certificate is of utmost importance to the efficient working of a medical-legal investigative system.

Cause of Death

This section must be completed by the medical examiner or coroner. The cause-of-death section follows guidelines recommended by the World Health Organization. An important feature is the reported underlying cause of death determined by the medical examiner or coroner and defined as:

1. the disease or injury that initiated the train of morbid events leading directly to death, or

2. the circumstances of the accident or violence that produced the fatal injury. In addition to the underlying cause of death, this section provides for reporting the entire sequence of events leading to death as well as other conditions significantly contributing to death.

The cause-of-death section is designed to elicit the opinion of the medical certifier. Causes of death on the death certificate represent a medical opinion that might vary among individual medical-legal officers. A properly completed cause-of-death section provides an etiological explanation of the order, type, and association of events resulting in death. The initial condition that starts the etiological sequence is specific if it does not leave any doubt as to why it developed. For instance, sepsis is not specific because a number of different conditions may have resulted in sepsis, whereas Human immunodeficiency virus infection is specific.

In certifying the cause of death, any disease, abnormality, injury, or poisoning, if believed to have adversely affected the decedent, should be reported. If the use of alcohol and/or other substance, a smoking history, or a recent pregnancy, injury, or surgery was believed to have contributed to death, then this condition should be reported. The conditions present at the time of death may be completely unrelated, arising independently of each other; or they may be causally related to each other, that is, one condition may lead to another which in turn leads to a third condition, and so forth. Death may also result from the combined effect of two or more conditions.

The mechanism of death, such as cardiac or respiratory arrest, should not be reported as it is a statement not specifically related to

403

the disease process, and it merely attests to the fact of death. The mechanism of death therefore provides no additional information on the cause of death.

The cause-of-death section consists of two parts. The first part is for reporting the sequence of events leading to death, proceeding backwards from the final disease or condition resulting in death. So, each condition in Part I should cause the condition above it. A specific cause of death should be reported in the last entry in Part I so there is no ambiguity about the etiology of this cause. Other significant conditions that contributed to the death, but did not lead to the underlying cause, are reported in Part II.

In addition, there are questions relating to autopsy, manner of death (for example, accident), and injury. The cause of death should include information provided by the pathologist if an autopsy or other type of post mortem examination is done. For deaths that have microscopic examinations pending at the time the certificate is filed, the additional information should be reported as soon as it is available. If the medical examiner or coroner has any questions about the procedure for doing this, contact the registrar.

The completion of the cause-of-death section for a medical-legal case requires careful consideration due to special problems that may be involved. The medical-legal case may depend upon toxicological examination for its ultimate cause-of-death certification (a situation not encountered as frequently in ordinary medical practice). Occasionally the medical examiner or coroner must deal with death certifications in which the cause of death is not clear, even after autopsy and toxicological examination. Despite these special problems that the medical examiner or coroner may encounter in dealing with causes of death, it is important that the medical certification be as accurate and complete as circumstances allow.

For statistical and research purposes, it is important that the causes of death and, in particular, the underlying cause of death, be reported as specifically and as precisely as possible. Careful reporting results in statistics for both underlying and multiple causes of death (i.e., all conditions mentioned on a death certificate) reflecting the best medical opinion.

Every cause-of-death statement is coded and tabulated in the statistical offices according to the latest revision of the *International Classification of Diseases*. When there is a problem with the reported cause of death (e.g., when a causal sequence is reported in reverse order), the rules provide a consistent way to select the most likely underlying cause. However, it is better when rules designed to compensate for poor reporting are not invoked, so that the rules are confirming the physician's statement rather than imposing assumptions about what the physician meant.

Statistically, mortality research focuses on the underlying cause of death because public health interventions seek to break the sequence of causally related medical conditions as early as possible. However, all cause information reported on death certificates is important and is analyzed.

Chapter 56

If Death Occurs While Traveling

Obtaining U.S. Department of State Assistance

When a U.S. citizen dies outside the United States, the deceased person's family members, domestic partner, or legal representative should notify U.S. consular officials at the Department of State. Consular personnel are available 24 hours a day, 7 days a week, to provide assistance to U.S. citizens for overseas emergencies.

- If a family member, domestic partner, or legal representative is in the foreign country with the deceased U.S. citizen, he or she should contact the nearest U.S. embassy or consulate for assistance. Contact information for U.S. embassies, consulates, and consular agencies overseas may be found at the Department of State website.

- If a family member, domestic partner, or legal representative is located in the United States or Canada, he or she should call the Department of State's Office of Overseas Citizens Services in Washington, DC, from 8 am to 8 pm Eastern Time, Monday through Friday, at 888-407-4747 (toll-free) or 202-501-4444. For emergency assistance after working hours or on weekends and holidays, call the Department of State switchboard

This chapter includes text excerpted from "Death during Travel," Centers for Disease Control and Prevention (CDC), July 10, 2015.

at 202-647-4000 and ask to speak with the Overseas Citizens Services duty officer. In addition, the U.S. embassy closest to or in the country where the U.S. citizen died can provide assistance.

Emergency services provided by U.S. consular officials can include advising the family, domestic partner, or legal representative about disposing of the remains and personal effects of the deceased. Preparing and returning human remains to the United States can be an expensive and lengthy process. The Department of State does not pay for these expenses; they are the responsibility of the deceased person's family, domestic partner, or legal representative. Consular officials may also serve as provisional conservators of the deceased person's estate, if no other legal representative is present in the foreign country where the death occurred.

Importation of Human Remains for Interment or Cremation

General Guidance

Except for cremated remains, human remains intended for interment (placement in a grave or tomb) or cremation after entry into the United States must be accompanied by a death certificate stating the cause of death. A death certificate is an official document signed by a coroner, healthcare provider, or other official authorized to make a declaration of cause of death. Death certificates written in a language other than English must be accompanied by an English translation.

Remains of a Person Known or Suspected to Have Died from a Quarantinable Communicable Disease

Federal quarantine regulations (42 CFR Part 71.55) state that the remains of a person who is known or suspected to have died from a quarantinable communicable disease may not be brought into the United States unless the remains are cremated, properly embalmed and placed in a hermetically sealed casket, or accompanied by a Centers for Disease Control and Prevention (CDC) permit to allow importation of human remains, issued by the CDC director.

Quarantinable communicable diseases include cholera, diphtheria, infectious tuberculosis, plague, smallpox, yellow fever, viral hemorrhagic fevers (Lassa, Marburg, Ebola, Crimean-Congo, or others not yet isolated or named), severe acute respiratory syndromes, and influenza caused by novel or re-emergent influenza viruses that are causing or have the potential to cause a pandemic. A hermetically sealed casket is one that is airtight and secured against the escape of microorganisms. It should be accompanied by valid documentation certifying that it is hermetically sealed.

If a CDC permit is obtained to allow importation of human remains, CDC may impose additional conditions for importation. Permits for the importation of human remains of a person known or suspected to have died from a quarantinable communicable disease may be obtained from CDC's Division of Global Migration and Quarantine by calling the CDC Emergency Operations Center at 770-488-7100. A copy of the CDC permit must accompany the human remains at all times during shipment.

Remains of a Person Who Died of Any Cause Other than a Quarantinable Communicable Disease

When the cause of death is anything other than a quarantinable communicable disease, the remains may be cleared, released, and authorized for entry into the United States if one of the following conditions is met:

1. The remains meet the standards for importation found in 42 CFR 71.55: the remains are cremated or properly embalmed and placed in a hermetically sealed casket or are accompanied by a permit issued by the CDC director.

2. The remains are shipped in a leakproof container. A leakproof container is one that is puncture resistant and sealed so that there is no leakage of fluids outside the container during handling, storage, transport, or shipping.

CDC may also require additional measures, including detention, disinfection, disinfestation, fumigation, or other related measures, if there is evidence that the human remains are or may be infected or contaminated with a communicable disease and that such measures are necessary to prevent the introduction, transmission, or spread of communicable diseases into the United States.

Exportation of Human Remains

CDC places no restrictions on the exportation of human remains outside the United States, although other state and local regulations may apply. Exporters of human remains and travelers taking human remains out of the United States should be aware that the importation requirements of the destination country and the air carrier must be met. Information regarding these requirements may be obtained from the appropriate foreign embassy or consulate and the air carrier.

Chapter 57

Grief, Bereavement, and Coping with Loss

Bereavement and Grief

Bereavement is the period of sadness after losing a loved one through death.

Grief and mourning occur during the period of bereavement. Grief and mourning are closely related. Mourning is the way we show grief in public. The way people mourn is affected by beliefs, religious practices, and cultural customs. People who are grieving are sometimes described as bereaved.

Grief is the normal process of reacting to the loss.

Grief is the emotional response to the loss of a loved one. Common grief reactions include the following:

- Feeling emotionally numb.

- Feeling unable to believe the loss occurred.

- Feeling anxiety from the distress of being separated from the loved one.

- Mourning along with depression.

- A feeling of acceptance.

This chapter includes text excerpted from "Grief, Bereavement, and Coping with Loss (PDQ®)–Patient Version," National Cancer Institute (NCI), March 6, 2013.

Types of Grief Reactions

Anticipatory Grief

Anticipatory grief may occur when a death is expected.

Anticipatory grief occurs when a death is expected, but before it happens. It may be felt by the families of people who are dying and by the person dying. Anticipatory grief helps family members get ready emotionally for the loss. It can be a time to take care of unfinished business with the dying person, such as saying "I love you" or "I forgive you."

Like grief that occurs after the death of a loved one, anticipatory grief involves mental, emotional, cultural, and social responses. However, anticipatory grief is different from grief that occurs after the death. Symptoms of anticipatory grief include the following:

- Depression.

- Feeling a greater than usual concern for the dying person.

- Imagining what the loved one's death will be like.

- Getting ready emotionally for what will happen after the death.

Anticipatory grief may help the family but not the dying person.

Anticipatory grief helps family members cope with what is to come. For the patient who is dying, anticipatory grief may be too much to handle and may cause him or her to withdraw from others.

Anticipatory grief does not always occur.

Some researchers report that anticipatory grief is rare. Studies showed that periods of acceptance and recovery usually seen during grief are not common before the patient's actual death. The bereaved may feel that trying to accept the loss of a loved one before death occurs may make it seem that the dying patient has been abandoned.

Also, grief felt before the death will not decrease the grief felt afterwards or make it last a shorter time.

Normal Grief

Normal or common grief begins soon after a loss and symptoms go away over time.

During normal grief, the bereaved person moves toward accepting the loss and is able to continue normal day-to-day life even though it is hard to do. Common grief reactions include:

- Emotional numbness, shock, disbelief, or denial. These often occur right after the death, especially if the death was not expected.

- Anxiety over being separated from the loved one. The bereaved may wish to bring the person back and become lost in thoughts of the deceased. Images of death may occur often in the person's everyday thoughts.

- Distress that leads to crying; sighing; having dreams, illusions, and hallucinations of the deceased; and looking for places or things that were shared with the deceased.

- Anger.

- Periods of sadness, loss of sleep, loss of appetite, extreme tiredness, guilt, and loss of interest in life. Day-to-day living may be affected.

In normal grief, symptoms will occur less often and will feel less severe as time passes. Recovery does not happen in a set period of time. For most bereaved people having normal grief, symptoms lessen between 6 months and 2 years after the loss.

Many bereaved people will have grief bursts or pangs.

Grief bursts or pangs are short periods (20–30 minutes) of very intense distress. Sometimes these bursts are caused by reminders of the deceased person. At other times they seem to happen for no reason.

Grief is sometimes described as a process that has stages.

There are several theories about how the normal grief process works. Experts have described different types and numbers of stages that people go through as they cope with loss. At this time, there is not enough information to prove that one of these theories is more correct than the others.

Although many bereaved people have similar responses as they cope with their losses, there is no typical grief response. The grief process is personal.

Complicated Grief

There is no right or wrong way to grieve, but studies have shown that there are patterns of grief that are different from the most common. This has been called complicated grief.

Complicated grief reactions that have been seen in studies include:

- Minimal grief reaction: A grief pattern in which the person has no, or only a few, signs of distress or problems that occur with other types of grief.

- Chronic grief: A grief pattern in which the symptoms of common grief last for a much longer time than usual. These symptoms are a lot like ones that occur with major depression, anxiety, or post-traumatic stress.

Factors that Affect Complicated Grief

Researchers study grief reactions to try to find out what might increase the chance that complicated grief will occur.

Studies have looked at how the following factors affect the grief response:

Whether the death is expected or unexpected.

It may seem that any sudden, unexpected loss might lead to more difficult grief. However, studies have found that bereaved people with high self-esteem and/or a feeling that they have control over life are likely to have a normal grief reaction even after an unexpected loss. Bereaved people with low self-esteem and/or a sense that life cannot be controlled are more likely to have complicated grief after an unexpected loss. This includes more depression and physical problems.

The personality of the bereaved.

Studies have found that people with certain personality traits are more likely to have long-lasting depression after a loss. These include people who are very dependent on the loved one (such as a spouse), and people who deal with distress by thinking about it all the time.

The religious beliefs of the bereaved.

Some studies have shown that religion helps people cope better with grief. Other studies have shown it does not help or causes more distress. Religion seems to help people who go to church often. The positive effect on grief may be because church-goers have more social support.

Whether the bereaved is male or female.

In general, men have more problems than women do after a spouse's death. Men tend to have worse depression and more health problems than women do after the loss. Some researchers think this may be because men have less social support after a loss.

The age of the bereaved.

In general, younger bereaved people have more problems after a loss than older bereaved people do. They have more severe health problems, grief symptoms, and other mental and physical symptoms. Younger bereaved people, however, may recover more quickly than older bereaved people do, because they have more resources and social support.

The amount of social support the bereaved has.

Lack of social support increases the chance of having problems coping with a loss. Social support includes the person's family, friends, neighbors, and community members who can give psychological, physical, and financial help. After the death of a close family member, many people have a number of related losses. The death of a spouse, for example, may cause a loss of income and changes in lifestyle and day-to-day living. These are all related to social support.

Treatment of Grief

Normal grief may not need to be treated.

Most bereaved people work through grief and recover within the first 6 months to 2 years. Researchers are studying whether bereaved people experiencing normal grief would be helped by formal treatment. They are also studying whether treatment might prevent complicated grief in people who are likely to have it.

For people who have serious grief reactions or symptoms of distress, treatment may be helpful.

Complicated grief may be treated with different types of psychotherapy (talk therapy).

Researchers are studying the treatment of mental, emotional, social, and behavioral symptoms of grief. Treatment methods include discussion, listening, and counseling.

Complicated grief treatment (CGT) is a type of grief therapy that was helpful in a clinical trial.

Complicated grief treatment (CGT) has three phases:

- The first phase includes talking about the loss and setting goals toward recovery. The bereaved are taught to work on these two things.

415

- The second phase includes coping with the loss by retelling the story of the death. This helps bereaved people who try not to think about their loss.

- The last phase looks at progress that has been made toward recovery and helps the bereaved make future plans. The bereaved's feelings about ending the sessions are also discussed.

In a clinical trial of patients with complicated grief, CGT was compared to interpersonal psychotherapy (IPT). IPT is a type of psychotherapy that focuses on the person's relationships with others and is helpful in treating depression. In patients with complicated grief, the CGT was more helpful than IPT.

Cognitive behavioral therapy (CBT) for complicated grief was helpful in a clinical trial.

Cognitive behavioral therapy (CBT) works with the way a person's thoughts and behaviors are connected. CBT helps the patient learn skills that change attitudes and behaviors by replacing negative thoughts and changing the rewards of certain behaviors.

A clinical trial compared CBT to counseling for complicated grief. Results showed that patients treated with CBT had more improvement in symptoms and general mental distress than those in the counseling group.

Depression related to grief is sometimes treated with drugs.

There is no standard drug therapy for depression that occurs with grief. Some healthcare professionals think depression is a normal part of grief and doesn't need to be treated. Whether to treat grief-related depression with drugs is up to the patient and the healthcare professional to decide.

Clinical trials of antidepressants for depression related to grief have found that the drugs can help relieve depression. However, they give less relief and take longer to work than they do when used for depression that is not related to grief.

Chapter 58

Working through Grief

What Is Grief?

Grief is the normal response of sorrow, emotion, and confusion that comes from losing someone or something important to you. It is a natural part of life. Grief is a typical reaction to death, divorce, job loss, a move away from family and friends, or loss of good health due to illness.

How Does Grief Feel?

Just after a death or loss, you may feel empty and numb, as if you are in shock. You may notice physical changes such as trembling, nausea, trouble breathing, muscle weakness, dry mouth, or trouble sleeping and eating.

You may become angry—at a situation, a particular person, or just angry in general. Almost everyone in grief also experiences guilt. Guilt

This chapter contains text excerpted from the following sources: Text beginning with the heading "What Is Grief?" is excerpted from "How to Deal with Grief," Substance Abuse and Mental Health Services Administration (SAMHSA), U.S. Department of Health and Human Services (HHS), January 2001. Reviewed October 2016; Text under the heading "Treatment of Grief" is excerpted from "Treatment of Grief," National Cancer Institute (NCI), March 6, 2013; Text under the heading "Coping with Grief" is excerpted from "Coping with Grief," *NIH News in Health*, National Institutes of Health (NIH), November 15, 2009. Reviewed October 2016.

is often expressed as "I could have, I should have, and I wish I would have" statements.

People in grief may have strange dreams or nightmares, be absent-minded, withdraw socially, or lack the desire to return to work. While these feelings and behaviors are normal during grief, they will pass.

How Long Does Grief Last?

Grief lasts as long as it takes you to accept and learn to live with your loss. For some people, grief lasts a few months. For others, grieving may take years.

The length of time spent grieving is different for each person. There are many reasons for the differences, including personality, health, coping style, culture, family background, and life experiences. The time spent grieving also depends on your relationship with the person lost and how prepared you were for the loss.

How Will I Know When I'm Done Grieving?

Every person who experiences a death or other loss must complete a four-step grieving process:

1. Accept the loss.
2. Work through and feel the physical and emotional pain of grief.
3. Adjust to living in a world without the person or item lost.
4. Move on with life.

The grieving process is over only when a person completes the four steps.

Coping with Grief

When someone you love dies, your world changes. You may feel numb, shocked or frightened. You may feel depressed and have trouble concentrating. You may feel guilty for being the one who is still alive. All of these feelings are normal. There is no right or wrong way to mourn.

Each year, about 2.5 million people die nationwide. Every death leaves behind an average of 4 or 5 grieving survivors. For most, extreme feelings of grief begin to fade within 6 months after the loss.

But some bereaved people may continue to struggle for years to move on with their lives.

It's often helpful to talk with family and friends about the person who's gone. People sometimes hesitate to mention a dead person's name or discuss the loss, because they don't want to cause pain. But it can help when people share their feelings.

Researchers have tried for decades to identify different stages of grief. They've found that the grieving process differs for every individual. It's affected by how attached you felt to the person who died; whether you were a parent, child or spouse; how the death occurred and other factors.

One study found that acceptance of a death comes surprisingly early for most bereaved people, usually within the first month after the loss. The researchers found that in the 2 years following a death, the most often-reported symptom is yearning for the person who died. Yearning is much more common than depression, anger and disbelief.

This study and many others have found that if symptoms aren't tapering off by 6 months after the loss, it may be a sign of a more serious problem, sometimes called complicated grief. People with complicated grief are at risk for major depression, substance abuse, post-traumatic stress disorder and suicidal thoughts and actions.

"Prolonged grief, or complicated grief, is seen in a small portion of bereaved individuals—about 10% or 20%. Their symptoms are disruptive to their lives and daily functioning," says Dr. Mary-Frances O'Connor, a psychologist at the University of California, Los Angeles. "These people may experience extreme yearning, loneliness and a feeling that life will never have any meaning. They may have intrusive thoughts and feel ongoing anger or bitterness over the death."

O'Connor's brain imaging studies have found differences in brain activity between bereaved people with complicated grief and those who are coping well with their loss. Both groups showed pain-related brain activity when they looked at photos of their loved ones. But only those with complicated grief showed activation in parts of the brain's reward-processing centers.

"That may seem strange. But other studies have shown that when people are very attached to their loved ones, they feel rewarded when they are with them," O'Connor says. People with complicated grief may still feel very attached, and so feel "rewarded" by seeing photos of their loved ones. Those who adapt well, O'Connor suggests, have somehow accepted the reality that the person is not physically with them anymore. "They still feel sad, but they no longer yearn for the person in the same way," she says.

419

Complicated grief is difficult to treat. Some evidence suggests that a specialized talk therapy can help people with complicated grief improve faster and better than traditional talk therapy. This experimental therapy, called complicated grief treatment, involves vividly recalling the death with a trained grief counselor and having an imaginary conversation with the person who died. Researchers are now testing whether complicated grief treatment might work even better in combination with antidepressants or other approaches.

Some studies show that people who've been caregivers for a relative with a long-term illness may adapt relatively quickly to the death. Dr. Richard Schulz, a social psychologist at the University of Pittsburgh, studies caregivers for relatives with Alzheimer disease. He and his colleagues found that most did remarkably well after their loved one died. "Their level of depression, which was very high during the caregiving phase before the death, returned to almost normal levels within 6 months after the death," Schulz says.

People caring for someone with a long-term illness may begin the grieving process while their loved one is still alive. "The death may mark the end of suffering for the care-givers and the patients," Schulz says. "The death also eliminates much of the burden associated with daily care in the home. It frees up time, so the person can now re-engage in social contacts they might have had prior to taking on the caregiver role."

But Schulz's research also found that about 1 in 5 caregivers had persistent, severe depression and other troubling symptoms more than 6 months after the death. Many of those who struggled to adapt were either highly depressed before the death or had positive feelings about their caregiving role.

Treating depression before the death seemed to help caregivers cope afterward. People also did better if they'd participated in a program that helped them cope while their relative was still alive.

"The program provided group support, information about the disease and other resources," says Schulz. "It was not designed to help people after the death, but that was an unexpected benefit. The quality of the caregiving experience may have helped them prepare for the death indirectly."

Some studies have found that when patients, doctors and family members directly address the prospect of death before it happens, it helps survivors after the death. "If you're in a long-term disease situation where death is likely, it's helpful to engage in end-of-life care planning, to make it easier to deal with the death once it occurs," says Schulz.

NIH-funded (National Institute of Health) scientists continue to study different aspects of the grieving process and to search for new treatments. Researchers are also looking at how cultural attitudes and beliefs about death can affect grief and mourning.

Remember, although the death of a loved one can feel overwhelming, most people can make it through the grieving process with the support of family and friends. Take care of yourself, accept offers of help or companionship from those around you, and be sure to get additional help or counseling if you need it.

It may take time. The process will be difficult. But you can eventually adjust to life after someone you love has died.

Part Nine

Mortality Statistics

Chapter 59

Life Expectancy: Global Trends

The world is on the brink of a demographic milestone. Since the beginning of recorded history, young children have outnumbered their elders. In about five years' time, however, the number of people aged 65 or older will outnumber children under age 5. Driven by falling fertility rates and remarkable increases in life expectancy, population aging will continue, even accelerate. The number of people aged 65 or older is projected to grow from an estimated 524 million in 2010 to nearly 1.5 billion in 2050, with most of the increase in developing countries.

The remarkable improvements in life expectancy over the past century were part of a shift in the leading causes of disease and death. At the dawn of the 20th century, the major health threats were infectious and parasitic diseases that most often claimed the lives of infants and children. Currently, non communicable diseases that more commonly affect adults and older people impose the greatest burden on global health.

In today's developing countries, the rise of chronic noncommunicable diseases such as heart disease, cancer, and diabetes reflects changes in lifestyle and diet, as well as aging. The potential economic and societal costs of non communicable diseases of this type rise sharply with age and have the ability to affect economic growth. A World Health

This chapter includes text excerpted from "Global Health and Aging," National Institute on Aging (NIA), National Institutes of Health (NIH), October 2011. Reviewed October 2016.

Organization (WHO) analysis in 23 low- and middle-income countries estimated the economic losses from three noncommunicable diseases (heart disease, stroke, and diabetes) in these countries would total US$83 billion between 2006 and 2015.

Reducing severe disability from disease and health conditions is one key to holding down health and social costs. The health and economic burden of disability also can be reinforced or alleviated by environmental characteristics that can determine whether an older person can remain independent despite physical limitations. The longer people can remain mobile and care for themselves, the lower are the costs for long-term care to families and society.

Because many adult and older-age health problems were rooted in early life experiences and living conditions, ensuring good child health can yield benefits for older people. In the meantime, generations of children and young adults who grew up in poverty and ill health in developing countries will be entering old age in coming decades, potentially increasing the health burden of older populations in those countries. With continuing declines in death rates among older people, the proportion aged 80 or older is rising quickly, and more people are living past 100. The limits to life expectancy and lifespan are not as obvious as once thought. And there is mounting evidence from cross-national data that—with appropriate policies and programs—people can remain healthy and independent well into old age and can continue to contribute to their communities and families.

The potential for an active, healthy old age is tempered by one of the most daunting and potentially costly consequences of ever-longer life expectancies: the increase in people with dementia, especially Alzheimer disease. Most dementia patients eventually need constant care and help with the most basic activities of daily living, creating a heavy economic and social burden. Prevalence of dementia rises sharply with age. An estimated 25–30 percent of people aged 85 or older have dementia. Unless new and more effective interventions are found to treat or prevent Alzheimer disease, prevalence is expected to rise dramatically with the aging of the population in the United States and worldwide.

Aging is taking place alongside other broad social trends that will affect the lives of older people. Economies are globalizing, people are more likely to live in cities, and technology is evolving rapidly. Demographic and family changes mean there will be fewer older people with families to care for them. People today have fewer children, are less likely to be married, and are less likely to live with older generations. With declining support from families, society will need better information and tools to ensure the well-being of the world's growing number of older citizens.

Humanity's Aging

In 2010, an estimated 524 million people were aged 65 or older—8 percent of the world's population. By 2050, this number is expected to nearly triple to about 1.5 billion, representing 16 percent of the world's population. Although more developed countries have the oldest population profiles, the vast majority of older people—and the most rapidly aging populations—are in less developed countries. Between 2010 and 2050, the number of older people in less developed countries is projected to increase more than 250 percent, compared with 71 percent increase in developed countries.

This remarkable phenomenon is being driven by declines in fertility and improvements in longevity. With fewer children entering the population and people living longer, older people are making up an increasing share of the total population. In more developed countries, fertility fell below the replacement rate of two live births per woman by the 1970s, down from nearly three children per woman around 1950. Even more crucial for population aging, fertility fell with surprising speed in many less developed countries from an average of six children in 1950 to an average of two or three children in 2005. In 2006, fertility was at or below the two-child replacement level in 44 less developed countries.

Most developed nations have had decades to adjust to their changing age structures. It took more than 100 years for the share of France's population aged 65 or older to rise from 7 percent to 14 percent. In contrast, many less developed countries are experiencing a rapid increase in the number and percentage of older people, often within a single generation. For example, the same demographic aging that unfolded over more than a century in France will occur in just two decades in Brazil. Developing countries will need to adapt quickly to this new reality. Many less developed nations will need new policies that ensure the financial security of older people, and that provide the health and social care they need, without the same extended period of economic growth experienced by aging societies in the West. In other words, some countries may grow old before they grow rich.

In some countries, the sheer number of people entering older ages will challenge national infrastructures, particularly health systems. This numeric surge in older people is dramatically illustrated in the world's two most populous countries: China and India. China's older population —those over age 65—will likely swell to 330 million by 2050 from 110 million today. India's current older population of 60 million is projected to exceed 227 million in 2050, an increase of nearly 280 percent from today. By the middle of this century, there could be 100 million Chinese over the age of 80. This is an amazing achievement considering that there were fewer than 14 million people this age on the entire planet just a century ago.

Living Longer

The dramatic increase in average life expectancy during the 20th century ranks as one of society's greatest achievements. Although most babies born in 1900 did not live past age 50, life expectancy at birth now exceeds 83 years in Japan—the current leader—and is at least 81 years in several other countries. Less developed regions of the world have experienced a steady increase in life expectancy since World War II, although not all regions have shared in these improvements. (One notable exception is the fall in life expectancy in many parts of Africa because of deaths caused by the Human immunodeficiency virus/Acquired immune deficiency syndrome (HIV/AIDS) epidemic.) The most dramatic and rapid gains have occurred in East Asia, where life expectancy at birth increased from less than 45 years in 1950 to more than 74 years today.

These improvements are part of a major transition in human health spreading around the globe at different rates and along different pathways. This transition encompasses a broad set of changes that include a decline from high to low fertility; a steady increase in life expectancy at birth and at older ages; and a shift in the leading causes of death and illness from infectious and parasitic diseases to noncommunicable diseases and chronic conditions. In early nonindustrial societies, the risk of death was high at every age, and only a small proportion of people reached old age. In modern societies, most people live past middle age, and deaths are highly concentrated at older ages.

The victories against infectious and parasitic diseases are a triumph for public health projects of the 20th century, which immunized millions of people against smallpox, polio, and major childhood killers like measles. Even earlier, better living standards, especially more nutritious diets and cleaner drinking water, began to reduce serious infections and prevent deaths among children. More children were surviving their vulnerable early years and reaching adulthood. In fact, more than 60 percent of the improvement in female life expectancy at birth in developed countries between 1850 and 1900 occurred because more children were living to age 15, not because more adults were reaching old age. It wasn't until the 20th century that mortality rates began to decline within the older ages. Research for more recent periods shows a surprising and continuing improvement in life expectancy among those aged 80 or above.

The progressive increase in survival in these oldest age groups was not anticipated by demographers, and it raises questions about how high the average life expectancy can realistically rise and about the potential length of the human lifespan. While some experts assume that life expectancy must be approaching an upper limit, data on life expectancies between 1840 and 2007 show a steady increase averaging about three months of life per year. The country with the highest average life expectancy has varied over time. In 1840 it was Sweden and today it is Japan—but the pattern is strikingly similar. So far there is little evidence that life expectancy has stopped rising even in Japan.

The rising life expectancy within the older population itself is increasing the number and proportion of people at very old ages. The "oldest old" (people aged 85 or older) constitute 8 percent of the world's 65-and-over population: 12 percent in more developed countries and 6 percent in less developed countries. In many countries, the oldest old are now the fastest growing part of the total population. On a global level, the 85-and-over population is projected to increase 351 percent between 2010 and 2050, compared to a 188 percent increase for the population aged 65 or older and a 22 percent increase for the population under age 65.

The global number of centenarians is projected to increase 10-fold between 2010 and 2050. In the mid-1990s, some researchers estimated that, over the course of human history, the odds of living from birth to age 100 may have risen from 1 in 20,000,000 to 1 in 50 for females in low- mortality nations such as Japan and Sweden. This group's longevity may increase even faster than current projections assume—previous population projections often underestimated decreases in mortality rates among the oldest old.

New Disease Patterns

The transition from high to low mortality and fertility that accompanied socioeconomic development has also meant a shift in the leading causes of disease and death. Demographers and epidemiologists describe this shift as part of an "epidemiologic transition" characterized by the waning of infectious and acute diseases and the emerging importance of chronic and degenerative diseases. High death rates from infectious diseases are commonly associated with the poverty, poor diets, and limited infrastructure found in developing countries. Although many developing countries still experience high child mortality from infectious and parasitic diseases, one of the major epidemiologic trends of the current century is the rise of chronic and degenerative diseases in countries throughout the world—regardless of income level.

Evidence from the multicountry Global Burden of Disease project and other international epidemiologic research shows that health problems associated with wealthy and aged populations affect a wide and expanding swath of world population. Over the next 10 to 15 years, people in every world region will suffer more death and disability from such non communicable diseases as heart disease, cancer, and diabetes than from infectious and parasitic diseases. The myth that non communicable diseases affect mainly affluent and aged populations was dispelled by the project, which combines information about mortality and morbidity from every world region to assess the total health burden from specific diseases. The burden is measured by estimating the loss of healthy years of life due to a specific cause based on detailed epidemiological information. In 2008, noncommunicable diseases accounted for an estimated 86 percent of the burden of disease in high-income countries, 65 percent in middle-income countries, and a surprising 37 percent in low-income countries.

By 2030, noncommunicable diseases are projected to account for more than one-half of the disease burden in low-income countries and more than three-fourths in middle-income countries. Infectious and parasitic diseases will account for 30 percent and 10 percent, respectively, in low- and middle-income countries. Among the 60-and-over population, noncommunicable diseases already account for more than 87 percent of the burden in low-, middle-, and high-income countries.

But the continuing health threats from communicable diseases for older people cannot be dismissed, either. Older people account for a growing share of the infectious disease burden in low-income countries. Infectious disease programs, including those for HIV/AIDS, often neglect older people and ignore the potential effects of population aging. Yet, antiretroviral therapy is enabling more people with HIV/AIDS to survive to older ages. And, there is growing evidence that older people are particularly susceptible to infectious diseases for a variety of reasons, including immunosenescence (the progressive deterioration of immune function with age) and frailty. Older people already suffering from one chronic or infectious disease are especially vulnerable to additional infectious diseases. For example, type 2 diabetes and tuberculosis are well- known "comorbid risk factors" that have serious health consequences for older people.

Chapter 60

Mortality Trends in the United States

Key Findings

Data from the National Vital Statistics System, Mortality:

* Life expectancy for the U.S. population in 2014 was unchanged from 2013 at 78.8 years.

* The age-adjusted death rate decreased 1.0% to 724.6 deaths per 100,000 standard population in 2014 from 731.9 in 2013.

* The 10 leading causes of death in 2014 remained the same as in 2013. Age-adjusted death rates significantly decreased for 5 leading causes and significantly increased for 4 leading causes.

* The infant mortality rate decreased 2.3% to a historic low of 582.1 infant deaths per 100,000 live births. The 10 leading causes of infant death in 2014 remained the same as in 2013.

This chapter presents 2014 United States final mortality data on deaths and death rates by demographic and medical characteristics. These data provide information on mortality patterns among U.S. residents by such variables as sex, race and ethnicity, and cause of

This chapter includes text excerpted from "Mortality in the United States, 2014," Centers for Disease Control and Prevention (CDC), November 6, 2015.

death. Information on mortality patterns is key to understanding changes in the health and well-being of the U.S. population. Life expectancy estimates, age-adjusted death rates by race and ethnicity and sex, the 10 leading causes of death, and the 10 leading causes of infant death were analyzed by comparing 2014 final data with 2013 final data.

How Long Can We Expect to Live?

Life expectancy at birth represents the average number of years that a group of infants would live if the group was to experience, throughout life, the age-specific death rates present in the year of birth. In 2014, life expectancy at birth was 78.8 years for the total U.S. population—81.2 years for females and 76.4 years for males, the same as in 2013. Life expectancy for females was consistently higher than life expectancy for males. In 2014, the difference in life expectancy between females and males was 4.8 years, the same as in 2013.

Life expectancy at age 65 for the total population was 19.3 years, the same as in 2013. Life expectancy at age 65 was 20.5 years for females, unchanged from 2013, and 18.0 years for males, a 0.1-year increase from 2013. The difference in life expectancy at age 65 between females and males decreased 0.1 year, to 2.5 years in 2014 from 2.6 years in 2013.

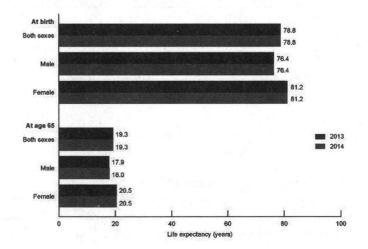

Figure 60.1. *Life Expectancy at Selected Ages, by Sex: United States, 2013 and 2014*

Which Population Groups Experienced Reductions in Mortality?

The age-adjusted death rate for the total population decreased 1.0% to a record low of 724.6 deaths per 100,000 standard population in 2014 from 731.9 in 2013. Age-adjusted death rates decreased significantly in 2014 from 2013 for non-Hispanic black males (2.1%), non-Hispanic black females (1.3%), non-Hispanic white males (0.5%), non-Hispanic white females (0.7%), Hispanic males (2.0%), and Hispanic females (2.5%).

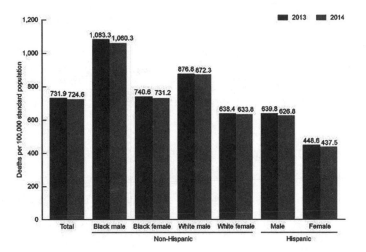

Figure 60.2. *Age-Adjusted Death Rates for Selected Populations: United States, 2013 and 2014*

What Are the Leading Causes of Death?

In 2014, the 10 leading causes of death—heart disease, cancer, chronic lower respiratory diseases, unintentional injuries, stroke, Alzheimer disease, diabetes, influenza and pneumonia, kidney disease, and suicide—remained the same as in 2013. The 10 leading causes accounted for 73.8% of all deaths in the United States in 2014.

From 2013 to 2014, age-adjusted death rates significantly decreased for 5 of the 10 leading causes of death and significantly increased for 4 leading causes. The rate decreased by 1.6% for heart disease, 1.2% for cancer, 3.8% for chronic lower respiratory diseases, 1.4% for diabetes, and 5.0% for influenza and pneumonia. The rate increased by 2.8% for unintentional injuries, 0.8% for stroke, 8.1% for Alzheimer disease, and 3.2% for suicide. The rate for kidney disease in 2014 remained the same as in 2013.

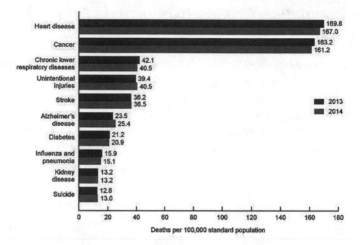

Figure 60.3. *Age-Adjusted Death Rates for the 10 Leading Causes of Death: United States, 2013 and 2014*

What Are the Leading Causes of Infant Death?

The infant mortality rate (IMR)—the ratio of infant deaths to live births in a given year—is generally considered a good indicator of the overall health of a population. IMR declined 2.3% to a record low 582.1 infant deaths per 100,000 live births in 2014 from 596.1 in 2013.

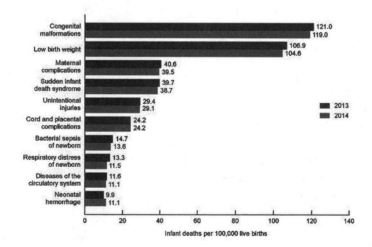

Figure 60.4. *Infant Mortality Rates for the 10 Leading Causes of Infant Death: United States, 2013 and 2014*

The 10 leading causes of infant death in 2014 accounted for 69.1% of all infant deaths in the United States. The leading causes remained the same as in 2013. For Respiratory distress of newborn, IMR decreased 13.5% to 11.5 infant deaths per 100,000 live births in 2014 from 13.3 in 2013. Mortality rates for other leading causes of infant death did not change significantly.

Summary

From 2013 to 2014, the age-adjusted death rate for the total population declined 1.0%, and life expectancy at birth remained unchanged at 78.8 years. In 2014, a total of 2,626,418 resident deaths were registered in the United States. The age-adjusted death rate declined for each major race and ethnicity group by sex. Significant decreases in mortality in 2014 compared with 2013 are consistent with long-term trends. Although year-to-year changes are usually relatively small, the age-adjusted death rate in the United States decreased 16.6% between 2000 and 2014.

The leading causes of death in 2014 remained the same as in 2013. Mortality significantly decreased for five leading causes and increased for four. Life expectancy at birth remained unchanged at 78.8 years as decreases in mortality for heart disease, cancer, chronic lower respiratory diseases, diabetes, and influenza and pneumonia were offset somewhat by increases in mortality from unintentional injuries, stroke, Alzheimer disease, and suicide.

In 2014, a total of 23,215 deaths occurred in children aged under 1 year, which was 225 fewer infant deaths than in 2013. IMR decreased 2.3% to a historic low. The leading causes of infant death were the same in 2014 as in 2013. The only significant change among leading causes of infant death was a 13.5% decrease in IMR for Respiratory distress of newborn.

Chapter 61

Leading Causes of Death in the United States

Chapter Contents

Section 61.1

Leading Causes of Death

This section includes text excerpted from "Deaths:
Final Data for 2014," Centers for Disease Control and
Prevention (CDC), June 30, 2016.

The 15 leading causes of death in 2014 accounted for 79.6% of all deaths in the United States. The leading causes of death in 2014 remained the same as in 2013. Causes of death are ranked according to the number of deaths; for ranking procedures, see Technical Notes. By rank, the 15 leading causes of death in 2014 were:

1. Diseases of heart (heart disease)

2. Malignant neoplasms (cancer)

3. Chronic lower respiratory diseases

4. Accidents (unintentional injuries)

5. Cerebrovascular diseases (stroke)

6. Alzheimer disease

7. Diabetes mellitus (diabetes)

8. Influenza and pneumonia

9. Nephritis, nephrotic syndrome and nephrosis (kidney disease)

10. Intentional self-harm (suicide)

11. Septicemia

12. Chronic liver disease and cirrhosis

13. Essential hypertension and hypertensive renal disease (hypertension)

14. Parkinson disease

15. Pneumonitis due to solids and liquids

The pattern of mortality varies greatly with age. As a result, the shifting age distribution of a population can significantly influence changes in crude death rates over time. Age-adjusted death rates, in contrast, eliminate the influence of such differences in the population age structure. Therefore, whereas causes of death are ranked according to the number of deaths, age-adjusted death rates are used to depict trends for leading causes of death in this report because they are better than crude rates for showing changes in mortality over time and among causes of death.

From 2013 to 2014, the age-adjusted death rate declined significantly for 6 of the 15 leading causes of death and increased for 5 leading causes. The age-adjusted death rate for the leading cause of death, heart disease, decreased 1.6%. The age-adjusted death rate for cancer decreased 1.2%. Deaths from these two diseases combined accounted for 45.9% of deaths in the United States in 2014. Except for a relatively small increase in 1993, mortality from heart disease has declined steadily since 1980 (Figure 61.1.). The age-adjusted death rate for cancer, the second leading cause of death, has shown a gradual but consistent downward trend since 1993.

Other leading causes of death that showed significant decreases in 2014 relative to 2013 were chronic lower respiratory diseases (3.8%), diabetes (1.4%), Influenza and pneumonia (5.0%), and hypertension (3.5%).

The age-adjusted death rate increased significantly between 2013 and 2014 for five leading causes: unintentional injuries (2.8%), stroke (0.8%), Alzheimer disease (8.1%), suicide (3.2%), and Chronic liver disease and cirrhosis (2.0%).

Observed changes from 2013 to 2014 in the age-adjusted death rate for Parkinson disease and Pneumonitis due to solids and liquids were not significant. Age-adjusted rates were unchanged in 2014 from 2013 for Septicemia and kidney disease.

Assault (homicide), the 17th leading cause of death in 2014, dropped from among the 15 leading causes of death in 2010 but is still a major issue for some age groups. In 2014, homicide remained among the 15 leading causes of death for age groups 1–4 (3rd), 5–14 (5th), 15–24 (3rd), 25–34 (3rd), 35–44 (5th), and 45–54 (13th).

Although Human immunodeficiency virus (HIV) disease has not been among the 15 leading causes of death since 1997, it is still considered a major public health problem for some age groups. Historically, for all ages combined, HIV disease mortality reached its highest level in 1995 after a period of increase from 1987 through 1994. Subsequently, the rate for this disease decreased an average of 33.0% per year from 1995 through 1998, and 6.3% per year from 1999 through 2014. In 2014, HIV disease remained among the 15 leading causes of death for age groups 15–24 (13th), 25–34 (8th), 35–44 (9th), 45–54 (11th), and 55–64 (14th).Among these age groups, the ranking of HIV disease changed between 2013 and 2014 only for those aged 45–54, dropping from 10th leading cause in 2013 to 11th leading cause in 2014.

Enterocolitis due to Clostridium difficile (C. difficile)—a predominantly antibiotic-associated inflammation of the intestines caused by C. difficile, a gram-positive, anaerobic, spore-forming bacillus—is of growing concern. The disease is often acquired in hospitals or other healthcare facilities with long-term patients or residents. The number of deaths from C. difficile climbed from 793 deaths in 1999 to a high of 8,085 deaths in 2011. In 2014, the number of deaths from C. difficile was 7,130, continuing to decline after a slight increase in 2011. In 2014, the age-adjusted death rate for this cause was 1.9 deaths per 100,000 U.S. standard population, a decrease of 9.5% from the rate in 2013. In 2014, C. difficile ranked as the 18th leading cause of death for the population aged 65 and over. Nearly 90% of deaths from C. difficile occurred among people aged 65 and over.

Changes in mortality levels by age and cause of death can have a major effect on changes in life expectancy. While changes in causes of death occurred in 2014 from 2013, life expectancy at birth for the total population did not change. Decreases in mortality from cancer, chronic lower respiratory diseases, and heart disease were offset by increases in mortality from unintentional injuries, Alzheimer disease, and suicide. Life expectancy at birth for both males and females did not change between 2013 and 2014. For males, decreases in mortality from cancer, heart disease, and Chronic lower respiratory diseases were offset by increases in mortality from unintentional injuries, Alzheimer disease, and suicide. Similarly for the female population, decreases in mortality from chronic lower respiratory diseases, cancer, and heart disease were offset by increases in mortality from Alzheimer disease, unintentional injuries, and stroke.

The relative risk of death in one population group compared with another can be expressed as a ratio. Ratios based on age-adjusted death rates show that males have higher rates than females for 13 of the 15 leading causes of death, with rates for males being at least twice as great as those for females for 4 of these leading causes. The largest ratio was for suicide (3.6). Other large ratios were evident for Parkinson disease (2.3), unintentional injuries and Chronic liver disease and cirrhosis (2.0 each), Pneumonitis due to solids and liquids

(1.9), heart disease (1.6), diabetes and kidney disease (1.5 each), cancer (1.4), Influenza and pneumonia (1.3), Chronic lower respiratory diseases and Septicemia (1.2 each), and hypertension (1.1). Age-adjusted rates were lower for males than for females for one leading cause, Alzheimer disease (0.7).

Age-adjusted death rates for the black population were higher than for the white population for 8 of the 15 leading causes of death. The largest ratio was for hypertension (2.1). Other causes for which the ratio was high include kidney disease (2.0), diabetes (1.9), Septicemia (1.8), stroke (1.4), heart disease (1.2), and cancer and Influenza and pneumonia (1.1 each). For 6 of the leading causes, age-adjusted rates were lower for the black population than for the white population. The smallest black-to-white ratio was for suicide (0.4); that is, the risk of dying from suicide was more than double for the white population than for the black population. Other conditions with a low black-to-white ratio were Parkinson disease (0.5), chronic liver disease and cirrhosis (0.6), chronic lower respiratory diseases (0.7), and unintentional injuries and Alzheimer disease (0.8 each).

Life expectancy for the white population in 2014 decreased 0.1 years to 79.0 years. This decrease was due to increases in mortality from unintentional injuries, Alzheimer disease, suicide, Chronic liver disease and cirrhosis, and stroke. These increases in mortality were offset by decreases for cancer, chronic lower respiratory diseases, and heart disease.

Life expectancy for the black population in 2014 increased 0.1 years to 75.6 years. This increase was due to decreases in mortality from cancer, heart disease, Septicemia, Chronic lower respiratory diseases, and diabetes. These decreases in mortality were offset by increases for congenital malformations, deformations and chromosomal abnormalities, Alzheimer disease, homicide, and Influenza and pneumonia leading to an increase in life expectancy of only 0.1 years.

The difference in life expectancy between the white and black populations narrowed from 3.6 years in 2013 to 3.4 years in 2014. The narrowing in the black-white life expectancy gap was due primarily to greater improvements in mortality for the black population than for the white population. For example, the black population experienced greater improvements in mortality from suicide; unintentional injuries, chronic liver disease and cirrhosis, and Chronic lower respiratory diseases.

Death rates for the AIAN population are not adjusted for misclassification. Given that the rates for the AIAN population are underestimated by about 30%, disparities in the age-adjusted death rates should

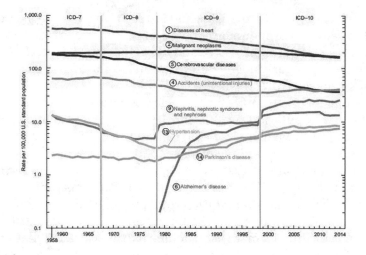

Figure 61.1. *Age-adjusted death rates for selected leading causes of death: United States, 1958–2014*

be interpreted with caution when making comparisons across races. For the API population, death rates are not adjusted for misclassification and are underestimated by about 7% due to underreporting on death certificates. Therefore, even though the level of underestimation for this population is not as great as for the AIAN population, similar caution should be exercised when interpreting rate disparities involving the API population and other races.

Death rates for the population of Hispanic origin are not adjusted for misclassification. Because these rates are both unadjusted for misclassification and underestimated by about 5.0%, caution should be exercised when interpreting rate disparities in the Hispanic and non-Hispanic populations.

Life table partitioning analysis indicates that the difference of 3.0 years in life expectancy between the Hispanic and non-Hispanic white populations is mostly explained by greater improvements in mortality from cancer, heart disease, Chronic lower respiratory diseases, unintentional injuries, and suicide experienced by the Hispanic population.

Section 61.2

Leading Causes of Death by Age, Race, and Sex

This section includes text excerpted from "Deaths: Final Data for 2014," Centers for Disease Control and Prevention (CDC), June 30, 2016.

Deaths and Death Rates

In 2014, a total of 2,626,418 resident deaths were registered in the United States—29,425 more deaths than in 2013. The crude death rate for 2014 (823.7 deaths per 100,000 population) was 0.3% higher than the 2013 rate (821.5).

The age-adjusted death rate in 2014 was 724.6 deaths per 100,000 U.S. standard population—a record low value that was 1.0% lower than the 2013 rate of 731.9. Age-adjusted death rates are constructs that show what the level of mortality would be if no changes occurred in the age composition of the population from year to year. Thus, age-adjusted death rates are better indicators than unadjusted (crude) death rates for examining changes in the risk of death over a period of time when the age distribution of the population is changing. Age-adjusted death rates also are better indicators of relative risk when comparing mortality across geographic areas or between sex or race subgroups of the population that have different age distributions. Since 1980, the age-adjusted death rate has decreased significantly every year except 1983, 1985, 1988, 1993, 1999, 2005, 2008, and 2013.

Race—In 2014, age-adjusted death rates for the major race groups were:

- White population: 725.4 deaths per 100,000 U.S. standard population

- Black population: 849.3

In 2014, the age-adjusted death rate for the black population was 1.2 times that for the white population. The average risk of death for the black population was 17.1% higher than for the white population.

From 1960 through 1982, rates for the black and white populations declined by similar percentages (22.6% and 26.5%, respectively). From 1983 through 1988, rates diverged, increasing 3.5% for the black population and decreasing 2.0% for the white population. The disparity in age-adjusted death rates between the black and white populations was greatest from 1988 through 1996 (1.4 times greater for the black population). Since 1996, the disparity between the two populations has narrowed, as the age-adjusted rate for the black population declined 27.9% while the rate for the white population declined 16.5%.

Age (years)	All races			White[1]			Black[1]			American Indian or Alaska Native[1,2]			Asian or Pacific Islander[1,3]		
	Both sexes	Male	Female	Both sexes	Male	Female	Both sexes	Male	Female	Both sexes	Male	Female	Both sexes	Male	Female
All ages							Percent change								
Crude	0.3	0.9	-0.3	0.4	1.1	-0.3	0.6	0.4	0.7	4.2	4.0	4.4	-1.2	-1.8	-0.6
Age-adjusted	-1.0	-1.0	-1.1	-0.8	-0.7	-1.0	-1.3	-1.8	-1.0	0.4	-0.6	1.1	-4.2	-5.3	-3.5
Under 1 year[4]	-1.1	-1.8	-0.2	-1.4	-2.7	0.2	-0.9	0.5	-2.5	15.1	3.3	34.8	-2.2	-6.0	2.8
1-4	-5.9	-6.6	-4.9	-6.4	-9.2	-2.5	0.0	3.9	-4.5	-8.3	-1.2	-20.0	-28.7	-25.9	-32.1
5-14	-2.3	2.1	-6.3	-1.6	0.7	-5.7	2.9	7.1	-3.4	0.9	1.7	-0.9	-18.0	-10.8	-26.1
15-24	1.1	1.3	0.6	1.0	1.4	0.0	0.8	-0.1	3.2	6.7	5.9	9.3	4.3	5.9	0.6
25-34	2.2	2.3	1.8	3.8	3.9	3.6	-2.7	-3.0	-2.6	0.4	3.7	-5.9	-1.0	-0.2	-3.5
35-44	1.9	1.4	2.8	2.6	2.2	3.1	0.5	-1.2	3.2	6.5	8.2	3.8	-5.7	-6.2	-4.7
45-54	-0.3	-0.8	0.5	0.0	-0.6	0.8	-0.5	-1.0	0.3	2.7	0.4	5.9	-4.0	-3.7	-4.5
55-64	1.2	0.9	1.7	1.5	1.2	1.9	0.0	-1.0	1.3	2.2	5.0	-1.7	-0.3	0.4	-1.4
65-74	-0.9	-0.5	-1.4	-0.8	-0.4	-1.4	-1.0	-0.6	-1.5	1.4	-0.9	4.1	-1.3	-1.7	-0.5
75-84	-1.8	-1.9	-1.8	-1.6	-1.6	-1.7	-2.0	-3.0	-1.4	-1.4	-3.0	0.1	-5.2	-5.9	-4.7
85 and over	-1.8	-1.8	-2.0	-1.6	-1.4	-1.8	-2.4	-2.7	-2.3	-2.6	-4.7	-1.4	-5.7	-8.7	-3.6

[1]Multiple-race data were reported by 46 states and the District of Columbia in 2014 and by 42 states and the District of Columbia in 2013. The multiple-race data for these reporting areas were bridged to the single-race categories of the 1977 OMB standards for comparability with other reporting areas; see Technical Notes.
[2]Includes Aleut and Eskimo persons.
[3]Includes Chinese, Filipino, Hawaiian, Japanese, and other Asian or Pacific Islander persons.
[4]Death rates for "Under 1 year" (based on population estimates) differ from infant mortality rates (based on live births).

Figure 61.2. *Percentage change in death rates and age-adjusted death rates in 2014 from 2013, by age, race, and sex: United States*

In 2014, age-adjusted death rates decreased for white males (0.7%), white females (1.0%), black males (1.8%), and black females (1.0%).

In general, age-adjusted death rates declined from 1980 through 2014 for white males and females and for black males and females. The rate decreased an average of 1.3% per year for white males, 0.7% for white females, 1.4% for black males, and 1.1% for black females during 1980–2014.

Rates for the American Indian or Alaska Native (AIAN) and Asian or Pacific Islander (API) populations should be interpreted with caution because of reporting problems regarding correct identification of race on both the death certificate and in population censuses and surveys.

Counts of deaths for the AIAN population are substantially under-reported (by about 30%) on the death certificate relative to self-reporting while alive. Thus, the age-adjusted death rates that are shown for the AIAN population do not lend themselves to valid comparisons against other races.

Year-to-year trends for the AIAN population present valid insight into changes in mortality affecting this group, if it is reasonable to assume that the level of underreporting of AIAN deaths has remained more or less constant over past years. The age-adjusted death rate for the AIAN population fluctuated from 1980 through 1999, peaking in 1993 at 796.4 deaths per 100,000 U.S. standard population. Since 1999, the rate has trended downward, declining 23.9% from 1999 to 2014. The rate for the AIAN population increased 0.4% from 2013 (591.7) to 2014 (594.1), although the change was not significant.

In 2014, the age-adjusted death rate for the API population was 388.3 deaths per 100,000 U.S. standard population. The level of underreporting of deaths for the API population (about 7%) is not as high as for the AIAN population, but this underreporting still creates enough of a challenge that any comparisons of this population with other races must be interpreted with caution. The age-adjusted death rate for the API population peaked at 586.5 in 1985. The rate fluctuated from 1985 through 1993 before starting a persistent downward trend, decreasing 31.4% from 1993 to 2014.

Hispanic origin—Problems of race and Hispanic-origin reporting affect Hispanic death rates and the comparison of rates for the Hispanic and non-Hispanic populations; see Technical Notes. Mortality for Hispanic persons is somewhat understated because of net underreporting of Hispanic origin on the death certificate (by an estimated 5%), while the non-Hispanic white and non-Hispanic black populations are not affected by problems of underreporting. Underreporting of Hispanic origin on the death certificate is relatively stable across age groups.

| | | | | | Age-adjusted death rate | | | |
| | | | | | | Percent change | Ratio | |
Rank[1]	Cause of death (based on ICD-10)	Number	Percent of total deaths	2014 crude death rate	2014	2013 to 2014	Male to female	Black[2] to white
...	All causes	2,626,418	100.0	823.7	724.6	-1.0	1.4	1.2
1	Diseases of heart .... (I00-I09,I11,I13,I20-I51)	614,348	23.4	192.7	167.0	-1.6	1.6	1.2
2	Malignant neoplasms .... (C00-C97)	591,699	22.5	185.6	161.2	-1.2	1.4	1.1
3	Chronic lower respiratory diseases .... (J40-J47)	147,101	5.6	46.1	40.5	-3.8	1.2	0.7
4	Accidents (unintentional injuries) .... (V01-X59,Y85-Y86)	136,053	5.2	42.7	40.5	2.8	2.0	0.8
5	Cerebrovascular diseases .... (I60-I69)	133,103	5.1	41.7	36.5	0.8	1.0	1.4
6	Alzheimer's disease .... (G30)	93,541	3.6	29.3	25.4	8.1	0.7	0.8
7	Diabetes mellitus .... (E10-E14)	76,488	2.9	24.0	20.9	-1.4	1.5	1.9
8	Influenza and pneumonia .... (J09-J18)	55,227	2.1	17.3	15.1	-5.0	1.3	1.1
9	Nephritis, nephrotic syndrome and nephrosis ...... (N00-N07, N17-N19,N25-N27)	48,146	1.8	15.1	13.2	0.0	1.5	2.0
10	Intentional self-harm (suicide) .... (*U03,X60-X84,Y87.0)	42,773	1.6	13.4	13.0	3.2	3.6	0.4
11	Septicemia .... (A40-A41)	38,940	1.5	12.2	10.7	0.0	1.2	1.8
12	Chronic liver disease and cirrhosis .... (K70,K73-K74)	38,170	1.5	12.0	10.4	2.0	2.0	0.6
13	Essential hypertension and hypertensive renal disease .... (I10,I12,I15)	30,221	1.2	9.5	8.2	-3.5	1.1	2.1
14	Parkinson's disease .... (G20-G21)	26,150	1.0	8.2	7.4	1.4	2.3	0.5
15	Pneumonitis due to solids and liquids .... (J69)	18,792	0.7	5.9	5.1	-1.9	1.9	1.0
...	All other causes .... (residual)	535,666	20.4	168.0	...	...	...	...

... Category not applicable.
[1]Based on number of deaths; see Technical Notes.
[2]Multiple-race data were reported by 46 states and the District of Columbia in 2014. The multiple-race data for these reporting areas were bridged to the single-race categories of the 1977 OMB standards for comparability with other reporting areas; see Technical Notes.

Figure 61.3. *Number of deaths, percentage of total deaths, death rates, and age-adjusted death rates for 2014, percentage change in age-adjusted death rates in 2014 from 2013, and ratio of age-adjusted death rates by sex and by race for the 15 leading causes of death for the total population in 2014: United States*

The age-adjusted death rate in 2014 was 523.3 for the Hispanic population (a decrease of 2.3% from the rate in 2013), 742.8 for the non-Hispanic white population (a decrease of 0.6%), and 870.7 for the non-Hispanic black population (a decreaseof1.6%).

The age-adjusted death rate decreased in 2014 from 2013 for Hispanic males (2.0%), Hispanic females (2.5%), non-Hispanic white males (0.5%), non-Hispanic white females (0.7%), non-Hispanic black males (2.1%), and non-Hispanic black females (1.3%).

Within the Hispanic population, the age-adjusted death rate for males was 1.4 times the rate for females in 2014. The male-to-female death rate ratio for the Hispanic population was unchanged from the ratio in 2013. The corresponding male-to-female ratio was 1.4 for the non-Hispanic white population and 1.5 for the non-Hispanic black population in 2014. The male-to-female ratios for non-Hispanic white and non-Hispanic black populations were also unchanged from 2013. Age-adjusted death rates in 2014 for selected Hispanic subgroups, in order of relative magnitude, were:

- Puerto Rican population: 633.2 deaths per 100,000 U.S. standard population

- Mexican population: 547.8

- Cuban population: 525.2

- Central and South American population: 346.8

Death Rates by Age and Sex

Age-specific death rates decreased significantly from 2013 to 2014 for age groups 1–4, 65–74, 75–84, and 85 and over. Age-specific death rates increased for age groups 25–34, 35–44 and 55–64. Changes in rates for the other age groups were not significant.

The death rate for males declined significantly for age groups 1–4, 75–84, and 85 and over. Significant increases in rates for males were for age groups 25–34, 35–44, and 55–64. Changes in the rates for males in other age groups were not significant. The death rates for females declined significantly for age groups 5–14, 65–74, 75–84, and 85 and over, while increasing for age groups 35–44 and 55–64.

Race—In 2014, age-specific death rates declined significantly for white males in age groups1–4, 75–84,and85and over, and increased for age groups 25–34, 35–44, and 55–64. For the black male population in 2014, death rates decreased for age groups 75–84 and 85 and over. For API males, rates decreased for age groups 75–84 and 85 and over. For AIAN males, rates did not change significantly for any age group. Other observed changes for males by race were not statistically significant.

For white females, age-specific death rates decreased significantly in 2014 for those aged 65–74, 75–84, and 85 and over, and increased significantly for those aged 25–34, 35–44, and 55–64. For black females in 2014, the only statistically significant change was a decrease for age group 85 and over. For API females, rates decreased for age groups 1–4, 5–14, 75–84, and 85 and over. The only significant change in rates for AIAN females was an increase for those under 1 year. Other observed changes for females by race were not statistically significant.

Hispanic origin—For the total Hispanic population in 2014 compared with 2013, age-specific death rates decreased significantly for age groups 1–4, 65–74, 75–84, and 85 and over. Rates for Hispanic males decreased for age groups 1–4, 65–74, 75–84, and 85 and over, and increased for ages 35–44. For Hispanic females, rates decreased for age groups 75–84 and 85 and over. Other observed changes were not statistically significant.

Non-Hispanic origin—For the total non-Hispanic white population in 2014 compared with 2013, age-specific death rates decreased significantly for age groups 65–74, 75–84, and 85 and over, and increased for those aged 25–34, 35–44, and 55–64. Rates for non-Hispanic white males decreased for age groups under 1 year, 75–84, and 85 and over, and increased for those aged 25–34, 35–44, and 55–64. For non-Hispanic white females, rates decreased for age groups 65–74, 75–84, and 85 and over, and increased for those aged 25–34, 35–44, 45–54, and 55–64.

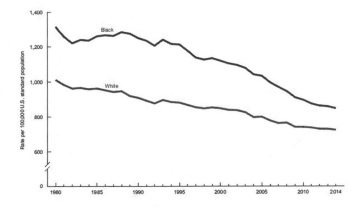

Figure 61.4. *Age-adjusted death rates, by race: United States, 1980–2014*

For the total non-Hispanic black population in 2014 compared with 2013, age-specific death rates decreased significantly for age groups 25–34, 65–74, 75–84, and 85 and over. Rates for non-Hispanic black males decreased for age groups 75–84 and 85 and over. For non-Hispanic black females, rates decreased for age groups 65–74, 75–84, and 85 and over. Other observed changes were not statistically significant.

Chapter 62

Life Expectancy at Birth

Life expectancy at birth represents the average number of years that a group of infants would live if the group was to experience throughout life the age-specific death rates present in the year of birth.

Life table data shown in this report for data years 2001–2014 are based on a revised methodology first presented with final data reported for 2008. The life table methodology was revised by changing the smoothing technique used to estimate the life table functions at the oldest ages. This revision improves on the methodologies used previously.

The methods used to produce life expectancies by Hispanic origin are based on death rates adjusted for misclassification. In contrast, the age-specific and age-adjusted death rates shown in this report for the Hispanic population are not adjusted for misclassification of Hispanic origin. Thus, the report shows Hispanic deaths and death rates as collected by the registration areas; these match those produced using the mortality data file.

Life tables were generated for both sexes and by each sex for the following populations:

- Total U.S. population

- Black population

- White population

This chapter includes text excerpted from "Deaths: Final Data for 2014," Centers for Disease Control and Prevention (CDC), June 30, 2016.

Age (years)	All origins[1]			Hispanic			Non-Hispanic[2]			Non-Hispanic white[3]			Non-Hispanic black[3]		
	Both sexes	Male	Female	Both sexes	Male	Female	Both sexes	Male	Female	Both sexes	Male	Female	Both sexes	Male	Female
All ages							Percent change								
Crude	0.3	0.9	-0.3	1.3	2.0	0.6	0.3	0.9	-0.2	0.6	1.3	0.0	0.3	0.1	0.4
Age-adjusted	-1.0	-1.0	-1.1	-2.3	-2.0	-2.5	-0.9	-0.9	-1.0	-0.6	-0.5	-0.7	-1.6	-2.1	-1.3
Under 1 year[4]	-1.1	-1.8	-0.2	0.6	1.4	-0.4	-1.6	-2.7	-0.2	-1.9	-3.8	0.6	-1.4	-0.6	-2.4
1-4	-5.9	-6.6	-4.9	-10.1	-13.0	-6.5	-4.8	-4.6	-4.6	-4.6	-7.4	-1.0	0.3	4.2	-4.0
5-14	-2.3	2.1	-6.3	2.8	6.8	-2.0	-2.9	0.6	-7.8	-4.0	-1.4	-7.5	2.2	7.2	-3.8
15-24	1.1	1.3	0.6	3.8	3.4	6.3	0.6	0.7	-0.5	0.5	1.1	-1.3	0.0	-0.7	1.6
25-34	2.2	2.3	1.8	2.2	3.7	-0.2	2.2	2.0	1.9	4.1	3.9	4.3	-3.0	-3.1	-3.0
35-44	1.9	1.4	2.8	2.7	4.3	0.3	1.9	1.0	3.2	2.7	1.9	3.8	0.5	-1.4	3.3
45-54	-0.3	-0.8	0.5	-2.1	-2.0	-2.3	0.1	-0.6	1.0	0.6	-0.1	1.6	-0.8	-1.6	0.3
55-64	1.2	0.9	1.7	-0.2	-1.2	1.4	1.3	1.1	1.7	1.7	1.5	2.0	-0.3	-1.3	1.0
65-74	-0.9	-0.5	-1.4	-2.0	-3.2	-0.3	-0.8	-0.3	-1.5	-0.7	-0.2	-1.4	-1.3	-0.9	-1.8
75-84	-1.8	-1.9	-1.8	-3.1	-2.7	-3.5	-1.7	-1.9	-1.7	-1.4	-1.5	-1.5	-2.4	-3.3	-1.8
85 and over	-1.8	-1.8	-2.0	-3.5	-2.6	-4.2	-1.7	-1.7	-1.8	-1.4	-1.3	-1.6	-2.6	-3.1	-2.5

[1]Figures for origin not stated are included in "All origins" but not distributed among specified origins.
[2]Includes races other than white and black.
[3]Race categories are consistent with the 1977 Office of Management and Budget (OMB) standards. Multiple-race data were reported by 46 states and the District of Columbia in 2014 and by 42 states and the District of Columbia in 2013; see Technical Notes. The multiple-race data for these reporting areas were bridged to the single-race categories of the 1977 OMB standards for comparability with other reporting areas; see Technical Notes.
[4]Death rates for "Under 1 year" (based on population estimates) differ from infant mortality rates (based on live births).

Figure 62.1. *Percentage change in death rates and age-adjusted death rates in 2014 from 2013, by age, Hispanic origin, race for non-Hispanic population, and sex: United States*

- Hispanic population

- Non-Hispanic white population

- Non-Hispanic black population

In 2014, life expectancy at birth for the U.S. population was 78.8 years, unchanged since 2012. The trend in U.S. life expectancy since 1900 has been one of gradual improvement, with occasional single-year decreases. In 2014, life expectancy was the same as in 2013 for females (81.2 years) and males (76.4 years). From 1900 through the late 1970s, the gap in life expectancy between the sexes widened, from 2.0 to 7.8 years (data prior to 1975 are not shown). Since its peak in the 1970s, the gap between sexes has been narrowing. In 2014, the difference in life expectancy between the sexes was 4.8 years, unchanged since 2010.

Life expectancy increased 0.1 years for the black population in 2014 to 75.6 years compared with 2013 (75.5). Life expectancy for the white population decreased 0.1 years to 79.0 years. The difference in life expectancy between the white and black populations in 2014 was 3.4 years. The white-black gap has been narrowing gradually, from a peak of 7.1 years in 1993 to the current record low.

This continues a long-term decline in the white-black difference in life expectancy that was interrupted from 1983 through 1993 when the gap widened.

Life expectancy for white males has increased or remained the same nearly every year since 1975. In contrast, life expectancy for black males declined every year from 1985 through 1989, then resumed the

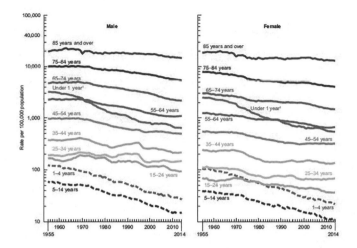

Figure 62.2. *Death rates, by age and sex: United States, 1955–2014*

long-term trend of increase for most years from 1990 through 2014. For white females, life expectancy increased in most years from 1975 through 1998. In 1999, life expectancy for white females briefly fell slightly below 1998's then-record high but began to increase again in 2001. From 1989 through 1992, during 1994, and from 1996 through 1998, life expectancy for black females increased. In 1999, life expectancy for black females declined, as it did for white females, only to begin climbing again in 2000. Life expectancy for white and black females has remained unchanged since 2012.

Life expectancy for the Hispanic population was 81.8 years in 2014, an increase of 0.2 years compared with 2013. Life expectancy figures for the Hispanic population have been available starting with data for 2006. Since that year, life expectancy for the Hispanic population has increased by 1.5 years. In 2014, life expectancy for the Hispanic female population was 84.0 years, a 0.2-year increase from 2013. Life expectancy for the Hispanic male population in 2014 was 79.2 years, a 0.1-year increase from 2013. The difference in life expectancy between the sexes for the Hispanic population was 4.8 years, a 0.1-year increase from the 2013 gap.

Life expectancy for the non-Hispanic white population was 78.8 years in 2014, a decrease of 0.1 years compared with 2013. For non-Hispanic white males, life expectancy did not change (76.5 years), while for non-Hispanic white females, life expectancy decreased 0.1 years to 81.1 years.

451

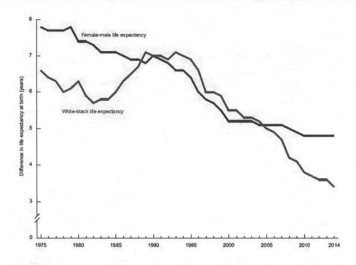

Figure 62.3. *Differences in female-male and white-black life expectancy: United States, 1975–2014*

Life expectancy for the non-Hispanic black population was 75.2 years in 2014, an increase of 0.1 years compared with 2013. For non-Hispanic black males, life expectancy increased 0.2 years to 72.0, while life expectancy for non-Hispanic black females remained unchanged since 2012 (78.1 years).

Among the six Hispanic origin-race-sex groups in 2014, Hispanic females had the highest life expectancy at birth (84.0 years), followed by non-Hispanic white females (81.1), Hispanic males (79.2), non-Hispanic black females (78.1), non-Hispanic white males (76.5), and non-Hispanic black males (72.0).

Life expectancy data by race include persons of Hispanic and non-Hispanic origin; life expectancy data by Hispanic origin include persons of any race. Life expectancy is higher when the Hispanic population is included in the race group. For example, life expectancy was 75.6 years for the black population, but was 75.2 for the non-Hispanic black population. Similarly, life expectancy for the white population was 79.0, but was 78.8 for the non-Hispanic white population.

Life expectancy for both males and females was more than 2 years higher for the Hispanic population than for the non-Hispanic white and non-Hispanic black populations. Various hypotheses have been proposed to explain favorable mortality outcomes among Hispanic persons. The most prevalent hypotheses are the healthy migrant effect, which argues that Hispanic immigrants are selected for their good health and robustness; the "salmon bias" effect, which posits that U.S. residents of Hispanic origin may return to their country of origin to die or when ill; and the "cultural effects," which argues that culturally influenced family structure, lifestyle behaviors, and social networks may confer a protective barrier against the negative effects of low socioeconomic and minority status.

Life tables shown in this report may be used to compare life expectancies at selected ages from birth to 100 years. For example, on the basis of mortality experienced in 2014, a person aged 50 could expect to live an average of 31.6 more years, for a total of 81.6 years. A person aged 65 could expect to live an average of 19.3 more years, for a total of 84.3, and a person aged 85 could expect to live an average of 6.6 more years, for a total of 91.6.

Chapter 63

Infant and Maternal Mortality Trends and Disparities

Birth/Infant Death Data Set and Preliminary Mortality Data File

Data from the Linked Birth/Infant Death Data Set and Preliminary Mortality Data File, National Vital Statistics System

- The U.S. infant mortality rate did not decline from 2000 to 2005.

- Data from the preliminary mortality file suggest a 2% decline in the infant mortality rate from 2005 to 2006.

- The U.S. infant mortality rate is higher than those in most other developed countries, and the gap between the U.S. infant mortality rate and the rates for the countries with the lowest infant mortality appears to be widening.

- The infant mortality rate for non-Hispanic black women was 2.4 times the rate for non-Hispanic white women. Rates were also elevated for Puerto Rican and American Indian or Alaska Native women.

This chapter includes text excerpted from "Recent Trends in Infant Mortality in the United States," Centers for Disease Control and Prevention (CDC), November 6, 2015.

- Increases in preterm birth and preterm-related infant mortality account for much of the lack of decline in the U.S. infant mortality rate from 2000 to 2005.

Infant mortality is one of the most important indicators of the health of a nation, as it is associated with a variety of factors such as maternal health, quality and access to medical care, socioeconomic conditions, and public health practices. The U.S. infant mortality rate generally declined throughout the 20th century. In 1900, the U.S. infant mortality rate was approximately 100 infant deaths per 1,000 live births, while in 2000, the rate was 6.89 infant deaths per 1,000 live births. However, the U.S. infant mortality rate did not decline significantly from 2000 to 2005, which has generated concern among researchers and policy makers.

What Is the Recent Trend in Infant Mortality?

In 2005, the U.S. infant mortality rate was 6.86 infant deaths per 1,000 live births, not significantly different than the rate of 6.89 in 2000, based on data from the linked birth/infant death data set. Data from the preliminary mortality file estimate an infant mortality rate of 6.71 for 2006, a 2% decline from the final rate in 2005. The 2000–2005 plateau in the U.S. infant mortality rate represents the first period of sustained lack of decline in the U.S. infant mortality rate since the 1950s. The Healthy People 2010 target goal for the U.S. infant mortality rate is 4.5 infant deaths per 1,000 live births. The current U.S. rate is about 50% higher than the goal. The impact of infant mortality is considerable: There are more than 28,000 deaths to children under 1 year of age each year in the United States.

How Does the United States Compare with Other Developed Countries in Infant Mortality?

In 2004 (the latest year that data are available for all countries), the United States ranked 29th in the world in infant mortality, tied with Poland and Slovakia. Infant mortality rates were generally lowest (below 3.5 per 1,000) in selected Scandinavian (Sweden, Norway, and Finland) and East Asian (Japan, Hong Kong, and Singapore) countries. In 2004, 22 countries had infant mortality rates below 5.0. The United States' international ranking fell from 12th in 1960 to 23rd in 1990, and to 29th in 2004. International comparisons of infant mortality can be affected by differences in reporting of fetal and infant deaths. However, it appears unlikely that differences in reporting are the primary explanation for the United States relatively low international ranking.

Are There Differences in Infant Mortality Rates between Racial and Ethnic Groups?

In 2005, there was a more than threefold difference in infant mortality rates by race and ethnicity, from a high of 13.63 for non-Hispanic black women to a low of 4.42 for Cuban women. Infant mortality rates were above the U.S. average for non-Hispanic black, Puerto Rican (8.30), and American Indian or Alaska Native (8.06) women. These differences may relate in part to differences in risk factors for infant mortality such as preterm and low birthweight delivery, socioeconomic status, access to medical care, etc. However, many of the racial and ethnic differences in infant mortality remain unexplained. The infant mortality rate did not change significantly for any race/ethnicity group from 2000 to 2005. The only race/ethnicity group to achieve the Healthy People 2010 target goal (4.5) as of 2005 was the Cuban population (4.42).

How Has the Increase in Preterm Births Affected the U.S. Infant Mortality Rate?

Preterm birth (births at less than 37 completed weeks of gestation) is a key risk factor for infant death. The percentage of preterm births has increased rapidly in the United States in recent years. From 2000 to 2005, the percentage of preterm births increased from 11.6% to 12.7%-a 9% increase. From 2000 to 2005, increases occurred for each preterm gestational age grouping. For example, the percentage of very preterm births (less than 32 weeks of gestation) increased by 5%-from 1.93% in 2000 to 2.03% in 2005. From 2000 to 2005, the increase was most rapid for infants born in the late preterm period (34–36 weeks of gestation). The percentage of late preterm births increased by 11%-from 8.2% in 2000 to 9.1% in 2005. The overall percentage of preterm births has increased in the United States since the mid-1980s. Although a portion of the increase is due to increases in multiple births, the percentage of preterm births also increased among single births.

What Is the Impact of Preterm-Related Causes of Death?

In 2005, 36.5% of infant deaths in the United States were due to preterm-related causes of death, a 5% increase since 2000 (34.6%).

Preterm-related causes were those where the cause of death was a direct consequence of preterm birth, and 75% or more of total infant deaths attributed to that cause were preterm. From 2000 to 2005, the percentage of infant deaths from preterm-related causes increased significantly for non-Hispanic white, non-Hispanic black, Asian or Pacific Islander, and Mexican mothers. The impact of preterm-related infant mortality was high for all racial and ethnic groups. However, some groups were disproportionately affected. For example, nearly half (46%) of infant deaths to non-Hispanic black women, and 41% of infant deaths to Puerto Rican women were preterm-related, compared with 32% for non-Hispanic white women.

U.S. Infant Mortality Rate—Summary

Despite the dramatic decline in infant mortality during the 20th century, the U.S. infant mortality rate appears to have plateaued in the first few years of the 21st century.

The U.S. infant mortality rate is higher than rates in most other developed countries. The relative position of the United States in comparison to countries with the lowest infant mortality rates, appears to be worsening. In 2004, the United States ranked 29th in the world in infant mortality, tied with Poland and Slovakia. Previously, the United States' international ranking in infant mortality was 12th in 1960 and 23rd in 1990. There are large differences in infant mortality rates by race and ethnicity. Non-Hispanic black, American Indian or Alaska Native, and Puerto Rican women have the highest infant mortality rates; rates are lowest for Asian or Pacific Islander, Central and South American, and Cuban women.

Preterm birth has a considerable impact on the U.S. infant mortality rate. The plateau in the U.S. infant mortality rate from 2000 to 2005 is due to an increase in the percentage of infants born preterm (including very preterm and late preterm), together with a lack of decline in the infant mortality rate for very preterm infants. There has also been an increase in the relative impact of preterm-related causes of death. In 2005, 36.5% of infant deaths in the United States were due to preterm-related causes of death, a 5% increase since 2000. The impact of preterm-related causes of death was even higher for non-Hispanic black and Puerto Rican women.

Chapter 64

Childhood Risk of Injury-Related Death

Injury Deaths

- On average, 12,175 children 0 to 19 years of age died each year in the United States from an unintentional injury.

- Males had higher injury death rates than females.

- The death rate for males was almost two times the rate for females, and males had a higher injury death rate compared to females in all childhood age groups.

- Injuries due to transportation were the leading cause of death for children.

- The highest death rates were among occupants of motor vehicles in traffic.

- There were also a substantial number of pedestrian and pedalcyclist deaths among children.

- Combining all unintentional injury deaths among those between 0 and 19 years, motor vehicle traffic–related deaths were the leading cause.

This chapter includes text excerpted from "CDC Childhood Injury Report," Centers for Disease Control and Prevention (CDC), December 23, 2015.

- The leading causes of injury death differed by age group.

- For children less than 1 year of age, two–thirds of injury deaths were due to suffocation.

- Drowning was the leading cause injury death for those 1 to 4 years of age.

- For children 5 to 19 years of age, the most injury deaths were due to being an occupant in a motor vehicle traffic crash.

- Risk for injury death varied by race.

- Injury death rates were highest for American Indian and Alaska Natives and were lowest for Asian or Pacific Islanders.

- Overall death rates for whites and African–Americans were approximately the same.

- Injury death rates varied by state depending upon the cause of death.

- Overall, states with the lowest injury death rates were in the northeast. Fire and burn death rates were highest in some of the southern states.

- Death rates from transportation–related injuries were highest in some southern states and some states of the upper plains, while lowest rates occurred in states in the northeast region.

- For injury causes with an overall low burden, death rates greatly varied by age.

- The poisoning death rate for those older than 15 years of age was at least five times the rates of the younger age groups, and the suffocation death rate for infants was over 16 times the rates for all older age groups.

Nonfatal Injuries

- An estimated 9.2 million children annually had an initial emergency department visit for an unintentional injury.

- Males generally had higher nonfatal injury rates than females.

- For children 1 to 19 years of age, nonfatal injury rates were higher among males than females, while the rates were approximately the same for those under 1 year.

- Injuries due to falls were the leading cause of nonfatal injury.

- Each year, approximately 2.8 million children had an initial emergency department visit for injuries from a fall.

- For children less than 1 year of age, falls accounted for over 50% of nonfatal injuries.

- The majority of nonfatal injuries are from five causes.

- Falls was the leading cause of nonfatal injury for all age groups less than 15.

- For children ages 0 to 9, the next two leading causes were being stuck by or against an object and animal bites or insect stings.

- For children 10 to 14 years of age, the next leading causes were being struck by or against an object and overexertion.

- For children 15 to 19 years of age, the three leading causes of nonfatal injuries were being struck by or against an object, falls, and motor vehicle occupant injuries.

- Nonfatal injury rates varied by age group.

- Nonfatal suffocation rates were highest for those less than 1 year of age.

- Rates for fires or burns, and drowning were highest for children 4 years and younger.

- Children 1 to 4 years of age had the highest rates of nonfatal falls and poisoning.

- Injury rates related to motor vehicles was highest in children 15 to 19 years of age.

Chapter 65

Work-Related Fatalities

Preliminary Results

A preliminary total of 4,679 fatal work injuries were recorded in the United States in 2014, an increase of 2 percent over the revised count of 4,585 fatal work injuries in 2013, according to results from the Census of Fatal Occupational Injuries (CFOI) conducted by the U.S. Bureau of Labor Statistics (BLS). The preliminary rate of fatal work injury for U.S. workers in 2014 was 3.3 per 100,000 full-time equivalent (FTE) workers; the revised rate for 2013 was also 3.3.

Revised 2014 data from CFOI will be released in the late spring of 2016. Over the last 5 years, net increases to the preliminary count have averaged 173 cases, ranging from a low of 84 in 2011 (up 2 percent) to a high of 245 in 2012 (up 6 percent).

Key preliminary findings of the 2014 Census of Fatal Occupational Injuries:

- The number of fatal work injuries in private goods-producing industries in 2014 was 9 percent higher than the revised 2013 count but slightly lower in private service-providing industries. Fatal injuries were higher in mining (up 17 percent), agriculture (up 14 percent), manufacturing (up 9 percent), and construction (up 6 percent). Fatal work injuries for government workers were lower (down 12 percent).

This chapter includes text excerpted from "National Census of Fatal Occupational Injuries in 2014," U.S. Bureau of Labor Statistics (BLS), September 17, 2015.

- Falls, slips, and trips increased 10 percent to 793 in 2014 from 724 in 2013. This was driven largely by an increase in falls to a lower level to 647 in 2014 from 595 in 2013.

- Fatal work injuries involving workers 55 years of age and over rose 9 percent to 1,621 in 2014 up from 1,490 in 2013. The preliminary 2014 count for workers 55 and over is the highest total ever reported by CFOI.

- After a sharp decline in 2013, fatal work injuries among self-employed workers increased 10 percent in 2014 from 950 in 2013 to 1,047 in 2014.

- Women incurred 13 percent more fatal work injuries in 2014 than in 2013. Even with this increase, women accounted for only 8 percent of all fatal occupational injuries in 2014.

- Fatal work injuries among Hispanic or Latino workers were lower in 2014, while fatal injuries among non-Hispanic white, black or African-American, and Asian workers were all higher.

- In 2014, 797 decedents were identified as contracted workers, 6 percent higher than the 749 fatally-injured contracted workers reported in 2013. Workers who were contracted at the time of their fatal injury accounted for 17 percent of all fatal work injury cases in 2014.

- The number of fatal work injuries among police officers and police supervisors was higher in 2014, rising from 88 in 2013 to 103 in 2014, an increase of 17 percent.

Worker Characteristics

Fatal injuries to self-employed workers rose 10 percent in 2014 to 1,047, up from 950 in 2013. Although higher than in 2013, the 2014 preliminary total for self-employed workers is about the same as the 10- year average for the series. Fatal injuries among wage and salary workers remained at about the same level as in 2013.

Fatal work injuries involving workers age 45 to 54 years, 55 to 64 years, and 65 years of age and over all increased in 2014 compared to 2013 totals. The number of workers 55 years and over who were fatally injured in 2014 increased 9 percent to 1,621, the highest annual total since the inception of the fatality census in 1992. Workers of a wide variety of ages are included in the 2014 CFOI counts—8 workers under the age of 16 are included as well as 8 workers age 90 and over.

Fatal injuries among women rose 13 percent in 2014 to 359 from 319 in 2013. Fatal work injuries among men in 2014 were slightly higher than the previous year. Consistent with previous years, men accounted for 92 percent of all fatal occupational injuries.

Fatal work injuries among Hispanic or Latino workers fell 3 percent to 789 in 2014, compared to 817 in 2013. Fatal work injuries were higher among non-Hispanic white, non-Hispanic black or African-American, and non-Hispanic Asian workers.

Overall, there were 827 fatal work injuries involving foreign-born workers in 2014. These 827 foreign-born workers came from over 80 different countries, of which the greatest share (334 or 40 percent) was born in Mexico. Of the 789 fatal work injuries incurred by Hispanic or Latino workers, 503 (64 percent) involved foreign-born workers. Of the 134 fatal work injuries incurred by non-Hispanic Asian workers, 116 (87 percent) involved foreign-born workers.

Type of Incident

In 2014, fatal work injuries due to transportation incidents were slightly higher – 1,891, up from 1,865 in 2013. Overall, transportation incidents accounted for 40 percent of fatal workplace injuries in 2014. Within the transportation event category, roadway incidents constituted 57 percent of the fatal work injury total in 2014. The second largest number of transportation fatalities in 2014 involved pedestrian vehicular incidents (17 percent). Fatalities resulting from pedestrian vehicular incidents were up 6 percent from last year's revised count (313 in 2014 up from 294 in 2013). Rail vehicle incidents also increased in 2014, rising 34 percent to 55 fatal injuries from 41 in 2013.

(Note that roadway incident counts presented in this release are expected to rise when updated 2014 data are released in the late spring of 2016 because key source documentation detailing specific transportation-related incidents has not yet been received.)

Fatal work injuries due to violence and other injuries by persons or animals were lower in 2014, with 749 deaths in 2014 compared to 773 in 2013. The number of workplace homicides was about the same as the total in 2013, but workplace suicides decreased slightly in 2014, from 282 to 271. Among the workplace homicides in which women were the victims, the greatest share of assailants were relatives or domestic partners (32 percent of those homicides). In workplace homicides involving men, robbers were the most common type of assailant (33 percent).

465

Fatal falls, slips, and trips were up 10 percent in 2014 from the previous year. Falls to lower level were up 9 percent to 647 from 595 in 2013, and falls on the same level increased 17 percent. In 532 of the 647 fatal falls to lower level, the height of the fall was known. Of those cases in which the height of fall was known, four-fifths involved falls of 30 feet or less (427) while about two-thirds (340) involved falls of 20 feet or less.

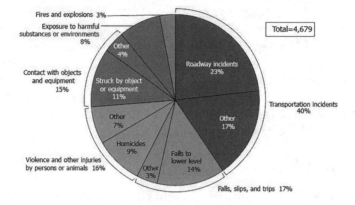

Figure 65.1. *Fatal occupational injuries by major event, 2014*

Work-related injury deaths due to contact with objects and equipment were down slightly from the revised 2013 number (721 to 708). The largest proportion of fatal injuries in this category (34 percent) occurred when workers were struck by falling objects or equipment. The next largest share (28 percent) involved injuries in which decedents were struck by powered vehicles in nontransport situations (e.g., struck by a rolling vehicle or by a vehicle that had tipped over while on jacks).

Fatal work injuries due to fires decreased 35 percent from 82 in 2013 to 53 in 2014. Fatal injuries resulting from explosions, however, increased 25 percent to 84 cases, led by an increase in explosions of pressure vessels, piping, or tires.

A total of 372 workers were killed in 163 multiple fatality incidents (events where more than one worker was killed).

Occupation

Transportation and material moving occupations accounted for the largest share (28%) of fatal occupational injuries of any occupation group. Fatal work injuries in this group rose 3 percent to 1,289 in 2014, the highest total since 2008. Drivers/sales workers and truck drivers accounted for nearly 2 out of every 3 fatal injuries in this group (835 of the 1,289 fatal injuries in 2014). In this group, drivers/sales workers increased 74 percent to 54 in 2014, and heavy and tractor-trailer drivers had their highest total since 2008 (725 fatalities in 2014).

Fatal work injuries in construction and extraction occupations increased 5 percent (40 cases) in 2014 to 885. This is the highest total for this occupation group since 2008. The fatal injury rate for workers in construction and extraction occupations was 11.8 per 100,000 FTE workers in 2014 and 12.2 per 100,000 FTE workers in 2013. Fatal injuries among construction trades workers increased 3 percent in 2014 to 611 fatalities, the highest count since 2009. Fatal work injuries to construction laborers, the occupation within construction trades workers with the highest number of fatalities, decreased by 14 cases in 2014 to 206. Conversely, the number of fatally-injured electricians increased by 14 cases in 2014 to 78.

The number of fatal work injuries among protective service occupations decreased 15 percent in 2014 to 211 fatalities, a series low for this occupation group. This was led by a drop in fatalities among firefighters and first-line supervisors of firefighting and prevention workers, down 51 percent to 35 in 2014. Fatal injuries to police officers and first-line supervisors of police and detectives, however, increased 17 percent to 103 in 2014.

Fatalities among farming, fishing, and forestry occupations rose 9 percent to 253 in 2014. The increase was led by fatalities involving agricultural workers (up 12 percent to 143) and fatalities involving logging workers (up 31 percent to 77).

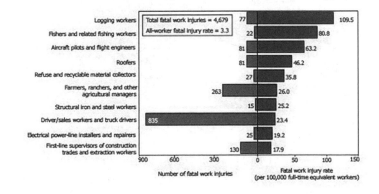

Figure 65.2. *Civilian occupations with high fatal work injury rates, 2014*

Fatal injuries to resident military personnel declined to 55 from 71 in 2013.

Industry

In the private sector, a total of 4,251 fatal work injuries were recorded in 2014, 4 percent higher than the revised total of 4,101 in 2013. Goods-producing industries were up 9 percent in 2014. Totals were higher for private mining, quarrying, and oil and gas extraction (up 17 percent); agriculture, forestry, fishing and hunting (up 14 percent); manufacturing (up 9 percent); and construction (up 6 percent).

Construction fatalities rose to 874 in 2014 from 828 in 2013. The number of fatal work injuries in construction in 2014 was the highest reported total since 2008. The fatal injury rate for workers in the private construction industry was 9.5 per 100,000 FTE workers in 2014 and 9.7 per 100,000 FTE workers in 2013. Heavy and civil engineering construction recorded a series low of 138 fatal injuries in 2014, down from 165 in 2013.

Agriculture, forestry, fishing and hunting fatalities were 14 percent higher in 2014 at 568 compared to 500 in 2013. Fatal injuries in forestry and logging rose to 92 in 2014 from 81 in 2013 and the highest total since 2008. Agriculture, forestry, fishing and hunting recorded the highest fatal injury rate of any industry sector at 24.9 fatal work injuries per 100,000 FTE workers in 2014.

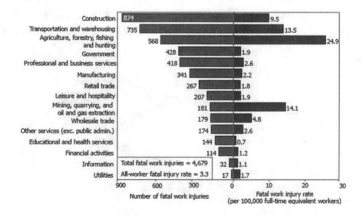

Figure 65.3. *Number and rate of fatal occupational injuries by industry sector, 2014*

Fatal work injuries in the private mining, quarrying, and oil and gas extraction sector were 17 percent higher in 2014, rising to 181 from 155 in 2013, and the fatal injury rate also increased to 14.1 per 100,000 FTE workers in 2014 from 12.4 per 100,000 FTE workers in 2013. While coal mining recorded smaller numbers of fatal work injuries in 2014, the number of fatal work injury cases in oil and gas extraction industries were 27 percent higher in 2014, rising to 142 in 2014 from 112 in 2013. Oil and gas extraction industries include oil and gas extraction (North American Industry Classification System [NAICS] 21111), drilling oil and gas wells (NAICS 213111), and support activities for oil and gas operations (NAICS 213112).

Service-providing industries in the private sector decreased slightly from 2013. Fatal work injuries in transportation and warehousing accounted for 735 fatal work injuries in 2014, almost unchanged from the revised 2013 count of 733 fatalities. Financial activities rose 31 percent, while wholesale trade fell 11 percent.

Fatal occupational injuries among government workers fell 12 percent to a series low of 428 fatal work injuries in 2014, down from 484 in 2013. Federal government work fatalities, which fell 29 percent to 92 in 2014 from 129 in 2013, accounted for most of the decline.

Contracted Workers

In 2014, the number of fatal occupational injuries incurred by contracted workers was 797, or 17 percent of all fatal injuries, compared to 749 (16 percent) reported in 2013. Falls to a lower level accounted for 33 percent of contracted worker deaths while struck by object or equipment (17 percent), pedestrian vehicular incidents (12 percent), and exposure to electricity (9 percent) incidents were also frequent events among contracted workers. These four types of incidents each constituted a greater share of fatalities among contracted workers than they did for all workers.

Fatally-injured contracted workers were most often contracted by a firm in the private construction industry sector (164 or 21 percent of all contracted workers). They were also frequently contracted by a government entity (148 or 19 percent) and by firms in the private financial activities (81 or 10 percent); private mining, quarrying, and oil and gas extraction (72 or 9 percent); and private manufacturing (70 or 9 percent) industry sectors.

Over half of all contracted workers (415 workers) were working in construction and extraction occupations when fatally injured. Decedents in this occupation group were most often employed as construction laborers (108); electricians (48); first-line supervisors of construction trades and extraction workers (44); roofers (42); and painters, construction and maintenance (25). Among contracted workers who were employed outside the construction and extraction occupation group, the largest number of fatal occupational injuries was incurred by heavy and tractor-trailer truck drivers (76 workers); landscaping and groundskeeping workers (21); security guards (17); tree trimmers and pruners (16); heating, air conditioning, and refrigeration mechanics and installers (15); and excavating and loading machine and dragline operators (13).

Chapter 66

Suicide Facts and Statistics

Suicide

- Suicide was the tenth leading cause of death for all ages in 2013.

- There were 41,149 suicides in 2013 in the United States—a rate of 12.6 per 100,000 is equal to 113 suicides each day or one every 13 minutes.

- Based on data about suicides in 16 National Violent Death Reporting System states in 2010, 33.4% of suicide decedents tested positive for alcohol, 23.8% for antidepressants, and 20.0% for opiates, including heroin and prescription pain killers.

- Suicide results in an estimated $51 billion in combined medical and work loss costs.

Nonfatal Suicidal Thoughts and Behavior

- Among adults aged ≥18 years in the United States during 2013:

  - An estimated 9.3 million adults (3.9% of the adult U.S. population) reported having suicidal thoughts in the past year.

  - The percentage of adults having serious thoughts about suicide was highest among adults aged 18 to 25 (7.4%), followed

This chapter includes text excerpted from "Suicide," Centers for Disease Control and Prevention (CDC), September 11, 2015.

by adults aged 26 to 49 (4.0%), then by adults aged 50 or older (2.7%).

- An estimated 2.7 million people (1.1%) made a plan about how they would attempt suicide in the past year.

- The percentage of adults who made a suicide plan in the past year was higher among adults aged 18 to 25 (2.5%) than among adults aged 26 to 49 (1.35%) and those aged 50 or older (0.6%).

- An estimated 1.3 million adults aged 18 or older (0.6%) attempted suicide in the past year. Among these adults who attempted suicide, 1.1 million also reported making suicide plans (0.2 million did not make suicide plans).

- Among students in grades 9–12 in the United States during 2013:

  - 17.0% of students seriously considered attempting suicide in the previous 12 months (22.4% of females and 11.6% of males).

  - 13.6% of students made a plan about how they would attempt suicide in the previous 12 months (16.9% of females and 10.3% of males).

  - 8.0% of students attempted suicide one or more times in the previous 12 months (10.6% of females and 5.4% of males).

  - 2.7% of students made a suicide attempt that resulted in an injury, poisoning, or an overdose that required medical attention (3.6% of females and 1.8% of males).

Gender Disparities

- Males take their own lives at nearly four times the rate of females and represent 77.9% of all suicides.

- Females are more likely than males to have suicidal thoughts.

- Suicide is the seventh leading cause of death for males and the fourteenth leading cause for females.

- Firearms are the most commonly used method of suicide among males (56.9%).

- Poisoning is the most common method of suicide for females (34.8%).

Racial and Ethnic Disparities

- Suicide is the eighth leading cause of death among American Indians/Alaska Natives across all ages.

- Among American Indians/Alaska Natives aged 10 to 34 years, suicide is the second leading cause of death.

- The suicide rate among American Indian/Alaska Native adolescents and young adults ages 15 to 34 (19.5 per 100,000) is 1.5 times higher than the national average for that age group (12.9 per 100,000).

- The percentages of adults aged 18 or older having suicidal thoughts in the previous 12 months were 2.9% among blacks, 3.3% among Asians, 3.6% among Hispanics, 4.1% among whites, 4.6% among Native Hawaiians /Other Pacific Islanders, 4.8% among American Indians/Alaska Natives, and 7.9% among adults reporting two or more races.

- Among Hispanic students in grades 9–12, the prevalence of having seriously considered attempting suicide (18.9%), having made a plan about how they would attempt suicide (15.7%), having attempted suicide (11.3%), and having made a suicide attempt that resulted in an injury, poisoning, or overdose that required medical attention (4.1%) was consistently higher than white and black students.

Age Group Differences

- Suicide is the third leading cause of death among persons aged 10–14, the second among persons aged 15–34 years, the fourth among persons aged 35–44 years, the fifth among persons aged 45–54 years, the eighth among person 55–64 years, and the seventeenth among persons 65 years and older.

- In 2011, middle-aged adults accounted for the largest proportion of suicides (56%), and from 1999–2010, the suicide rate among this group increased by nearly 30%.

- Among adults aged 18–22 years, similar percentages of full-time college students and other adults in this age group had suicidal thoughts (8.0 and 8.7%, respectively) or made suicide plans (2.4 and 3.1%).

- Full-time college students aged 18–22 years were less likely to attempt suicide (0.9 vs. 1.9 percent) or receive medical attention as a result of a suicide attempt in the previous 12 months (0.3 vs. 0.7%).

Nonfatal, Self-Inflicted Injuries

- In 2013, 494,169 people were treated in emergency departments for self-inflicted injuries.

- Nonfatal, self-inflicted injuries (including hospitalized and emergency department treated and released) resulted in an estimated $10.4 billion in combined medical and work loss costs.

Chapter 67

Alcohol-Attributable Deaths

Alcohol Use and Your Health

Drinking too much can harm your health. Excessive alcohol use led to approximately 88,000 deaths and 2.5 million years of potential life lost (YPLL) each year in the United States from 2006–2010, shortening the lives of those who died by an average of 30 years. Further, excessive drinking was responsible for 1 in 10 deaths among working-age adults aged 20–64 years. The economic costs of excessive alcohol consumption in 2010 were estimated at $249 billion, or $2.05 a drink.

What Is a "Drink"?

In the United States, a standard drink contains 0.6 ounces (14.0 grams or 1.2 tablespoons) of pure alcohol. Generally, this amount of pure alcohol is found in:

- 12-ounces of beer (5% alcohol content).

- 8-ounces of malt liquor (7% alcohol content).

- 5-ounces of wine (12% alcohol content).

This chapter contains text excerpted from the following sources: Text under the heading "Alcohol Use and Your Health" is excerpted from "Fact Sheets—Alcohol Use and Your Health," Centers for Disease Control and Prevention (CDC), June 29, 2016; Text beginning with the heading "Alcohol Deaths" is excerpted from "Alcohol Deaths," Centers for Disease Control and Prevention (CDC), June 30, 2014.

- 1.5-ounces of 80-proof (40% alcohol content) distilled spirits or liquor (e.g., gin, rum, vodka, whiskey).

What Is Excessive Drinking?

Excessive drinking includes binge drinking, heavy drinking, and any drinking by pregnant women or people younger than age 21.

- Binge drinking, the most common form of excessive drinking, is defined as consuming

- For women, 4 or more drinks during a single occasion.

- For men, 5 or more drinks during a single occasion.

- Heavy drinking is defined as consuming

- For women, 8 or more drinks per week.

- For men, 15 or more drinks per week.

Most people who drink excessively are not alcoholics or alcohol dependent.

What Is Moderate Drinking?

The Dietary Guidelines for Americans defines moderate drinking as up to 1 drink per day for women and up to 2 drinks per day for men. In addition, the Dietary Guidelines do not recommend that individuals who do not drink alcohol start drinking for any reason.

However, there are some people who should not drink any alcohol, including those who are:

- Younger than age 21.

- Pregnant or may be pregnant.

- Driving, planning to drive, or participating in other activities requiring skill, coordination, and alertness.

- Taking certain prescription or over-the-counter medications that can interact with alcohol.

- Suffering from certain medical conditions.

- Recovering from alcoholism or are unable to control the amount they drink.

By adhering to the Dietary Guidelines, you can reduce the risk of harm to yourself or others.

Alcohol Deaths

Drinking too much can harm your health. One in 10 deaths among working-age adults aged 20–64 years are due to excessive alcohol use. Excessive alcohol use is a leading cause of preventable death. This dangerous behavior accounted for approximately 88,000 deaths per year from 2006–2010, and accounted for 1 in 10 deaths among working-age adults aged 20–64 years. Excessive alcohol use shortened the lives of those who died by about 30 years. These deaths were due to health effects from drinking too much over time, such as breast cancer, liver disease, and heart disease, and health effects from consuming a large amount of alcohol in a short period of time, such as violence, alcohol poisoning, and motor vehicle crashes.

A study, published in Preventing Chronic Disease, found that nearly 70% of deaths due to excessive drinking involved working-age adults, and about 70% of the deaths involved males. The study also found that about 5% of the deaths involved people younger than age 21. The impact of these deaths affects the nation's economy and the sustainability of families. Excessive drinking cost the United States about $224 billion, or $1.90 per drink, in 2006, and about 40% of these costs were paid by government. Most of these costs were due to lost productivity, including reduced earnings among excessive drinkers as well as deaths due to excessive drinking among working age adults.

Chapter 68

Disparities in Deaths from Stroke

Despite steady decreases in U.S. stroke mortality over the past several decades, stroke remained the fourth leading cause of death during 2010–2012 and the fifth leading cause in 2013. Most studies have focused on the excess mortality experienced by black persons compared with white persons and by residents of the southeastern states, referred to as the Stroke Belt. Few stroke mortality studies have focused on Asian or Pacific Islander and Hispanic persons or have explored urban–rural differences. The report provides updated information about stroke mortality among U.S. Residents aged 45 and over during 2010–2013 by age, race and ethnicity, income, urban–rural residence, and residence inside or outside the Stroke Belt.

Stroke Mortality among Adults Aged 45 and Over Varied by Race and Hispanic Origin and Sex during 2010–2013. Deaths per 100,000 Population

- The age-adjusted stroke death rate for non-Hispanic black men aged 45 and over (154.8 deaths per 100,000 population) was 54% higher than the rate for non-Hispanic white men, 67% higher

This chapter includes text excerpted from "Differences in Stroke Mortality among Adults Aged 45 and Over: United States, 2010–2013," Centers for Disease Control and Prevention (CDC), July 2015.

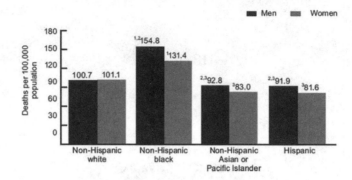

Figure 68.1. *Age-adjusted stroke death rates among men and women aged 45 and over, by race and Hispanic origin: average annual, 2010–2013*

than the rate for non-Hispanic Asian or Pacific Islander men, and 68% higher than the rate for Hispanic men of the same age (Figure 68.1.).

- The rate for non-Hispanic black women (131.4 per 100,000 population) was 30% higher than the rate for non-Hispanic white women, 58% higher than the rate for non-Hispanic Asian or Pacific Islander women, and 61% higher than the rate for Hispanic women of the same age.

- Non-Hispanic Asian or Pacific Islander and Hispanic men and women had the lowest age-adjusted stroke death rates (men: 92.8 and 91.9 per 100,000 population; women: 83.0 and 81.6).

- Non-Hispanic white men and women aged 45 and over had similar age-adjusted stroke death rates (100.7 and 101.1 deaths per 100,000 population). Men in the other race-ethnicity groups had higher age-adjusted stroke death rates than women of the same race and ethnicity (12% to 18% higher).

The Age Distribution of Stroke Deaths Varied by Race and Hispanic Origin during 2010–2013.

- More than one-fourth of the stroke deaths among non-Hispanic black persons aged 45 and over (28.6%) occurred to those in the youngest age group (45–64). By contrast, the portion of stroke deaths in this age group among the other race?ethnicity groups ranged from one-tenth among non-Hispanic white persons (10.0%) to less than one-fourth among Hispanic persons (22.4%).

- The portion of stroke deaths in the oldest age group (85 and over) was largest among non-Hispanic white persons (nearly one-half or 47.4%) and smallest among non-Hispanic black persons (one-fourth or 24.9%).

- The percent distribution of stroke deaths by age was similar among non-Hispanic Asian or Pacific Islander and Hispanic persons.

Stroke Mortality among Persons Aged 45 and Over Decreased with Increasing County Median Household Income during 2010–2013.

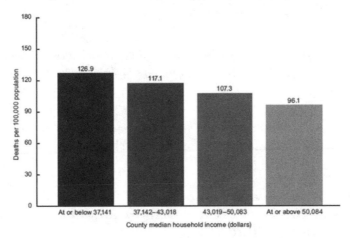

Figure 68.2. *Age-adjusted stroke death rates among persons aged 45 and over, by county median household income quartile: average annual, 2010–2013*

- The age-adjusted stroke death rate for persons aged 45 and over decreased as county median household income increased (Figure 68.2.).

- The age-adjusted stroke death rate for persons residing in counties in the lowest median household income quartile was 32% higher than the rate for persons residing in counties in the highest quartile (126.9 compared with 96.1 deaths per 100,000 population).

During 2010–2013, Stroke Mortality among Persons Aged 45 and Over Increased as Place of Residence Became More Rural.

- Among persons aged 45 and over, age-adjusted stroke death rates were highest in nonmetropolitan counties (micropolitan

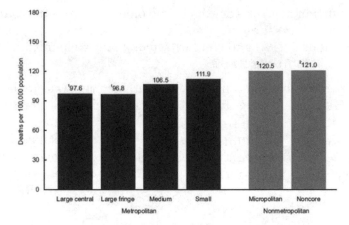

Figure 68.3. *Age-adjusted stroke death rates among persons aged 45 and over, by urbanization level of county of residence: average annual, 2010–2013*

and noncore: 120.5 and 121.0 deaths per 100,000 population) and lowest in large central and large fringe metro counties (97.6 and 96.8) (Figure 68.3.).

Among Persons Aged 45 and Over, Stroke Mortality inside and outside the Stroke Belt Varied by Race and Hispanic Origin during 2010–2013.

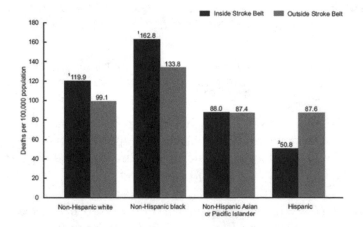

Figure 68.4. *Age-adjusted stroke death rates among persons aged 45 and over, by residence inside or outside the Stroke Belt and race and Hispanic origin: average annual, 2010–2013*

- Non-Hispanic black and non-Hispanic white persons aged 45 and over residing inside the Stroke Belt experienced excess stroke mortality compared with their counterparts residing outside the Stroke Belt (22% and 21% higher mortality) (Figure 68.4).

- The age-adjusted stroke death rate for non-Hispanic Asian or Pacific Islander persons residing inside the Stroke Belt did not differ from the rate for those residing outside the Stroke Belt (88.0 compared with 87.4 deaths per 100,000 population).

- In contrast to the other population groups, Hispanic persons residing inside the Stroke Belt had substantially lower stroke mortality than Hispanic persons residing outside the Stroke Belt (50.8 compared with 87.6 deaths per 100,000 population).

Summary

An overarching goal of the *Healthy People 2020* initiative is "to achieve health equity, eliminate disparities, and improve the health of all groups" in the United States. Despite significant declines in stroke mortality in recent decades, stroke continues to be one of the leading causes of death in the United States, and sociodemographic and geographic disparities persist. Consequently, there is an ongoing need to monitor the current magnitude and patterns of stroke mortality. The report describes current variations in stroke mortality by age, race and Hispanic origin, median household income, urbanization level of county of residence, and residence inside or outside the Stroke Belt.

During 2010–2013, stroke mortality among persons aged 45 and over varied by age and race and Hispanic origin. Non-Hispanic black persons had a markedly higher stroke death rate than any of the three other race-ethnicity groups, and a greater portion of their stroke deaths occurred at younger ages. Non-Hispanic Asian or Pacific Islander and Hispanic persons had lower rates than either non-Hispanic black or non-Hispanic white persons. For non-Hispanic white persons, a larger portion of stroke deaths occurred among those aged 85 and over, and a smaller portion occurred among those aged 45–64 compared with the other race-ethnicity groups. Except among non-Hispanic white persons, men had higher stroke death rates than women. Disparities in stroke mortality also were observed by place of residence. Stroke mortality was higher for persons residing in counties with lower median household income than for persons residing in counties with higher median household income. Persons residing in nonmetropolitan counties (micropolitan and noncore) had the highest stroke mortality rates; those residing in the most urban counties (large central and large fringe metro) had the lowest rates. Excess stroke mortality was observed for non-Hispanic white and non-Hispanic black residents of the Stroke

Belt but not for non-Hispanic Asian or Pacific Islander and Hispanic persons. Asian or Pacific Islander persons residing inside the Stroke Belt had a stroke death rate similar to those residing outside, while Hispanic persons residing inside the Stroke Belt had a much lower stroke death rate than those residing outside.

Part Ten

Additional Help and Information

Chapter 69

Glossary of End-of-Life Terms

accelerated death benefit (ADB): A life insurance policy feature that lets you use some of the policy's death benefit prior to death.

activities of daily living (ADLs): Basic actions that independently functioning individuals perform on a daily basis.

acute care: Recovery is the primary goal of acute care. Physician, nurse, or other skilled professional services are typically required and usually provided in a doctor's office or hospital. Acute care is usually short term.

adult day services: Services provided during the day at a community-based center. Programs address the individual needs of functionally or cognitively impaired adults. These structured, comprehensive programs provide social and support services in a protective setting during any part of a day, but not 24-hour care. Many adult day service programs include health-related services.

advanced directive: Legal document that specifies whether you would like to be kept on artificial life support if you become permanently unconscious or are otherwise dying and unable to speak for yourself. It also specifies other aspects of healthcare you would like under those circumstances.

This glossary contains terms excerpted from documents produced by several sources deemed reliable.

Alzheimer disease: Progressive, degenerative form of dementia that causes severe intellectual deterioration. First symptoms are impaired memory, followed by impaired thought and speech, and finally complete helplessness.

annuity: A contract in which an individual gives an insurance company money that is later distributed back to the person over time. Annuity contracts traditionally provide a guaranteed distribution of income over time, until the death of the person or persons named in the contract or until a final date, whichever comes first.

arthritis: Disease involving inflammation of a joint or joints in the body.

assessment: In healthcare, a process used to learn about a patient's condition. This may include a complete medical history, medical tests, a physical exam, a test of learning skills, tests to find out if the patient is able to carry out the tasks of daily living, a mental health evaluation, and a review of social support and community resources available to the patient.

assisted living facility: Residential living arrangement that provides individualized personal care, assistance with Activities of Daily Living, help with medications, and services such as laundry and housekeeping. Facilities may also provide health and medical care, but care is not as intensive as care offered at a nursing home.

benefits: Monetary sum paid by an insurance company to a recipient or to a care provider for services that the insurance policy covers.

board and care home: Residential private homes designed to provide housing, meals, housekeeping, personal care services, and supports to frail or disabled residents. At least one caregiver is on the premises at all times. In many states, Board and Care Homes are licensed or certified and must meet criteria for facility safety, types of services provided, and the number and type of residents they can care for.

cardiopulmonary resuscitation (CPR): Combination of rescue breathing (mouth-to-mouth resuscitation) and chest compressions used if someone isn't breathing or circulating blood adequately. CPR can restore circulation of oxygen-rich blood to the brain.

caregiver: A caregiver is anyone who helps care for an elderly individual or person with a disability who lives at home. Caregivers usually provide assistance with activities of daily living and other essential activities like shopping, meal preparation, and housework.

charitable remainder trust (CRT): Special tax-exempt irrevocable trust written to comply with federal tax laws and regulations. You transfer cash or assets into the trust and may receive some income from it for life or a specified number of years (not to exceed 20).

chronically ill: Having a long-lasting or recurrent illness or condition that causes you to need help with Activities of Daily Living and often other health and support services. The condition is expected to last for at least 90 consecutive days.

cognitive impairment: Deficiency in short or long-term memory, orientation to person, place and time, deductive or abstract reasoning, or judgment as it relates to safety awareness. Alzheimer Disease is an example of a cognitive impairment.

community-based services: Services and service settings in the community, such as adult day services, home delivered meals, or transportation services. Often referred to as home- and community-based services, they are designed to help older people and people with disabilities stay in their homes as independently as possible.

continuing care retirement communities (CCRC): Retirement complex that offers a range of services and levels of care. Residents may move first into an independent living unit, a private apartment, or a house on the campus. The CCRC provides social and housing-related services and often also has an assisted living unit and an on-site or affiliated nursing home. If and when residents can no longer live independently in their apartment or home, they move into assisted living or the CCRC's nursing home.

dehydration: A condition caused by the loss of too much water from the body. Severe diarrhea or vomiting can cause dehydration.

dementia: Deterioration of mental faculties due to a disorder of the brain.

depression: A mental condition marked by ongoing feelings of sadness, despair, loss of energy, and difficulty dealing with normal daily life. Other symptoms of depression include feelings of worthlessness and hopelessness, loss of pleasure in activities, changes in eating or sleeping habits, and thoughts of death or suicide.

diagnosis: The process of identifying a disease by the signs and symptoms

disabled: For Medicaid eligibility purposes, a disabled person is someone whose physical or mental condition prevents him or her from doing enough work or the type of work needed for self-support. The condition must be expected to last for at least a year or be expected to result in death. Persons receiving disability benefits through Supplemental Security Income (SSI), Social Security, or Medicare automatically meet this criterion.

disorder: In medicine, a disturbance of normal functioning of the mind or body. Disorders may be caused by genetic factors, disease, or trauma.

durable power of attorney: Legal document that gives someone else the authority to act on your behalf on matters that you specify. The power can be specific to a certain task or broad to cover many financial duties. You can specify if you want the power to start immediately or upon mental incapacity. For the document to be valid, you must sign it before you become disabled.

group home (also called Board and Care Home): Residential private homes designed to provide housing, meals, housekeeping, personal care services, and supports to frail or disabled residents. At least one caregiver is onsite at all times. In many states, group homes are licensed or certified and must meet criteria for facility safety, types of services provided, and the number and type of residents they can care for.

high blood pressure: Blood pressure is the force of blood pushing against your blood vessel walls. High blood pressure is when that force, as measured by a blood pressure cuff, is elevated above normal limits.

homemaker: Licensed Homemaker Services provides "hands-off" care such as helping with cooking and running errands. Often referred to as "Personal Care Assistants" or "Companions." This is the rate charged by a non-Medicare certified, licensed agency.

hospice care: Short-term, supportive care for individuals who are terminally ill (have a life expectancy of six months or less). Hospice care focuses on pain management and emotional, physical, and spiritual support for the patient and family. It can be provided at home or in a hospital, nursing home, or hospice facility. Medicare typically pays for hospice care. Hospice care is not usually considered long-term care.

incontinence: Inability to maintain control of bowel and bladder functions as well as the inability to perform associated personal hygiene such as caring for a catheter or colostomy bag. Continence is one of the six Activities of Daily Living.

informal caregiver: Any person who provides long-term care services without pay.

living will: Legal document that specifies whether you would like to be kept on artificial life support if you become permanently unconscious or are otherwise dying and unable to speak for yourself. It also specifies other aspects of healthcare you would like under those circumstances.

long-term care facility: (also called Long Nursing Home or Convalescent Care Facility) Licensed facility that provides general nursing care to those who are chronically ill or unable to take care of daily living needs.

long-term care insurance: Insurance policy designed to offer financial support to pay for long-term care services.

long-term care services: Services that include medical and non-medical care for people with a chronic illness or disability. Long-term care helps meet health or personal needs. Most long-term care services assists people with Activities of Daily Living, such as dressing, bathing, and using the bathroom.

long-term care: Services and supports necessary to meet health or personal care needs over an extended period of time.

Medicaid: Joint federal and state public assistance program for financing healthcare for low-income people. It pays for healthcare services for those with low incomes or very high medical bills relative to income and assets. It is the largest public payer of long-term care services.

medical power of attorney: Legal document that allows you to name someone to make healthcare decisions for you if, for any reason and at any time, you become unable to make or communicate those decisions for yourself.

Medicare: Federal program that provides hospital and medical expense benefits for people over age 65, or those meeting specific disability standards. Benefits for nursing home and home health services are limited.

multidisciplinary: In medicine, a term used to describe a treatment planning approach or team that includes a number of doctors and other healthcare professionals who are experts in different specialties (disciplines).

nursing home: Licensed facility that provides general nursing care to those who are chronically ill or unable to take care of daily living needs.

osteoporosis: Bone disease characterized by a reduction in bone density. Bones become porous and brittle as a result of calcium loss. People with osteoporosis are more vulnerable to breaking bones.

personal care: Non-skilled service or care, such as help with bathing, dressing, eating, getting in and out of bed or chair, moving around, and using the bathroom.

respite care: Temporary care which is intended to provide time off for those who care for someone on a regular basis. Respite care is typically 14 to 21 days of care per year and can be provided in a nursing home, adult day service center, or at home by a private party.

side effect: A problem that occurs when treatment affects healthy tissues or organs. Some common side effects of cancer treatment are fatigue, pain, nausea, vomiting, decreased blood cell counts, hair loss, and mouth sores.

skilled care: Nursing care such as help with medications and caring for wounds, and therapies such as occupational, speech, respiratory, and physical therapy. Skilled care usually requires the services of a licensed professional such as a nurse, doctor, or therapist.

spend down: Requirement that an individual spend most of his or her income and assets to pay for care before he or she can satisfy Medicaid's financial eligibility criteria.

supplemental security income (SSI): Program administered by the Social Security Administration (SSA) that provides financial assistance to needy persons who are disabled or aged 65 or older. Many states provide Medicaid without further application to persons who are eligible for SSI.

symptom: An indication that a person has a condition or disease. Some examples of symptoms are headache, fever, fatigue, nausea, vomiting, and pain.

transfer of assets: Giving away property for less than it is worth or for the sole purpose of becoming eligible for Medicaid. Transferring assets during the look back period results in disqualification for Medicaid payment of long-term care services for a penalty period.

Chapter 70

Support Groups for End-of-Life Issues

American Association of Suicidology (AAS)
5221 Wisconsin Ave. N.W.
Washington, DC 20015
Toll-Free: 1-800-273-TALK
(1-800-273-8255)
Phone: 202-237-2280
Fax: 202-237-2282
Website: www.suicidology.org

American Cancer Society (ACS)
250 Williams St. N.W.
Atlanta, GA, 30303
Toll-Free: 800-227-2345
Phone: 404-320-3333
Website: www.cancer.org

Compassionate Friends
1000 Jorie Blvd., Ste. 140
Oak Brook, IL 60523
Toll-Free: 877-969-0010
Phone: 630-990-0010
Fax: 630-990-0246
Website: www.
compassionatefriends.org
E-mail: nationaloffice@
compassionatefriends.org

First Candle / SIDS Alliance
9 Newport Dr., Ste. 200
Forest Hill, MD 21050
Toll-Free: 800-221-7437
Phone: 410-653-8226
Fax: 410-653-8709
Website: www.firstcandle.org
E-mail: info@firstcandle.org

Resources in this chapter were compiled from several sources deemed reliable, October 2016.

GriefShare
P.O. Box 1739
Wake Forest, NC 27588-1739
Toll-Free: 800-395-5755
Phone: 919-562-2112
Website: griefshare.org
E-mail: info@griefshare.org

Leukemia & Lymphoma Society (LLS)
3 International Dr.
Ste. 200
Rye Brook, NY 10573
Toll-Free: 800-955-4572
Phone: 914-949-5213
Fax: 914-949-6691
Website: www.lls.org
Email: infocenter@lls.org

National Hospice and Palliative Care Organization (NHPCO)
1731 King St.
Alexandria, VA 22314
Toll-Free: 800-658-8898
Phone: 703-837-1500
Fax: 703-837-1233
Website: www.nhpco.org
E-mail: nhpco_info@nhpco.org

National SHARE Office
402 Jackson St.
St. Charles, MO 63301-3468
Toll-Free: 800-821-6819
Phone: 636-947-6164
Fax: 636-947-7486
Website: nationalshare.org
Email: info@nationalshare.org

Suicide Prevention Resource Center (SPRC)
43 Foundry Ave.
Waltham, MA 02453-8313
Toll-Free: 877-GET-SPRC
(877-438-7772)
TTY: 617-964-5448
Website: www.sprc.org
E-mail: info@sprc.org

Tragedy Assistance Program for Survivors, Inc. (TAPS)
3033 Wilson Blvd.
Ste. 630
Arlington, VA 22201
Toll-Free: 800-959-TAPS
(800-959-8277)
Phone: 202-588-8277
Fax: 571-385-2524
Website: www.taps.org
Email: info@taps.org

Well Spouse Foundation
63 W. Main St.
Ste. H
Freehold, NJ 07728
Toll-Free: 800-838-0879
Website: www.wellspouse.org

Yellow Ribbon
P.O. Box 644
Westminster, CO 80036-0644
Phone: 303-429-3530
Fax: 303-426-4496
Website: www.yellowribbon.org
E-mail: ask4help@yellowribbon.org

Chapter 71

Resources for Information about Death and Dying

Administration for Community Living (ACL)
330 C St. S.W.
Washington, DC 20201
Toll-Free: 800-677-1116
Phone: 202-401-4634
E-mail: aclinfo@acl.hhs.gov

AIDSinfo
P.O. Box 4780
Rockville, MD 20849-6303
Toll-Free: 1-800-HIV-0440
(1-800-448-0440)
TTY: 1-888-480-3739
Fax: 1-301-315-2818
Website: aidsinfo.nih.gov
E-mail: ContactUs@aidsinfo.nih.gov

ALS Association
1275 K St. N.W., Ste. 250
Washington, DC 20005
Phone: 202-407-8580
Fax: 202-464-8869
Website: www.alsa.org
E-mail: alsinfo@alsa-national.org

Alzheimer's Association
225 N. Michigan Ave.
Fl. 17
Chicago, IL 60601
Toll-Free: 1-800-272-3900
Phone: 312-335-8700
TDD: 312-335-5886
Fax: 1-866-699-1246
Website: www.alz.org
E-mail: info@alz.org

Resources in this chapter were compiled from several sources deemed reliable, October 2016.

Alzheimer's Disease Education and Referral Center (ADEAR)
P.O. Box 8250
Silver Spring, MD 20907-8250
Phone: 1-800-438-4380
Fax: 301-495-3334
Website: www.nia.nih.gov/alzheimers
E-mail: adear@nia.nih.gov

American Academy of Hospice and Palliative Medicine (AAHPM)
8735 W. Higgins Rd.
Ste. 300
Chicago, IL 60631
Phone: 847-375-4712
Fax: 847-375-6475
Website: aahpm.org
E-mail: info@aahpm.org

American Association of Retired People (AARP)
601 E St. N.W.
Washington, DC 20049
Toll-Free: 1-888-OUR-AARP
(1-888-687-2277)
Toll-Free TTY: 1-877-434-7598
Website: www.aarp.org
E-mail: member@aarp.org

American Association of Suicidology (AAS)
5221 Wisconsin Ave. N.W.
Washington, DC 20015
Phone: 202- 237-2280
Fax: 202-237-2282
Website: www.suicidology.org
E-mail: info@suicidology.org

American Chronic Pain Association (ACPA)
P.O. Box 850
Rocklin, CA 95677
Phone: 1-800-533-3231
Fax: 916-652-8190
Website: theacpa.org
E-mail: ACPA@theacpa.org

American Pain Society (APS)
8735 W. Higgins Rd.
Ste. 300
Chicago, IL 60631
Phone: 847-375-4715
Website: americanpainsociety.org
E-mail: info@americanpainsociety.org

Americans for Better Care of the Dying (ABCD)
5568 General Washington Dr.
Alexandria, VA 22314-2866
Phone: 703-333-6960
Website: www.abcd-caring.org

Association for Death Education and Counseling (ADEC)
1 Parkview Plaza
Ste. 800
Oakbrook Terrace, IL 60181
Phone: 847-686-2240
Fax: 847-686-2251
Website: www.adec.org
E-mail: adec@adec.org

Association of Professional Chaplains (APC)
2800 W Higgins Rd., Ste. 295
Hoffman Estates, IL 60169
Phone: 847-240-1014
Fax: 847-240-1015
Website: www.
professionalchaplains.org
E-mail: info@
professionalchaplains.org

Bereaved Parents of the USA
5 Vanek Rd.
Poughkeepsie, NY 12603-5403
Website: bereavedparentsusa.
org

Cancer Care, Inc.
275 7th Ave.
New York, NY 10001
Toll-Free: 800-813-HOPE
(800-813-4673)
Phone: 212-712-8400
Fax: 212-712-8495
Website: www.cancercare.org
E-mail: info@cancercare.org

Caregiver Action Network
130 Connecticut Ave. N.W.
Ste. 500
Washington, DC 20036
Phone: 202-454-3970
E-mail: info@caregiveraction.org

Centers for Disease Control and Prevention (CDC)
1600 Clifton Rd.
Atlanta, GA 30329-4027
Toll-Free: 800-CDC-INFO
(800-232-4636)
TTY: 888-232-6348
Website: www.cdc.gov

Centers for Medicare and Medicaid Services (CMS)
7500 Security Blvd.
Baltimore, MD 21244
Toll-Free: 800-MEDICARE
(800-633-4227)
TTY: 877-486-2048
Website: www.cms.gov

Children's Hospice International (CHI)
500 Montgomery St.
Ste. 400
Alexandria, VA 22314
Phone: 1-703-684-0330
Website: www.chionline.org
E-mail: Info@CHIonline.org

Commission on Accreditation of Rehabilitation Facilities (CARF)
6951 E. Southpoint Rd.
Tucson, AZ 85756-9407
Toll-Free: 888- 281-6531
Fax: 520-318-1129
Website: www.carf.org

Compassion & Choices
P.O. Box 101810
Denver, CO 80250
Toll-Free: 800-247-7421
Website: www.
compassionandchoices.org

Compassionate Friends
1000 Jorie Blvd., Ste. 140
Oak Brook, IL 60523
Toll-Free: 877- 969-0010
Phone: 630-990-0010
Fax: 630-990-0246
Website: www.
compassionatefriends.org

Dougy Center for Grieving Children and Families
P.O. Box 86852
Portland, OR 97286
Toll-Free: 866-775-5683
Phone: 503-775-5683
Website: www.dougy.org
E-mail: help@dougy.org

Eldercare Locator
Administartion on Aging (AOA)
330 Independence Ave. S.W.
Washington, DC 20201
Toll-Free: 800-677-1116
Phone: 202-619-7501
Website: www.eldercare.gov

Family Caregiver Alliance (FCA)
785 Market St.
Ste. 750
San Francisco, CA 94103
Toll-Free: 800-445-8106
Phone: 415-434-3388
Website: www.caregiver.org
E-mail: eldercarelocator@
spherix.com

Federal Trade Commission (FTC)
600 Pennsylvania Ave. N.W.
Washington, DC 20580
Toll-Free: 1-877-FTC-HELP
(1-877-382-4357)
Phone: 202-326-2222
Toll-Free TDD: 866-653-4261
Website: www.ftc.gov
E-mail: info@caregiver.org

First Candle / SIDS Alliance
9 Newport Dr.
Ste. 200
Forest Hill, MD 21050
Toll-Free: 800-221-7437
Phone: 410-653-8226
Website: www.firstcandle.org
E-mail: info@firstcandle.com

Funeral Consumers Alliance (FCA)
33 Patchen Rd.
South Burlington, VT 05403
Toll-Free: 800-765-0107
Phone: 802-865-8300
Fax: 802-865-2626
Website: www.funerals.org

George Washington Institute for Spirituality and Health (GWish)
2600 Virginia Ave. N.W.
Ste. 300
Washington, DC 20037
Phone: 202-994-6220
Fax: 202-994-6413
Website: smhs.gwu.edu/gwish
E-mail: caring@gwish.org

Health in Aging Foundation
40 Fulton St.
18th Fl.
New York, NY 10038
Toll Free: 800-563-4916
Phone: 212-308-1414
Website: www.
healthinagingfoundation.org

Hospice Education Institute
3 Unity Sq.
P.O. Box 98
Machiasport, ME 04655-0098
Toll-Free: 800-331-1620
Phone: 207-255-8800
Fax: 207-255-8008
Website: www.hospiceworld.org
E-mail: hospiceall@aol.com

Hospice Foundation of America (HFA)
1707 L St. N.W.
Ste. 220
Washington, DC 20036
Toll-Free: 800-854-3402
Phone: 202-457-5811
Website: hospicefoundation.org

International Cemetery, Cremation & Funeral Association (ICCFA)
107 Carpenter Dr.
Ste. 100
Sterling, VA 20164
Toll-Free: 800-645-7700
Phone: 703-391-8400
Fax: 703-391-8416
Website: www.iccfa.com

Joint Commission on Accreditation of Healthcare Organizations
1515 W. 22nd St., Ste. 1300W
Oak Brook, IL 60523
Phone: 630-268-7400
Fax: 630-792-5005
Website: www.jcrinc.com
E-mail: info@jcrinc.com

National Association for Home Care (NAHC)
228 Seventh St. S.E.
Washington, DC 20003
Phone: 202-547-7424
Fax: 202-547-3540
Website: www.nahc.org
E-mail: hospice@nahc.org

National Association of Area Agencies on Aging (N4A)
1730 Rhode Island Ave. N.W.
Ste. 1200
Washington, DC 20036
Phone: 202-872-0888
Fax: 202-872-0057
Website: www.n4a.org
E-mail: info@n4a.org

National Association of Catholic Chaplains (NACC)
4915 S. Howell Ave.
Ste. 501
Milwaukee, WI 53207
Phone: 414-483-4898
Fax: 414-483-6712
Website: www.nacc.org
E-mail: info@nacc.org

National Association of States United for Aging and Disabilities (NASUAD)
1201 15th St. N.W.
Ste. 350
Washington, DC 20005
Phone: 202-898-2578
Fax: 202-898-2583
Website: www.nasuad.org
E-mail: info@nasuad.org

National Cancer Institute (NCI)
9609 Medical Center Dr.
Bethesda, MD 20892-9760
Toll-Free: 1-800-4-CANCER
(1-800-422-6237)
Toll-Free TTY: 800-332-8615
Website: www.cancer.gov
E-mail: cancergovstaff@mail.nih.gov

National Funeral Directors Association (NFDA)
13625 Bishop's Dr.
Brookfield, WI 53005
Toll-Free: 800-228-6332
Phone: 262-789-1880
Fax: 262-789-6977
Website: www.nfda.org
E-mail: nfda@nfda.org

National Hospice and Palliative Care Organization (NHPCO)
1731 King St.
Alexandria, VA 22314
Toll-Free: 800-658-8898
Phone: 703-837-1500
Fax: 703-837-1233
Website: www.nhpco.org
E-mail: nhpco_info@nhpco.org

National Institute on Aging (NIA)
31 Center Dr.
MSC 2292
Bethesda, MD 20892
Phone: 1-800-222-2225
TTY: 1-800-222-4225
Website: www.nia.nih.gov
E-mail: niaic@nia.nih.gov

National SHARE Office
402 Jackson St.
St. Charles, MO 63301-3468
Toll-Free: 800-821-6819
Phone: 636-947-6164
Fax: 636-947-7486
Website: nationalshare.org
Email: info@nationalshare.org

Safe Kids Worldwide
1255 23rd St. N.W.
Ste. 400
Washington, DC 20037-1151
Phone: 202-662-0600
Fax: 202-393-2072
Website: www.safekids.org

Social Security Administration (SSA)
Office of International Operations
P.O. Box 17769
Baltimore, MD 21235-7769
Toll-Free: 1-800-772-1213
Website: www.ssa.gov

Society of Critical Care Medicine (SCCM)
500 Midway Dr.
Mount Prospect, IL 60056
Phone: 1-847 827-6869
Fax: 847-439-7226
Website: www.sccm.org
E-mail: info@sccm.org

Substance Abuse and Mental Health Services Administration (SAMHSA)
5600 Fishers Ln.
Rockville, MD 20857
Toll-Free: 1-877-SAMHSA-7
(1-877-726-4727)
Toll-Free TDD: 800-487-4889
Website: www.samhsa.gov

Suicide Prevention Resource Center (SPRC)
43 Foundry Ave.
Waltham, MA 02453-8313
Toll-Free: 877-GET-SPRC
(877-438-7772)
Website: www.sprc.org
E-mail: info@sprc.org

U.S. Department of Labor (DOL)
200 Constitution Ave. N.W.
Washington, DC 20210
Phone: 1-866-4-USA-DOL
(1-866-487-2365)
Website: www.dol.gov

Visiting Nurse Associations of America (VNNA)
2121 Crystal Dr.
Ste. 750
Arlington, VA 22202
Toll-Free: 1-888-866-8773
Phone: 571-527-1520
Fax: 571-527-1521
Website: www.vnaa.org
E-mail: vnaa@vnaa.org

Yellow Ribbon
P.O. Box 644
Westminster, CO 80036-0644
Phone: 303-429-3530
Fax: 303-426-4496
Website: yellowribbon.org
E-mail: ask4help@yellowribbon.org

Index

Index

Page numbers followed by 'n' indicate a footnote. Page numbers in *italics* indicate a table or illustration.